Practicing Psychiatry in the Community

Community

A Manual

Practicing Psychiatry in the Community

A Manual

Edited by

Jerome V. Vaccaro, M.D.,
and
Gordon H. Clark, Jr., M.D., M.Div.

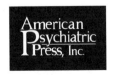

Washington, DC
London, England

Copyright © 1996 Jerome V. Vaccaro, M.D., and Gordon H. Clark, Jr., M.D., M.Div.
ALL RIGHTS RESERVED
Manufactured in the United States of America on acid-free paper
99 98 97 96   4 3 2 1
First Edition

American Psychiatric Press, Inc.
1400 K Street, N.W., Washington, DC   20005

Library of Congress Cataloging-in-Publication Data
Practicing psychiatry in the community: a manual / edited by Jerome V.
    Vaccaro and Gordon H. Clark, Jr.
        p. cm.
    Includes bibliographical references and index.
    ISBN 0-88048-663-5
    1. Community psychiatry. I. Vaccaro, Jerome V. II. Clark, Gordon H.,
1947–
    RC455.P696 1996
    362.2'2—dc20
                                                                95-39523
                                                                CIP

British Library Cataloguing in Publication Data
A CIP record is available from the British Library.

To our wives, Andra and Gail—
With love and gratitude for their abiding support.

Contents

Section III. Target Populations

Contributors

Leona L. Bachrach, Ph.D.
Research Professor of Psychiatry, Maryland Psychiatric Research Center, University of Maryland School of Medicine, Baltimore, Maryland; and Visiting Professor, Department of Psychiatry, University of Toronto, Toronto, Ontario, Canada, and University of Arizona, Tucson, Arizona.

Stephen J. Bartels, M.D.
Associate Professor of Psychiatry, Dartmouth Medical School; and Research Associate, New Hampshire–Dartmouth Psychiatric Research Center, Lebanon, New Hampshire.

Deborah R. Becker, M.Ed.
Research Associate, Department of Community and Family Medicine, Dartmouth Medical School; and Research Associate, New Hampshire–Dartmouth Psychiatric Research Center, Lebanon, New Hampshire.

Michael J. Bohn, M.D.
Assistant Professor, Department of Psychiatry, University of Wisconsin Medical School, Madison, Wisconsin.

Orlando J. Cartaya, M.D.
Staff Psychiatrist, Santa Monica West Community Mental Health Center, Santa Monica, California; and Assistant Clinical Professor of Psychiatry, University of California, Los Angeles School of Medicine, Los Angeles, California.

Richard Chung, M.D.
Vice President and Chief Clinical Officer, Medco Behavioral Care Systems, St. Louis, Missouri; and Associate Clinical Professor of Psychiatry, University of Hawaii, Honolulu, Hawaii.

Gordon H. Clark, Jr., M.D., M.Div.
President and Medical Director, Integrated Behavioral Health Services; Medical Director, Behavioral Health Network of Maine; Medical Director, Augusta Mental Health Institute; Associate Medical Director, Maine Department of Mental Health and Mental Retardation; Assistant Clinical Professor of Psychiatry, University of Pittsburgh School of Medicine; Founding President, American Association of Community Psychiatrists; Fellow, American Psychiatric Association.

Karen "Kip" Cunningham, M.D., Pharm.D.
Chief Resident in Psychiatry, Santa Monica West Mental Health Center, University of California, Los Angeles, Los Angeles, California.

David L. Cutler, M.D.
Professor of Psychiatry and Director, Public Psychiatry Training Program, Oregon Health Sciences University, Portland, Oregon.

Kathleen Daly, M.D., M.P.H.
Assistant Professor of Psychiatry, University of California, Los Angeles, Los Angeles, California; and Medical Director, West Los Angeles Veterans Affairs Medical Center Community Support Program, West Los Angeles, California.

Ronald J. Diamond, M.D.
Associate Professor of Psychiatry and Director, Acute Psychiatry Service, Department of Psychiatry, University of Wisconsin Medical School; and Medical Director, Mental Health Center of Dane County, Madison, Wisconsin.

Robert E. Drake, M.D., Ph.D.
Professor of Psychiatry, Dartmouth Medical School, and Director, New Hampshire–Dartmouth Psychiatric Research Center, Lebanon, New Hampshire.

Burr S. Eichelman, M.D., Ph.D.
Professor and Chairman, Department of Psychiatry and Behavioral Science, Temple University School of Medicine, Philadelphia, Pennsylvania.

Spencer Eth, M.D.
Clinical Professor of Psychiatry, School of Medicine, University of Southern California; Associate Professor of Clinical Psychiatry, School of Medicine, University of California, Los Angeles, California; and Associate Chief of Psychiatry, Veterans Affairs Medical Center, Los Angeles, California.

Robert M. Factor, M.D., Ph.D.
Professor of Psychiatry and Director of Residency Education, Department of Psychiatry, University of Wisconsin Medical School; Medical Director, Emergency Services Unit, Mental Health Center of Dane County, Madison, Wisconsin; and Medical Director, Intensive Psychiatric Community Care, VA Medical Center, Madison, Wisconsin.

Sally L. Godard, M.D.
Adjunct Assistant Professor of Psychiatry, Oregon Health Sciences University, Portland, Oregon.

Robert M. Goisman, M.D.
Director, Outpatient Training and Research, Massachusetts Mental Health Center, Boston, Massachusetts; and Assistant Professor of Psychiatry, Harvard Medical School, Boston, Massachusetts.

Charles R. Goldman, M.D.
Professor and Director, Public Psychiatry Training Program, Department of Neuropsychiatry and Behavioral Science, University of South Carolina School of Medicine,Columbia, South Carolina.

Anne C. Hartwig, J.D., Ph.D.
Consultant, Center for Social Policy and Community Development, Temple University, Philadelphia, Pennsylvania.

Timothy Howell, M.D., M.A.
Associate Professor (CHS), Departments of Psychiatry and Medicine, University of Wiconsin School of Medicine, Madison, Wisconsin; and Director, Geriatric Psychiatry Fellowship Program, University of Wisconsin Hospital/Madison Veterans Administration Hospital, Madison, Wisconsin.

Marvin Karno, M.D.
Professor of Psychiatry and Director of the Social and Community Psychiatry Division, University of California, Los Angeles, School of Medicine, Los Angeles, California.

Martin Kaufman, M.D.
Staff Psychiatrist, St. Luke Medical Center, Berlin, New Hampshire.

Harriet P. Lefley, Ph.D.
Professor of Psychiatry and Behavioral Sciences, Department of Psychiatry, University of Miami School of Medicine, Miami, Florida.

Gregory B. Leong, M.D.
Associate Professor of Clinical Psychiatry, University of Missouri–Columbia School of Medicine; and Chief, Psychiatry, Harry S. Truman Memorial Veterans Hospital, Columbia, Missouri.

William R. McFarlane, M.D.
Chief of Psychiatry, Maine Medical Center, Portland, Maine; Professor
of Psychiatry, University of Vermont, Burlington, Vermont; and Lecturer
in Psychiatry, Columbia University of Physicians and Surgeons, New York,
New York.

Hunter McQuistion, M.D.
Assistant Clinical Professor of Psychiatry, New York University, New
York, New York.

Arthur Merrell, M.D.
Staff Psychiatrist, Southeast Wyoming Mental Health Center, Cheyenne,
Wyoming.

Kenneth Minkoff, M.D.
Chief of Psychiatry, Choate Health Systems, Inc., Woburn, Massachu-
setts; and Assistant Professor of Psychiatry, Harvard Medical School,
Boston, Massachusetts.

H. Steven Moffic, M.D.
Professor, Vice Chairman, and Director of Development; Medical Director, Mental Health Managed Care Program; and Director, Mental Health
Clinic, Department of Psychiatry, Medical College of Wisconsin, Milwaukee, Wisconsin.

Deborah B. Pitts, M.B.A., O.T.R.
Deputy Chief, Community and Rehabilitative Psychiatry, West Los Angeles Veterans Affairs Medical Center, Los Angeles, California; and Director, Psychosocial Services, University of California, Los Angeles
Schizophrenia Clinical Program, Los Angeles, California.

David A. Pollack, M.D.
Adjunct Associate Professor of Psychiatry and Associate Director, Public
Psychiatry Training Program, Oregon Health Sciences University, Port-
land, Oregon.

Deborah Reed, M.D.
Assistant Professor of Clinical Psychiatry, and Medical Director, Older
Adult Outpatient Services, Northwestern University, Chicago, Illinois.

M. Steven Sager, M.D.
Director, Children and Family Services, Santa Monica West Mental Health Center, Santa Monica, California; Medical Director, Sector I, Children and Family Services Bureau, Los Angeles County Department of Mental Health; and Assistant Clinical Professor of Psychiatry, University of California, Los Angeles Department of Psychiatry and Biobehavioral Sciences, Los Angeles, California.

Ezra Susser, M.D., Dr.PH.
Associate Professor of Psychiatry, Columbia University, New York, New York.

William C. Torrey, M.D.
Assistant Professor of Psychiatry, Dartmouth Medical School, and Medical Director, West Central Community Support Services, Lebanon, New Hampshire.

Richard U'Ren, M.D.
Associate Professor of Psychiatry, Oregon Health Sciences University, and Consultant Psychiatrist, Robison Jewish Home, Portland, Oregon.

Jerome V. Vaccaro, M.D.
Associate Professor of Clinical Psychiatry and Director of Community Psychiatry Programs and the Schizophrenia Clinical Program, University of California, Los Angeles, School of Medicine, Los Angeles, California; Medical Director, Santa Monica West Mental Health Center, Santa Monica, California; and Chief, Community and Rehabilitative Psychiatry, West Los Angeles Veterans Affairs Medical Center, West Los Angeles, California.

Elie Valencia, J.D., M.A.
Assistant Clinical Professor of Public Health, Department of Psychiatry, Columbia University, New York, New York.

Lynn Verger, M.D.
Private practice in Geriatric Psychiatry, Hampton, Virginia.

Richard Warner, M.B., D.P.M.
Medical Director, Mental Health Center of Boulder County, Boulder, Colorado; Associate Clinical Professor, Department of Psychiatry, University of Colorado, Denver, Colorado; and Associate Professor-Adjunct, Department of Anthropology, University of Colorado, Boulder, Colorado.

William H. Wilson, M.D.
Adjunct Assistant Professor of Psychiatry and Associate Director, Public Psychiatry Training Program, Oregon Health Sciences University, Portland, Oregon.

Michael T. Witkovsky, M.D.
Assistant Professor, Department of Psychiatry, University of Wisconsin Medical School, Madison, Wisconsin.

Charlotte Wolleson, M.A.
Team Leader for Inpatient Services, Mental Health Center of Boulder County, Boulder, Colorado.

Alexander S. Young, M.D.
Associate Medical Director for Psychopharmacology at Santa Monica West Community Mental Health Center, Santa Monica, California; Associate Director, University of California, Los Angeles Schizophrenia Clinical Program; Robert Wood Johnson Clinical Scholar; and Assistant Clinical Professor of Psychiatry, University of California, Los Angeles, School of Medicine, Los Angeles, California.

A Glimpse of What's Inside

Jerome V. Vaccaro, M.D.
Gordon H. Clark, Jr., M.D., M.Div.

This manual is organized into four main sections: an *Overview,* in which we present historical and conceptual issues relevant to contemporary psychiatric practice in community settings; *The Treatment Continuum,* to highlight that special attribute of community psychiatry—namely, its emphasis on continuity of care; *Target Populations,* to capture the community psychiatry innovation of addressing the needs of groups of individuals rather than the narrower focus on the individual patient; and *Special Topics,* to include the many areas embraced by community psychiatry in today's changing mental health care environment.

The Treatment Continuum

In this section authors explore the varied environments in which community psychiatric services may be offered. Chung et al. survey the expanse of outpatient treatment, focusing on the ways in which managed care and health care reform have affected the provision of outpatient services in community settings. Factor and Diamond highlight the importance of a well-designed and carefully implemented system of crisis resolution services. Vaccaro and Pitts write about the contemporary generation of psychiatric rehabilitation programs, which are technologically advanced and superior to their early community mental health beginnings. Warner and Wolleson demonstrate that effective alternatives to acute inpatient care have been within the mainstream of community psychiatry for some time. Daly et al. highlight the important and changing role that inpatient units occupy in our treatment continuum.

Target Populations

In this section the target populations that have been the focus of community mental health programs for some time and those whose identification and focus are more recent are featured. Although many child psychiatrists practice what can only be described as truly community-based psychiatry, their presence in formal community mental health settings has been less than many clinicians would desire. There appears to be a resurgence in interest in community child psychiatry, marked by increased recruitment and more liaisons between academic child psychiatry programs and community mental health settings. Sager provides a summary of the various roles occupied by today's community child psychiatrist.

The needs of the mentally ill–developmentally disabled population have been relegated to the "back burner," or even completely off the stove, in most community mental health settings. Torrey provides a clear and compelling case for the inclusion of this population in our care system, along with very useful and practical guidelines for their care. Vaccaro and Young address the comprehensive treatment and rehabilitation needs of what has become the primary group served in most community mental health settings: those individuals with severe and disabling mental illnesses. The authors provide a blueprint for services for this previously neglected population. Bohn and Witkovsky provide readers with necessary information about the treatment of patients who suffer from substance-related disorders. Minkoff, who has been a beacon for the recognition of patients with dual diagnoses and a pioneer in their treatment, provides a clear view of these patients. He proposes ways in which the best of both treatment worlds be combined successfully to improve outcome.

The spectrum of human immunodeficiency virus–related psychiatric disorders has received deserved recognition over the past several years.

However, most community mental health settings lack clear direction in the provision of treatment services for this population. Goisman provides the rationale and guidelines for involvement of the community psychiatrist in this important area. Valencia et al. offer a clear model for engaging the homeless mentally ill individual in productive treatment and rehabilitation efforts in their insightful chapter. In the next two chapters, Eichelman and Hartwig explore the field of violence and its relationship to mental disorder and community mental health. This section concludes with consideration of the newly charted waters of geropsychiatry as it applies to community mental health in a chapter authored by Verger and Howell.

Special Topics

For many of us, community mental health settings are the most creative and exciting arenas for professional satisfaction. In this section authors explore some of the opportunities presented in these settings. Until relatively recently, consideration of the contemporary role for the community psychiatrist has been an underexplored area. Young and Clark discuss this essential topic in their chapter and offer clear guidelines for community psychiatric practice. In many ways multidisciplinary teamwork has been the heart and soul of community mental health work. Diamond, who has been deeply immersed in the practice of community psychiatry, offers insightful advice about ways to make teamwork successful and rewarding.

Goldman and Lefley explain the ways in which families and professionals can offer assistance to one another that improves patient outcome and makes the work of psychiatrists more efficient. McFarlane and Cunningham then chart the course for formal interventions that empower families to assist their ill relatives in productive, respectful ways. Moffic, long an authority on cultural psychiatry, organizes his experience and knowledge into principles for serving ethnically and culturally diverse populations in community mental health settings.

Community mental health and rural areas have had a long and conflicted relationship. Reed and Merrell speak to the challenge and joy of working in rural settings. Since it was first explicated by Gerald Caplan, community consultation has been one of the most productive, yet most challenged, areas of community psychiatric practice. U'Ren et al. revive interest in this important area in their compelling chapter. Forensic issues have assumed a growing role in community psychiatric practice, and Leong and Eth provide the community psychiatrist with the material needed to confront the challenges posed in this arena. The importance of training and education in community psychiatry cannot be overstated. Cutler et al. have been at the forefront of community psychiatric training for many years and collect their successes into a useful chapter for the psychiatrist wishing to improve an existing program or create one anew. This section concludes with Drake et al.'s user-friendly guide to the development of a research program in a community setting.

Foreword

Marvin Karno, M.D.

Jerome Vaccaro and Gordon H. Clark, Jr., have produced a practitioner's manual that both reflects and illuminates the complex tasks confronting today's community psychiatrist. The authors they have selected are current practitioners who write for practitioners. The settings of the emergency department, the outpatient clinic, the hospital ward, and rural as well as urban communities are examined for their special demands on community practice.

Mentally disordered children, adolescents, and elderly persons; those infected with the human immunodeficiency virus; homeless mentally ill individuals; developmentally disabled or chemically dependent persons; patients with dual diagnoses; and violent as well as chronically mentally ill individuals are the populations currently requiring skilled clinical care by the community psychiatrist. These diverse populations each require the focused clinical attention provided by specific chapters in this book.

Finally, the issues of cultural diversity; the principles of effective collaboration with advocacy and family/self-help groups; the role of the multidisciplinary team; and ethical, legal, training, and research issues at play in the domain of contemporary community psychiatric practice are vigorously explored in this manual by some of the most active, articulate, and expert current practitioners.

This manual should become a standard text in university medical school psychiatric residency training programs and in resurgent fellowship training programs in community psychiatry. It should also be available to every psychiatrist in community practice in the United States. As the United States moves ahead to the likely provision of psychiatric care for all severely mentally disordered members of our society, this manual may well become indispensable to all clinically active psychiatrists.

Section I

Overview

Chapter 1

The First 30 Years: A Historical Overview of Community Mental Health

Leona L. Bachrach, Ph.D.
Gordon H. Clark, Jr., M.D., M.Div.

Defining community psychiatry is no simple matter. Part of the difficulty comes from the fact that the field is undergoing a redefinition of its mission (Residency Training Committee 1991). However, a portion of the difficulty is also semantic in nature. The psychiatric literature has frequently neglected to distinguish between community psychiatry and community mental health, a situation that has led to confusion among both psychiatrists and other mental health professionals.

How may these terms be differentiated? Community psychiatry, which in the United States is often equated with social psychiatry (Schwartz 1972), refers generally to the "application of the theory and practice of psychiatry in noninstitutional and creatively nontraditional settings" (Group for the Advancement of Psychiatry 1983). It is frequently, but by no means exclusively, practiced in service settings that are fully or partially funded with public monies. The Residency Training Committee (1991) of the American Association of Community Psychiatrists (AACP) submitted a statement delimiting the scope of community psychiatry, and although this definition still awaits ratification, it notes that the field's concern is basically with "the particular biological and psychological dimensions of each individual patient in his/her immediate sociocultural context."

Community mental health, by contrast, has a broader scope and may be understood as the supportive framework for a "population-based, prevention-oriented, primarily publicly funded mental health system" (Borus 1978)— a definition that suggests clear links with the field of public health. In the United States, community mental health has frequently, and somewhat inaccurately, been identified with a short-lived federal effort during the 1960s and 1970s to endorse and fund comprehensive mental health services.

Indeed, under the umbrella of that federal initiative, community psychiatry and community mental health were, for a number of years, closely intertwined. Both sought to improve the life circumstances of individual patients, but they were also preoccupied with concepts such as primary prevention and community activism. Thus, in Kety's (1974) words, community psychiatry had "branched out well beyond mental illness into problems that it . . . [was] not especially qualified to handle—community, national, and international affairs; poverty; politics; and criminality." Kety saw this as problematic and wrote, "In each of these areas, we have responsibilities as citizens and human beings, [but] we have yet to demonstrate any special competence as psychiatrists."

Nor was Kety the only psychiatrist to be concerned with such a broad focus for community psychiatry. Zusman (1975) wrote that "community psychiatrists are bound to be amateurs working in complex areas where it would seem professional skills are very much needed." Sociologists expressed concern as well (Dunham 1976). Dinitz and Beran's (1971) observation that community mental health had "set for itself a boundaryless goal: the improvement of the whole man and every man, in his total environment" applied also to community psychiatry.

Such criticisms were in many ways prophetic. Community psychiatry has in more recent years turned increasingly toward the treatment of illness and away from efforts to modify the social milieu. At the same time, however, it has retained its appreciation of the cultural influences that affect psychiatric service need and service delivery.

Historical Antecedents

The early roots of American community psychiatry, which date back to the 18th and 19th centuries, have been explored and documented in a variety of excellent sources (see, for example, Aldrich 1972; Dunham 1976; Group for the Advancement of Psychiatry 1983; Langsley 1980b; Schwab and Schwab 1978; Talbott 1983; Yolles 1969). In this chapter we focus on the more recent antecedents of contemporary community psychiatry, particularly those that prevailed during the third quarter of this century.

Pre-1960s Influences

Prior to the 1960s the care and treatment of mentally ill individuals in the United States had largely been the responsibility of individual states. Although there had been earlier attempts to involve the federal government, the precedent for decentralized responsibility was well established. In 1854, on the premise that he could find no constitutional authority for the federal government to become the "great almoner of public charity," President Franklin Pierce had vetoed legislation to make federal land grants available for the development of public mental hospitals (Task Panel on Community Mental Health Centers Assessment 1978).

However, as the 1960s approached, new directions in service planning and service delivery for mentally ill individuals began to emerge. These were buttressed by reported successes in the practice of military psychiatry, the appearance of new psychoactive medications, the increasing popularity of public health concepts, the emergence of civil rights ideology, and a general climate of optimism throughout the country. Pressures on the federal government to become involved in issues of social concern, which had started during the 1930s, were increasing; and this, together with the availability of funding for social programs at the conclusion of World War II, provided a supportive environment for new initiatives.

The influence of military psychiatry is of considerable importance in this regard (Lamb 1988; Langsley 1980b; Smith and Hart 1975), although it is often overlooked. Certain principles that had been found to be productive in the treatment of psychiatric casualties during World War II emerged as focal points for service planning. These principles had proven effective both in returning many members of the armed forces to active military duty and in facilitating their eventual recovery.

A first principle of military psychiatry, proximity, was based on the idea that treatment should take place as close as possible to the location where symptoms were exhibited. This was coupled with a second principle, immediacy, which held that early identification and treatment of psychiatric disorders could lead to more favorable outcomes. A third principle, simplicity, held that a major part of psychiatric intervention should consist of rest, nourishment, and social support; and a fourth, expectancy, supported the idea that a patient's prompt return to former functioning was entirely feasible (Lamb 1988). It was tacitly assumed that these principles could be directly transferred to the civilian domain. Indeed, community psychiatry's endorsement of such concepts as early diagnosis and intervention to effect the prompt remission of symptoms and treatment in environments as close as possible to patients' homes held a clear relationship to these military principles.

These principles were actually reinforced by other events. The post–World War II years witnessed a growing interest in such public health strategies as primary preventive interventions and rehabilitative treatments (Bellak 1969; Bloom 1986; Lamb 1988). There was increasing confidence that psychiatric illness could largely be eliminated if early symptoms could be treated promptly and that in those cases where illness could not actually be prevented, rehabilitative strategies could arrest its course. There was even a belief that rehabilitation could largely restore mentally ill individuals to premorbid levels of functioning. These assumptions fit neatly into the prevailing social climate. This was an era during which a "can-do" attitude dominated American thought (Freedman 1967; Menninger 1989) and the civil rights of various disfranchised populations—including those persons resident in state mental hospitals—were being championed. In addition, new psychoactive medications, which could markedly reduce the symptomatology of hospitalized mental patients, were being marketed. It was increasingly easy to conclude that institutionalized mentally ill individuals, already perceived as living in inhumane and restrictive environments inappropriate for their needs, should be treated in community settings where they could function effectively with the help of medications.

It was, in short, a time for hope and change in American social policy (Dunham 1976), and this progressive climate was legitimized for mentally ill persons by the creation of a National Institute of Mental Health in 1949. From the beginning, the fledgling agency stressed both the inalienable rights of mentally ill persons and their legitimate claims on society, and it devoted a major portion of its efforts to the search for community-based alternatives to the hospitalization of severely mentally ill individuals (Bachrach and Lamb 1989).

The 1960s and Later

In 1955 the federal Mental Health Study Act, which authorized the formation of the Joint Commission on Mental Illness and Health, was passed. Among the recommendations appearing in the Commission's formal report, published in 1961, were that immediate care be made available to mental patients in community settings; that treatment of the major mental illnesses be recognized as the core responsibility of mental health service systems; that fully staffed, full-time mental health clinics be accessible to all people living in the United States; that large and remote state mental hospitals be replaced by smaller regional facilities; and that community-based aftercare and rehabilitation services for mentally ill individuals be greatly expanded.

In response, two significant federally inspired developments occurred in 1963, and they profoundly affected the course of community psychiatry in the United States. First, categorical Aid to the Disabled (ATD) became available to mentally ill individuals so that, for the first time, they were eligible for federal financial support in the community (Bachrach and Lamb 1989). Patients now had access to federal grants-in-aid, which were in some instances supplemented by state funds, and this enabled them to support themselves or be supported in the community at comparatively little cost to the states. In addition, many people found that they could earn additional income by taking mental patients into their homes. This provided needed alternative residences for mental patients.

ATD is known today as Supplemental Security Income (SSI) and is administered by the federal Social Security Administration. However, its distribution has been markedly curtailed since the 1980s (Okpaku 1988; Pear 1987), and mentally ill individuals have often had great difficulty in accessing its benefits. Because SSI is not an automatic entitlement, disabled individuals must undergo stringent eligibility tests to qualify and remain eligible for it.

The second significant federal development of 1963 was the passage of the Community Mental Health Centers Act, a response to President John F. Kennedy's (1963) famous message calling for a "bold new approach" in service delivery to mentally ill individuals. With enactment of this legislation and certain supplemental amendments passed during the late 1960s and 1970s, the federal government assumed unprecedented responsibility for persons disabled by mental illness. The community mental health initiative, which eventually resulted in the appropriation of $2.9 billion in federal monies to fund more than 750 community mental health centers (CMHCs) (U.S. General Accounting Office 1984), finally emerged as a fully legitimated federal endeavor that paralleled and, to a considerable degree became identified with, the ideals, hopes, and viewpoints of community psychiatry.

Even the text of President Kennedy's 1963 message held promise for a new kind of psychiatry:

> Private physicians, including general practitioners, psychiatrists, and other medical specialists . . . [will] all be able to participate directly and cooperatively in the work of the [community mental health] center. For the first time, a large proportion of our private practitioners will have the opportunity to treat their patients in a mental health facility served by an auxiliary professional staff that is directly and quickly available for outpatient and inpatient care.

As we will presently see, the optimism of these years was not sufficient to withstand the challenges that the federally inspired community mental health movement eventually encountered, and by the 1970s some serious problems had become widely recognized. President Jimmy Carter's Commission on Mental Health, established in 1977, tried to breathe new life into federal support for mental health services (President's Commission on Mental Health 1978), and in fact, a new and stronger commitment followed with passage of the Mental Health Systems Act of 1980. Funding for carrying out this legislation, however, was never appropriated; the Act was effectively rescinded shortly after President Ronald Reagan assumed office in January 1981.

Thus the federal government's involvement in the direct provision of mental health services in the United States was short-lived. It came to an abrupt end 18 years after it had begun, and there has been no substitute since. Although the federal government currently supports some community mental health demonstration projects and provides general health and human services block grants to the states, the level of federal funding has decreased drastically, and the mandated focus on mental health service delivery has been severely compromised (Bachrach 1991a; "Reagan's 1987 budget" 1986; U.S. General Accounting Office 1987).

Principles and Problems

It is important to examine more closely the ideological underpinnings of community psychiatry during the 1960s, because they formed, in Hegelian manner, a new synthesis that was even then moving inexorably toward further change. Community psychiatry, through its close alliance with community mental health, embraced a series of complex interrelated principles that defined its viewpoint and goals. These principles included, but were not limited to, the notions of geographical responsibility and equal access to care, community input and control, humanization of services, comprehensive services and continuity of care, primary prevention and rehabilitation, and professional egalitarianism.

Geographical Responsibility and Equal Access to Care

As originally conceived, the federal community mental health initiative sought to divide the United States into a series of precisely defined service areas so that all Americans might have equal and ready access to mental health services. There were to have been 1,500 such "catchment areas," each serving a base population of 75,000 to 200,000 local residents. Each was to contain a CMHC as its core mental health service agency. These centers were to identify residents' service needs, formulate plans to meet those needs, and provide relevant programs.

Geographical responsibility was, in fact, a concept intended to equalize access to mental health care. Prior to the 1960s there had been a two-class mental health system within which individuals with sufficient resources typically received private outpatient services, while those who were economically disadvantaged either received custodial state mental hospital inpatient services or else went totally unserved (Mollica 1983). Embedded in this differential was a marked imbalance in the availability of services according to race and ethnic origin. There was a belief that by dividing the country into geographical segments with manageable populations, communities would be able to provide all Americans with humane, readily available, high-quality mental health services, and that "catchmenting" would serve to abolish class distinctions through "unlimited access and universal entitlement" (Mollica 1983).

With the advent of CMHCs, many communities were in fact able to offer mental health care to their residents for the first time. Other communities could, and did, stretch existing offerings appreciably and broaden their target populations. At the same time, however, not all communities, and certainly not all Americans, shared in these benefits. Several problems arose almost immediately with catchmenting (President's Commission on Mental Health 1978), not the least of which was the increasing geographic mobility of the American population. Mentally ill individuals who were no longer institutionalized could, like other Americans, move around a great deal (Bachrach 1987b), and it became easy for service providers to question whether they should be treating people who had "just dropped into" their communities.

This difficulty is currently manifested in extreme form in service inequities for homeless mentally ill individuals (Bachrach 1984; Lamb 1988; Lamb et al. 1992). People who lack fixed addresses technically "belong" nowhere and so are not the responsibility of any particular community. Catchmenting thus effectively gives agencies permission to exclude these individuals on the grounds that they belong somewhere else, and it has given rise to a practice ironically called *Greyhound therapy,* in which people needing psychiatric services are provided with one-way bus tickets to another town (Cordes 1984; van Winkle 1980).

A second problem with catchmenting was its creation of artificial service area boundaries. It became increasingly evident that *catchment area* and *community* were not synonymous. Catchment areas were generally drawn up in conformance with previously established political districts, and in urban areas this sometimes meant that neighborhoods and "natural communities" were ignored. However, it was in smaller and more remote rural communities that some of the most difficult pragmatic issues came to the fore. To fulfill the requirements of a 75,000-person population minimum, it was necessary for some catchment areas to encompass huge geographic expanses (Task Panel on Rural Mental Health 1978), and most rural catchment areas exceeded 5,000 square miles in land area. A single catchment area in northern Arizona actually consisted of more than 60,000 square miles—an area roughly the size of all six New England states combined—and was bisected by the Grand Canyon.

Success was also mixed with respect to eliminating class distinctions in service provision. Although the new programs did in some places reach those racial, ethnic, and other minority populations that had previously been underserved or unserved, other kinds of inequities surfaced. For example, professional personnel employed in high-income catchment areas tended to have more intensive training and better academic preparation than those employed in low-income catchment areas (National Institute of Mental Health 1978). Once again, the situation in many rural communities reflected some of the more subtle issues associated with service delivery. Perhaps because they often lacked expertise in "grantsmanship" (Task Panel on Rural Mental Health 1978), rural catchment areas were relatively unsuccessful in competing for federal funding (Task Panel on Community Mental Health Centers Assessment 1978), and a disproportionate number of them were still totally unfunded when the federal community mental health initiative came to an end in 1981.

Mollica (1983) has argued persuasively that a two-class system of mental health care still prevails in the United States despite the federal community mental health effort. The state hospital, in spite of its apparent decline since the 1960s, "continues to be the principal facility for the acute inpatient care of the lower-class patient," and in fact, there has been a "pooling of the poorest patients at state facilities as middle-class and working-class patients have achieved financial access to private institutions."

Community Input and Control

Community input and governance were key features of the community mental health legislation and were especially emphasized in Public Law 94-63, the Community Mental Health Center amendment legislation of 1975. Under this law it was deemed essential that consumers should have input into the planning, operating, and monitoring processes of CMHCs. Apart from emphasizing the power of consumers, this legislation demanded greater flexibility on the part of service providers. Greater attention to the special needs and interests of ethnic minorities was also required (Ruiz and Tourlentes 1983).

Beyond such attention to consumer impact and needs, governance of CMHCs by citizens from within their respective catchment areas was legislatively mandated. The composition of the governing body as well as its specific oversight duties with regard to approval of policies, budget, and selection of a director for the CMHC are clearly spelled out in Public Law 94-63 (Ruiz and Tourlentes 1983).

Humanization of Services

One of the basic foundations of the federal community mental health initiative was its confidence that state mental hospitals, widely viewed as custodial warehouses, could be eliminated and replaced by community-based alternatives that would provide more humane care. During the 1960s the reductions in state hospital censuses were both rapid and marked as the result of stepped-up efforts to discharge patients. Thus, in 1962, immediately before passage of the federal Community Mental Health Centers Act, there had been some 515,000 patients residing in state hospitals. Twenty years later, in 1982, the count was down to 121,000, a drop of about 77% (National Institute of Mental Health, unpublished data).

However, during the same 20-year period, even as patients were being discharged en masse, admissions to state hospitals rose by more than 20%, and a significant percentage of these were readmissions (Bachrach 1986). State mental hospitals had thus become busy places where the same individuals were often admitted for brief stays—a situation that gave rise to the picture of those facilities as having uncontrollably revolving doors. Whether state hospital utilization had truly decreased depended on what criterion one chose to use! Moreover, there were questions about the extent to which the increasing utilization of community-based mental health services and the decreasing state hospital populations were truly paired events. Despite efforts at coordinating these services in some communities, there was little evidence, on a nationwide basis, that the patients no longer residing in state hospitals were the same ones who were admitted to community programs. To the contrary, there was good reason to believe that these facilities were serving entirely different patient populations and, moreover, that the most severely disabled individuals—those who were chronically mentally ill—were often totally unserved (Bachrach and Lamb 1989; Gronfein 1985; U.S. General Accounting Office 1977; Windle and Scully 1976). Langsley (1980a) has described this situation as one in which community mental health had "drifted away" from its "original purpose as defined by Kennedy, the treatment of the mentally ill."

In retrospect, it appears that part of the difficulty in reaching chronically mentally ill individuals may be explained by the increasing complexity of their service needs. Prior to the advent of community mental health, service planning for members of this population had been a relatively simple and uniform affair: most people who showed signs of severe mental illness were admitted to state mental hospitals, where their stays were generally of long duration, often for life. Although critics objected (and rightly so) to the content and quality of care that patients often received in those facilities, there was a simplicity and predictability to program design that was lost with the community mental health focus.

With the advent of community mental health, however, service planning itself became infinitely more complex. Chronic patients now had widely disparate residential and treatment histories, and they were presenting multiple challenges to community mental health planners. A major obstacle to effective care was the homogenization of services: planners often failed simply to recognize that there were many types of chronic patients, that these patients varied greatly in their capacities to adjust to life in the community, and that an extensive array of programs would be needed to meet their complex and diverse needs (Bachrach 1986).

Hence, "gatekeeping" emerged as a serious issue in the delivery of mental health services. Many programs ostensibly designed as initiatives for the most severely disabled patients in fact resisted admitting, or treating, these individuals and instead focused on providing services to people who were less impaired (Bachrach and Lamb 1989; Langsley 1980a, 1980b). Furthermore, instead of finding more humanized care in the community, chronic patients often discovered that they had no place to go. Caught between emasculated state hospitals, which had been forced by public outcry and diminished funding to reduce their services, and community agencies, which often acknowledged little responsibility to them, chronic mentally ill patients frequently became the casualties, not the beneficiaries, of community mental health care (Zusman and Lamb 1977).

The current situation of homeless mentally ill persons in the United States provides testimony that the goal of humanizing services has still been only partially fulfilled (Lamb 1984; Lamb et al. 1992). Although not all homeless individuals suffer from mental illnesses, those who do frequently experience a unique kind of eviction. The state hospitals that once might have served them are often no longer available to them, and the community alternatives that were to have been created for their care often have not materialized.

Comprehensive Services and Continuity of Care

With the passage of the original Community Mental Health Centers legislation in 1963, federal seed funds, for the first time in history, were made available for constructing and staffing community mental health programs in order to develop the five services considered essential to the provision of comprehensive care in the community: 1) 24-hour emergency services, 2) inpatient services, 3) partial hospitalization services, 4) outpatient services, and 5) preventive services in the form of community consultation and education. In 1975 Congress reaffirmed its commitment to the community mental health model by passing CMHC Amendment legislation that expanded to 12 the number of services considered essential, adding the following seven services to the original five: 6) services for children, 7) alcoholism services, 8) services for drug abusers, 9) services for elderly individuals, 10) preadmission screening of state mental hospital patients, 11) transitional housing, and 12) rehabilitation and aftercare (Barton and Barton 1983; Ruiz and Tourlentes 1983).

Community mental health ideology was largely based on an assumption that all the mental health needs of all community residents could—and indeed should—be met. In fact, the coordination of multiplex service efforts into a comprehensive system of care was one of the most fundamental concepts of the federal initiative (Aldrich 1972). "No longer," proclaimed a federal document, "will a patient face the choice between hospitalization and no treatment at all"; instead, the patient in a comprehensive community-based system of care could "enter or leave the [community mental health] center from any service component or be able to move from any service to any other service within the center" without interrupting the flow of his or her care (Person 1969).

Such a goal obviously presupposed mechanisms for linking agencies, for, with services no longer being offered in a single centralized location, many different providers would be involved in patient care. However, as Hansell (1978) noted, effective interagency communication and linkages were rare. Community-based mental health services, typically patterned after programs developed for "single-episode users of services," exhibited "a deficiency of interest in people with lifelong disorders" (Hansell 1978).

Indeed, CMHCs regularly encountered major difficulties as they strove to provide comprehensive care. With their prevailing emphasis on outpatient treatment and short-term interventions, these centers often expected patients to be sufficiently mobile and motivated to present themselves for treatment (Lamb 1988). They thus responded best to the needs of an essentially ambulatory and compliant population, not to those of severely disabled patients who required support and assistance in accessing services. Concern with such issues eventually led to a recognition of the importance of case management in community-based care. Case management, clearly a concept that is meant to redress the difficulties inherent in providing comprehensive care and continuity of care (Harris and Bachrach 1988), is essentially an affirmation of previously underestimated complexities, although it has often brought with it new bureaucratic complications (Franklin et al. 1987).

Primary Prevention and Rehabilitation

In the early years of community mental health, it was frequently assumed (and sometimes promised) that primary prevention strategies such as consultation and mental health education would result in a significant reduction in the incidence of major mental illness and would eventually dramatically limit the demand for conventional treatments (Lamb 1988; Langlsey 1980a, 1980b; Zusman and Lamb 1977). This position was advanced even though its theoretical foundation was somewhat shaky. Certainly, environmental manipulation may be expected to improve the life circumstances of mentally ill individuals and even to eliminate some varieties of personal unhappiness and stress, but it cannot be expected to eliminate the biochemical antecedents of mental illness.

Thus, it is not surprising that the answers to preventing schizophrenia and other major mental illnesses eluded the community mental health movement (Group for the Advancement of Psychiatry 1983), even though some patients, although not cured, benefited greatly from rehabilitative or tertiary prevention initiatives. Even in this regard, however, there was an excess of optimism in the early days of community mental health. Many proponents of rehabilitation at that time believed that, in those instances where illness could not itself be prevented, virtually all patients could still be restored to full social functioning if they could only have access to appropriate vocational and social opportunities in the community.

For a sizable number of mental patients, however, high levels of social functioning, competitive employment, and a return to society's mainstream proved to be unrealistic goals (Lamb 1988). Even today, given the current state of technology, there are some individuals whose rehabilitation (if that is even an appropriate term) is so slow that it must be conceptualized and measured incrementally (Bachrach 1987c). In fact, our continued insistence on "rehabilitating" some very severely disabled mentally ill individuals to full social and vocational functioning has sometimes done them more harm than good (Bachrach 1992).

Professional Egalitarianism

It is hardly surprising that a movement born during an era supporting civil rights and social activism, and nurtured by its values and concepts, subscribed to egalitarian goals. Egalitarianism in fact took several directions in community mental health: there were focused efforts to eliminate class distinctions in access to care, to involve local communities in the administration and delivery of mental health services, to involve patients themselves in the treatment process, and to equalize professional roles by creating multidisciplinary treatment teams. Because the first of these has been discussed previously and the next two have been accorded considerable attention elsewhere (see, for example, Bachrach 1991a; Lamb 1988), the following discussion deals only with the last.

Even though President Kennedy's message in 1963 had actually charged physicians with leadership in the new CMHCs, and even though it had stated specifically that physicians would be assisted in their efforts by "auxiliary treatment staff," community mental health became characterized by widely disparate viewpoints over who should be "in charge" of service delivery. Many nonpsychiatric service providers, understanding the call for multidisciplinary treatment to be a mandate to eradicate line authority in the care of mental patients, sought to eliminate invidious professional distinctions through "teamwork."

There is, however, an inherent inconsistency in the notions of teamwork and role interchangeability. Although teamwork is actually more compatible with concepts of hierarchy and complementarity than it is with role blurring (Bachrach 1988b; Jabitsky 1988), community mental health workers frequently attempted to level professional differences. Psychiatrists often found their clinical responsibilities assumed by others as their duties were increasingly limited to signing prescriptions, completing medical records, and verifying insurance forms.

Much to the detriment of patients' welfare, the significance of psychiatric illness as illness was frequently minimized, and this led to a more generalized deprofessionalization of mental health services (Doyle 1977; Fink and Weinstein 1979). The importance of professional judgment was often minimized, and greater value was placed on intuitive interpersonal skills in patient care than on training and expertise (Hopkin 1985).

The Diminishing Psychiatric Presence

Under these circumstances psychiatrists not only had to protect their professional turf, they also, more generally, had to justify their unique qualifications to practice. It is little wonder that CMHCs were becoming unattractive places for them to work (Berlin et al. 1981; Clark 1987a; Clark and Vaccaro 1987; Donovan 1982; Peterson 1981), and many chose to turn their energies elsewhere (Winslow 1979).

Thus, only 18% of CMHC psychiatrists surveyed in a national study expressed satisfaction with their positions, and only 21% stated their intention to continue working in those service sites (Reinstein 1976). The concerns raised by community psychiatrists during the 1970s were numerous and covered a wide array of grievances, such as inadequate input into administrative decisions, widespread interference with clinical autonomy, a curtailment of ongoing clinical relationships with patients, an absence of peer supports, inequitable compensation when compared with private practice psychiatrists' earnings, difficulties in functioning as members of multidisciplinary treatment teams, limited opportunities for continuing education, and low prestige and income as public employees (Clark 1987a; Langsley and Barter 1983; "Psychiatric exodus" 1978; Ribner 1980; Tucker et al. 1981).

The alliance between community mental health and community psychiatry—previously so strong that it was often difficult to tell them apart—was definitely unraveling. It was becoming increasingly difficult to attract new psychiatrists to work in the centers and to persuade those already there to stay. Thus, according to data from the National Institute of Mental Health, the percentage of all community mental health staff positions filled by psychiatrists dropped by 37% between 1970 and 1977—from 9.2% to 5.8%

(Thompson and Bass 1984)—and similar trends continued into the 1980s (Knox 1985). Statistics concerning psychiatric leadership within the centers were also revealing. In 1971 55% of CMHCs were headed by psychiatrists, but by 1985 the percentage had dropped to 8% (Knox 1985) as executive responsibilities continued to be taken over by psychologists, public administrators, lawyers, clergy, and laypersons ("Psychiatric exodus" 1978). Finally, the number of psychiatrists employed full time in CMHCs also fell (Bass 1978), a circumstance both reflecting and contributing to the diminution of psychiatric influence within those settings.

Thus, there was a serious drain of psychiatric expertise away from the centers. Perhaps more than any other single factor, the "boundarylessness" of community mental health ideology (Dinitz and Beran 1971) contributed to psychiatrists' increasing disaffection with CMHC practice. However, their growing individuation from community mental health care was more than mere guild interest; it was also rooted in a deep concern for the welfare of their patients—a concern that was validated in a report from the Inspector General of the U.S. Department of Health and Human Services indicating that perhaps as many as half of the federally funded CMHCs had failed to provide basic services to their target populations, particularly chronically mentally ill patients (Cody 1990; Hilts 1990; Moses 1990).

Toward a New Synthesis

Should the ideology of community mental health then be declared invalid for community psychiatry? That would seem to be neither warranted nor practicable, for although the principles supporting that movement had some serious drawbacks, they were still essential to community psychiatry's evolution in the United States. Thus, the principles are not so much to be perceived as wrong or invalid as they are to be regarded as tentative and temporary.

In point of fact, American community psychiatry is currently a field in search of a new equilibrium (Residency Training Committee 1991). Some of the tenets to which it subscribed during the heyday of community mental health are being discarded, others are being retained, and still others are being updated.

What has survived is in itself impressive as a legacy and as a foundation for future direction. Surely a major contribution of community mental health to the field of community psychiatry is an appreciation of citizens' basic rights to decent mental health care. Community mental health has also provided community psychiatry with a framework of hopefulness and optimism in caring for persons afflicted with mental illness. Community mental health's sensitivity to the effects of cultural circumstances on mental health service delivery continues to be reflected in the thinking of many, if not most, community psychiatrists today (Vaccaro 1988).Thus, community psychiatry's alliance with community mental health has led to a sensitivity, largely lacking in the past, to patients' various cultural identities and to the social and economic realities that often divide service provider and service recipient (Mollica 1983).

There is value for community psychiatry not only in what has been retained, but also in what has been discarded and what is being modified.The area of prevention provides an excellent example of changing perspectives. Community psychiatry, in acknowledging that there is presently no evidence that the incidence of major mental illness can be reduced through preventive interventions (American Medical Association Council on Scientific Affairs 1979; Group for the Advancement of Psychiatry 1983; Musto 1975; U.S. General Accounting Office 1977; Zusman and Lamb 1977), is clearly adopting a more realistic view of the potential of primary prevention. At the same time the field is becoming increasingly attuned to the possibilities of secondary prevention (i.e., early diagnosis and treatment to decrease the duration of acute illness) and tertiary prevention (i.e., rehabilitation to reduce residual disability), particularly for chronically mentally ill individuals. In fact, there currently is a more generalized appreciation of the unique needs of these most severely disabled individuals (Menninger 1989;Vaccaro 1986;Winston 1989), and this is one of the most encouraging outcomes of community psychiatry's efforts since the 1960s (Bachrach 1991b).

Emerging Emphases and Future Directions

Thus, despite the existence of problems in the alliance of community mental health and community psychiatry, and despite considerable skepticism on the part of some practicing community psychiatrists, parts of the community mental health ideology continue to hold appeal. Much of the enthusiasm that characterized community psychiatry during the early years of the community mental health movement has survived to the 1990s, even though the field generally acknowledges some earlier errors and even though the diminution of federal interest in mental health has curtailed program development (Bachrach 1988c, 1991a).There is still a widespread hope among community psychiatrists that services for mentally ill individuals will become more accessible, more comprehensive, more equitably distributed, and more humane.

Currently the federally funded, federally regulated CMHC program is no longer part of the mental health service scene in the United States. Except for the existence of a few time-limited demonstration projects, the federal monies that are devoted to community mental health efforts are funneled through state agencies that maintain substantial discretion over their disposition. Although members of some interest groups may decry the political forces that have emasculated federal concern with mental health service delivery, ironically enough, there has been some benefit for community psychiatry in this shift. No longer must community psychiatry be limited by the aforementioned aspects of community mental health ideology that curtailed psychiatric practice and often affected patient care adversely; the field is now free to redefine its scope and mission.

Thus, although most advocates would probably welcome more federal financial commitment and legitimation, there is at least an upside to the leanness of resources. Community psychiatrists, who at one time saw themselves as functioning primarily within the constraints of a federal community mental health effort, are currently considering how to apply their professional skills in a variety of service settings, not only CMHCs. This has led to increased optimism within the field, and much of this must be credited to the vitality of a new generation of community psychiatrists (Bachrach 1991b). Community psychiatry in the 1990s is attracting growing numbers of young, socially conscious physicians (Vaccaro 1986) who believe that psychiatry can and must respond to the treatment needs of psychiatrically unserved and underserved populations. They are attuned to concrete circumstances affecting psychiatric service demand, such as homelessness, demographic realities, and family burden.

In 1984 an organization was founded that is currently known as the American Association of Community Psychiatrists (AACP), a group intended to "provide mutual support" and develop "cohesive and politically effective" policies to "stem the tide of psychiatrists leaving community mental health centers" (Clark 1987b). Largely as the result of continuing efforts on the part of this new organization, the American Psychiatric Association in 1988 approved a series of guidelines for psychiatric practice in CMHCs (Clark 1990; *Guidelines for Psychiatric Practice in Community Mental Health Centers* 1991). These include model job descriptions for medical directors and staff psychiatrists, as well as guidelines for patient assessment, emergency intervention, and interdisciplinary clinical collaboration. It is clear that community psychiatrists are no longer passive and that they are adopting a firm stance toward the issues that affect the practice of their profession.

There has also been an increased emphasis on the need to define and delimit the responsibilities of community psychiatrists (Residency Training Committee 1991): vagueness and acquiescence are giving way to efforts to minimize role blurring and maximize the complementarity of professional disciplines, a position reflected in Tourlentes' (1981) statement that the "properly organized psychiatric team must not be an amorphous amoeba-like creature capable of moving in all directions. It should have a rational and consistent structure, predicated as much on significant professional differences as on incidental functional similarities"; thus, psychiatrists must not "compromise [their] medical responsibilities merely to please those who seek parity where none exists."

Such frankness and assertiveness on the part of community psychiatry were relatively rare in the early years of the community mental health movement, and they are currently accompanied by a reinforced commitment to biopsychosocial principles (Engel 1980; Liberman 1988; Residency Training Committee 1991) in which the patient's biological and psychosocial needs are simultaneously addressed.

Several related areas of special focus for the future development of community psychiatry may be noted.

First, efforts to attract psychiatrists to work in community-based service settings, whether these are CMHCs, outpatient facilities, inpatient psychiatric units in general hospitals, or nontraditional service sites such as railroad stations and shelters for homeless persons (Cohen 1990), must be increased. Sowers (1991) has suggested that the scope of community psychiatry even extends logically to the practice of public hospital psychiatry. Indeed, the emphasis on "outreach" as a valid psychiatric service concept is explored in Neal Cohen's (1990) *Psychiatry Takes to the Streets,* an edited volume whose metaphoric title aptly suggests the need for flexibility in the practice of community psychiatry.

Second, once recruited to work in these settings, community psychiatrists must be provided with incentives to stay there. In addition to adequate financial compensation, there must be full recognition of the unique qualifications of community psychiatrists to operate within a biopsychosocial framework in providing comprehensive care to mentally ill persons.

Third, there must be an increased effort in the area of specialty training to prepare psychiatrists for the important clinical tasks associated with community psychiatry (Talbott 1979). Training sites should, ideally, be places "where good psychiatry is practiced" (Rankin 1982), and it is important that a cadre of role models be developed (Dewey and Astrachan 1986). As Diamond et al. (1985) have aptly noted, "Learning is a matter of identification; in every profession students imitate the teachers whom they most respect. Skills and roles associated with community mental health need to be framed and modeled as 'high prestige,' a task which only skillful professionals can achieve." In this regard, affiliating community-based service sites with established medical schools has the potential for facilitating the recruitment and retention of community psychiatrists, as such liaisons can provide prestige and stimulate collegial relationships and opportunities for continuing education and research (Dewey and Astrachan 1985).

Finally, the effort to define and delimit appropriate clinical and administrative roles for community psychiatrists must be strengthened. Diamond et al. (1991) contributed to this effort by proposing a dichotomy: "essential" roles (including those of medical expert and legal or medical authority) and "nonessential but desirable" roles (including those of clinical assessor, generalist, teacher, and scholar). Although the specifics of this conceptual approach await consensus—Clark (1991) has argued that psychiatrists must assume an "overall clinical leadership role" that subsumes virtually all of these elements—it represents a framework within which to begin to order professional responsibilities.

One of the most promising prospects for the future lies in community psychiatrists' current efforts to build bridges with other branches of psychiatry, so that the concept of community-based treatment may be represented in mainstream psychiatric thinking. In 1986, for example, the American Psychiatric Association featured a symposium on the relationships between CMHCs and general hospital psychiatric units, an event to be marked for its unifying focus. Instead of concentrating on differences within psychiatry, this symposium attempted to promote pluralism within the profession and reduce fragmentation of services through mutual understanding and support (Bachrach 1987a).

There are, of course, problems to overcome, for some current agencies that call themselves CMHCs eschew psychiatry altogether (Bachrach 1988a). Other agencies, however, have been strengthened in their determination to encourage and enhance the psychiatric presence in service delivery. It has become the task of community psychiatrists to continue to solidify psychiatry's role in the latter service sites even as they lobby for psychiatric representation in those facilities that maintain an antimedical philosophy (Clark 1987b).

With such profound changes occurring in rapid succession, it is difficult to offer a summary judgment of the accomplishments of community psychiatry to date: it is probable that a more complete historical perspective is needed. However, the very search for new directions in the field is encouraging. It is interesting to note in this connection that the *Community Psychiatrist,* the AACP's quarterly newsletter, has assumed a determinedly eclectic focus in that it features regular contributions on psychotropic medications, psychobiology, medical issues, psychosocial rehabilitation, residency training, and concerns that affect the care of chronic mental patients and their families. The newsletter also routinely contains contributions from community psychiatrists from all regions of the United States, and its general tone suggests that something very like a grass roots movement is attracting such psychiatrists to the practice of community psychiatry.

Thus, whatever else it may be, community psychiatry in the United States is not stagnant. Thomas and Garrison wrote in 1975 that the CMHC "is clearly a structure in transition between a mental hospital and something else, the outlines of which are only emerging." Similar conclusions may be drawn regarding community psychiatry today. More than one criterion may be used to assess the field's success. If we choose not to dwell on its past problems but rather to support its strengthened efforts to humanize services through the application of progressive concepts, we may say with certainty that community psychiatry is not finished yet: it has an aggressive agenda for change as it applies the principles of psychiatric practice to work in community-based service settings.

References

Aldrich CK: The promise and problems of community mental health centers. J Med Soc N J 69:199–202, 1972

American Medical Association Council on Scientific Affairs: Evaluation of Community Mental Health Centers. Chicago, IL, American Medical Association, 1979

Bachrach LL: The homeless mentally ill and mental health services: an analytical review of the literature, in The Homeless Mentally Ill. Edited by Lamb HR. Washington, DC, American Psychiatric Association, 1984, pp 11–53

Bachrach LL: Deinstitutionalization: what do the numbers mean? Hosp Community Psychiatry 37:118–121, 1986

Bachrach LL: General hospitals and CMHCs: a commentary, in Leona Bachrach Speaks. New Directions for Mental Health Services, No 35. San Francisco, CA, Jossey-Bass, 1987a, pp 91–97

Bachrach LL: Geographic mobility among the homeless mentally ill. Hosp Community Psychiatry 38:27–28, 1987b

Bachrach LL: Measuring program outcomes in Tucson. Hosp Community Psychiatry 38:1151–1152, 1987c

Bachrach LL: Community mental health centers and other semantic concerns. Hosp Community Psychiatry 39:605–606, 1988a

Bachrach LL: Egalitarianism and the CMHC treatment team. Community Psychiatrist June 3:10–12, 1988b

Bachrach LL: Progress in community mental health. Community Ment Health J 24:3–6, 1988c

Bachrach LL: Community mental health centers in the USA, in Community Psychiatry: The Principles. Edited by Bennett D, Freeman H. Edinburgh, Scotland, Churchill Livingstone, 1991a, pp 543–569

Bachrach LL: Community psychiatry's changing role. Hosp Community Psychiatry 42:573–574, 1991b

Bachrach LL: Psychosocial rehabilitation and psychiatry in the care of long-term patients. Am J Psychiatry 149:1455–1463, 1992

Bachrach LL, Lamb HR: What have we learned from deinstitutionalization? Psychiatric Annals 19:12–21, 1989

Barton WE, Barton GM: Mental Health Administration: Principles and Practice. New York, Human Sciences Press, 1983

Bass RD: CMHC Staffing: Who Minds the Store? Rockville, MD, National Institute of Mental Health, 1978

Bellak L: Community mental health as a branch of public health, in Progress in Community Mental Health, Vol 1. Edited by Bellak L, Barten HH. New York, Grune & Stratton, 1969

Berlin RM, Kales JD, Humphrey FJ, et al: The patient care crisis in community mental health centers: a need for more psychiatric involvement. Am J Psychiatry 138:450–454, 1981

Bloom BL: Primary prevention: an overview, in Primary Prevention in Psychiatry: State of the Art. Edited by Barter JT, Talbott SW. Washington, DC, American Psychiatric Association, 1986, pp 3–12

Borus JF: Issues critical to the survival of community mental health. Am J Psychiatry 135:1029–1035, 1978

Clark GH: CMHCs and psychiatrists: a necessarily polemical review, in Community Psychiatry: Problems and Possibilities. Spring House, PA, McNeil Pharmaceuticals, 1987a, pp 5–21

Clark GH: Psychiatrists and community mental health centers. Hosp Community Psychiatry 38:113, 1987b

Clark GH: Assuring quality in community mental health centers: the need for psychiatric practice guidelines. Psychiatr Clin North Am 13:113–125, 1990

Clark GH: Psychiatrists' roles in CMHCs (letter). Hosp Community Psychiatry 42:1260, 1991

Clark GH, Vaccaro JV: Burnout among CMHC psychiatrists and the struggle to survive. Hosp Community Psychiatry 38:843–847, 1987

Cody P: CMHC administration studied amid alleged mismanagement. Psychiatr News November 19:1, 26, 1990

Cohen N (ed): Psychiatry Takes to the Streets: Outreach and Crisis Intervention for the Mentally Ill. New York, Guilford, 1990

Cordes C: The plight of the homeless mentally ill. APA Monitor, February 1984, pp 1, 13

Dewey L, Astrachan BM: Organizational issues in recruitment and retention of psychiatrists by CMHCs, in Community Mental Health Centers and Psychiatrists. Washington, DC, Joint Steering Committee of the American Psychiatric Association and the National Council of Community Mental Health Centers, 1985, pp 22–31

Diamond R, Cutler DL, Langsley DG, et al: Training, Recruitment, and Retention of Psychiatrists in CMHCs: Issues and Answers, in Community Mental Health Centers and Psychiatrists. Washington, DC, Joint Steering Committee of the American Psychiatric Association and the National Council of Community Mental Health Centers, 1985, pp 32–50

Diamond RJ, Stein LI, Susser E: Essential and nonessential roles for psychiatrists in community mental health centers. Hosp Community Psychiatry 42:187–189, 1991

Dinitz S, Beran N: Community mental health as a boundaryless and boundary-busting system. J Health Soc Behav 12:99–108, 1971

Donovan CM: Problems of psychiatric practice in community mental health centers. Am J Psychiatry 139:456–460, 1982

Doyle MC: Egalitarianism in a mental health center: an experiment that failed. Hosp Community Psychiatry 28:521–525, 1977

Dunham HW: Social Realities and Community Psychiatry. New York, Human Sciences Press, 1976

Engel GL: The clinical application of the biopsychosocial model. Am J Psychiatry 137:535–544, 1980

Fink PJ, Weinstein SP: Whatever happened to psychiatry: the deprofessionalization of community mental health centers. Am J Psychiatry 136:406–409, 1979

Franklin JL, Solovitz B, Mason M, et al: An evaluation of case management. Am J Public Health 77:674–678, 1987

Freedman AM: Historical and political roots of the Community Mental Health Centers Act. Am J Orthopsychiatry 37:487–494, 1967

Gronfein W: Incentives and intentions in mental health policy: a comparison of the Medicaid and Community Mental Health Programs. J Health Soc Behav 26:192–206, 1985

Group for the Advancement of Psychiatry: Community Psychiatry: A Reappraisal. New York, Mental Health Materials Center, 1983

Guidelines for Psychiatric Practice in Community Mental Health Centers. Am J Psychiatry 148:965–966, 1991

Hansell N: Services for schizophrenics: a lifelong approach to treatment. Hosp Community Psychiatry 29:105–109, 1978

Harris M, Bachrach LL (eds): Clinical Case Management. New Directions for Mental Health Services, No 40. San Francisco, CA, Jossey-Bass, 1988

Hilts PJ: Report is critical of mental clinics. New York Times, October 6, 1990, p 25

Hopkin JT: Psychiatry and medicine in the emergency room, in Emergency Psychiatry at the Crossroads. New Directions for Mental Health Services. Edited by Lipton FR, Goldfinger S. San Francisco, CA, Jossey-Bass, 1985, pp 47–53

Jabitsky IM: Psychiatric teams and the psychiatrist's authority in the New York State mental health system. NY State J Med 88:577–581, 1988

Joint Commission on Mental Illness and Health: Action for Mental Health. New York, Basic Books, 1961

Kennedy JF: Message from the President of the United States relative to mental illness and mental retardation. Washington, DC, 88th Congress, First Session, House of Representatives Document No 58, February 5, 1963

Kety SS: From rationalization to reason. Am J Psychiatry 131:957–963, 1974

Knox MD: National registry reveals profile of service provider. National Council News, September 1, 1985, p 1

Lamb HR (ed): The Homeless Mentally Ill. Washington, DC, American Psychiatric Association, 1984

Lamb HR: Community psychiatry and prevention, in The American Psychiatric Press Textbook of Psychiatry. Edited by Talbott JA, Hales RE, Yudofsky SC. Washington, DC, American Psychiatric Press, 1988

Lamb HR, Bachrach LL, Kass F (eds): Treating the Homeless Mentally Ill. Washington, DC, American Psychiatric Association, 1992

Langsley DG: The community mental health center: does it treat patients? Hosp Community Psychiatry 31:815–819, 1980a

Langsley DG: Community psychiatry, in Comprehensive Textbook of Psychiatry, Vol 3. Edited by Kaplan HI, Freedman AM. Baltimore, MD, Williams & Wilkins, 1980b

Langsley DG, Barter JT: Psychiatric roles in the community mental health center. Hosp Community Psychiatry 34:729–733, 1983

Liberman RP (ed): Psychiatric Rehabilitation of Chronic Mental Patients. Washington, DC, American Psychiatric Press, 1988

Menninger RW: Trends in American psychiatry: implications for psychiatry in Japan. Psychiatria et Neurologia Japonica 91:556–565, 1989

Mollica RF: From asylum to community. N Engl J Med 308:367–373, 1983

Moses S: CMHC grant programs face a full audit. APA Monitor, May 1990, pp 21–22

Musto DA: Whatever happened to "community mental health"? Public Interest 39:52–79, 1975

National Institute of Mental Health: Staffing Differences Between Federally Funded CMHCs Located in Low Income and High Income Catchment Areas, 1976. Division of Biometry and Epidemiology Memorandum No 30. Rockville, MD, National Institute of Mental Health, January 27, 1978

Okpaku SO: The psychiatrist and the Social Security Disability Insurance and Supplemental Security Income Programs. Hosp Community Psychiatry 39:879–883, 1988

Pear R: New Reagan policy to cut benefits for the aged, blind and disabled. New York Times, October 16, 1987, pp A1, B5

Person PH: A Statistical Information System for Community Mental Health Centers. Rockville, MD, National Institute of Mental Health, 1969

Peterson LG: On being a necessary evil at a mental health center. Hosp Community Psychiatry 32:644, 1981

President's Commission on Mental Health: Report to the President. Washington, DC, The White House, 1978

Psychiatric exodus from CMHCs: panel examines the causes and proposes some solutions. Hosp Community Psychiatry 29:407, 411, 414, 1978

Rankin RM: Response and critique. Community Mental Health J 18:17–18, 1982

Reagan's 1987 budget calls for further cuts in ADAMHA programs hit by Gramm-Rudman. Hosp Community Psychiatry 37:525, 1986

Reinstein MJ: Community mental health centers and the dissatisfied psychiatrist: results of an informal survey. Hosp Community Psychiatry 29:261–262, 1978

Residency Training Committee: Defining community psychiatry. Community Psychiatrist, Spring 1991, p 4

Ribner DS: Psychiatrists and community mental health: current issues and trends. Hosp Community Psychiatry 31:338–341, 1980

Ruiz P, Tourlentes TT: Community mental health centers, in Psychiatric Administration. Edited by JA Talbott. New York, Grune & Stratton, 1983

Schwab JJ, Schwab ME: Sociocultural Roots of Mental Illness: An Epidemiological Survey. New York, Plenum, 1978

Schwartz DA: Community mental health in 1972—an assessment, in Progress in Community Mental Health, Vol 2. Edited by Barten HH, Bellak L. New York, Grune & Stratton, 1972, pp 3–34

Smith WG, Hart DW: Community mental health: a noble failure? Hosp Community Psychiatry 26:581–583, 1975

Sowers W: The scope of community psychiatry includes public hospital practice. Community Psychiatrist, Summer 1991, pp 1–2

Talbott JA: Why psychiatrists leave the public sector. Hosp Community Psychiatry 30:778–782, 1979

Talbott JA: Trends in the delivery of psychiatric services, in Psychiatric Administration. Edited by JA Talbott. New York, Grune & Stratton, 1983

Task Panel on Community Mental Health Centers Assessment: in Reports Submitted to the President's Commission on Mental Health, Vol 2. Washington, DC, The White House, 1978

Task Panel on Rural Mental Health: in Reports Submitted to the President's Commission on Mental Health, Vol 3. Washington, DC, The White House, 1978, pp 1155–1190

Thomas CS, Garrison V: A general systems view of community mental health, in Progress in Community Mental Health, Vol 3. Edited by Bellak L, Barten HH. New York, Brunner/Mazel, 1975, pp 265–332

Thompson JW, Bass RD: Changing staffing patterns in community mental health centers. Hosp Community Psychiatry 35:1107–1114, 1984

Tourlentes TT: Psychiatric administration and medical responsibility. Adm Ment Health 9:154–158, 1981

Tucker GT, Turner J, Chapman R: Problems in attracting and retaining psychiatrists in rural areas. Hosp Community Psychiatry 43:118–120, 1981

U.S. General Accounting Office: Returning the Mentally Disabled to the Community: Government Needs to Do More (Report HRD-76-152). Washington, DC, U.S. General Accounting Office, 1977

U.S. General Accounting Office: States Have Made Few Changes in Implementing the Alcohol, Drug Abuse, and Mental Health Services Block Grant (Report HRD-84-52). Washington, DC, U.S. General Accounting Office, 1984

U.S. General Accounting Office: Block Grants: Proposed Formulas for Substance Abuse, Mental Health Provide More Equity (Report HRD-87-109BR). Washington, DC, General Accounting Office, 1987

Vaccaro JV: Residents' forum. Psychiatr News May:16, 31, 17, 1986,

Vaccaro JV: Culture and psychiatry. Community Psychiatrist 3:3, 1988

van Winkle WA: Bedlam by the bay. New West, December 1980, p 1

Windle C, Scully D: Community mental health centers and the decreasing use of state mental hospitals. Community Ment Health J 12:239–243, 1976

Winslow WW: The changing role of psychiatrists in community mental health centers. Am J Psychiatry 136:24–27, 1979

Winston LM: The community psychiatrist's leadership in psychosocial intervention. Community Psychiatrist, May 1989, p 9

Yolles SF: Past, present and 1980: trend projections, in Progress in Community Mental Health, Vol 1. Edited by Bellak L, Barten HH. New York, Grune & Stratton, 1969, pp 3–23

Zusman J: The philosophic basis for community and social psychiatry, in An Assessment of the Community Mental 1975 Health Movement. Edited by Barton WE, Sanborn CJ. Lexington, MA, Heath, 1975, pp 21–34

Zusman J, Lamb HR: In defense of community mental health. Am J Psychiatry 134:887–890, 1977

Chapter 2

Conceptual Issues for Contemporary Community Psychiatry Practice

Jerome V. Vaccaro, M.D.
Gordon H. Clark, Jr., M.D., M.Div.

In 1964 in his *Handbook of Community Psychiatry and Community Mental Health,* Bellak hailed community psychiatry as the "third psychiatric revolution." Inspired by the social changes of the day and the excitement of a new presidential administration, he and others saw new and expanding horizons opening up for psychiatry. He acknowledged the advent of psychotropic medications as making "community psychiatry a reality," making "it possible to develop and maintain the open ward, to treat psychotics in a general hospital setting, to reduce the length of hospitalization, and to provide for the aftercare and rehabilitation of the former mental patient in the community." He cautioned against the reductionistic assumption that mental illnesses would be found to have simple biological substrates that could be cured with the proverbial "magic pill." He further warned against the headlong rush toward the use of less experienced therapists to the exclusion of well-trained individuals. A reading of the book provides a glimpse into the heady early days of the community mental health movement, with its promise of revolutionizing mental health systems and the techniques used by community psychiatrists. Bellak's comments also reflect many contemporary concerns.

Many of the early expectations of the movement have been realized, whereas others have been discarded or given lower priority. Psychiatrists currently expect that most of their patients can be treated successfully in the community, medications are considered a mainstay in the treatment and rehabilitation of many mental disorders, and new psychopharmacological and psychosocial technologies have had their efficacy demonstrated. The diagnostic system has changed dramatically and is codified in DSM-IV (American Psychiatric Association 1994). Although psychiatrists accept that mental illnesses do not have simple biological explanations that are amenable to permanent correction, they understand that most mental disorders spring from a biological diathesis that is influenced by socioenvironmental stressors and that this interaction may lead to the production of symptoms. The cost-saving and population-focus thrusts of the community mental health movement have been appropriated by those who speak of an overhaul of the American health care system. In many ways, the promise of the early 1960s is with us again; the experiences of community psychiatry may offer significant guidance regarding future directions in mental health care delivery. In this chapter we provide an overview of contemporary conceptual issues facing community psychiatry and psychiatry in general. We suggest ways in which they may guide our practice over the coming decade, and offer some possibilities for where community psychiatry and community mental health may fit into our health care delivery systems.

From Catchment Areas to Target Populations

Perhaps the most notable and well-recognized achievement of the community mental health movement was its shifting of our focus away from the treatment of individual patients, toward targeting interventions to larger populations of individuals. Individuals living within a given catchment area then became the focal concern of clinicians. In its best applications, this emphasis resulted in the development of innovative approaches to help patients establish and then maintain themselves in the community. It also led to our reliance on alternative treatments and systems of care, contributing to the lessened reliance on hospitals for long-term care and reducing the lengths of hospital stay.

Stressing the catchment area did have its problems. Some have suggested that it led to diffuse efforts to correct a wide variety of social ills, for which we as mental health professionals are ill-equipped. This interest was spurred by findings of extensive levels of psychiatric symptoms among members of the general community, and by the interest of many professionals in the relationships among mental illnesses and various social stressors. In their most castigated sense, it is suggested that community mental health programs used public funding to support programs to enhance positive mental health and treatment of the "worried well and existentially unhappy," to the exclusion of individuals with disabling mental illnesses such as schizophrenia (Torrey et al. 1990). This situation is presently undergoing a dramatic shift. Partly due to redirection of public funding, "target populations" are more often discussed today than are catchment areas. In the early 1980s, data indicated that seriously mentally ill individuals represented less than 10% of most community mental health programs' client bases. Today that figure exceeds 50% in many settings.

Changes in the Funding Environment

The funding of community mental health programs has undergone dramatic change and has become extremely complex. During the 1970s and 1980s, states became the locus of control for most public mental health expenditures. This was partly occasioned by the dissolution of the branches of the National Institute of Mental Health charged with this service responsibility. Coincident with this change, most states developed separate administrative structures to deal with mental health and alcohol and drug abuse services. This partly was fueled by prevailing views of diagnostic reductionism that held that one could explain sets of psychiatric symptoms with a single diagnosis. In addition, the development of new approaches to treatment and the claiming of these treatments by various professional groups led to the view that one should treat one set of symptoms or one illness at a time.

Interestingly, many of the principles and practices developed for government oversight of community mental health programs are being utilized in the emerging managed health care industry. Another trend over the past decade has been the redirection of funding authority and responsibility from the federal government to state governments and now to local authorities. In fact, in the state of California an initiative termed "realignment" has been implemented so that county agencies control all state mental health funds, including those used for state hospital care. This climate is in keeping with the community mental health clinical principle of locating ultimate control over care as close as possible to the patient/clinician/family triad. Other initiatives include exploration of various capitated funding mechanisms for the care of chronically mentally ill individuals, and "case rate" or capitated funding strategies for other populations.

The Emergence of "Dual Diagnosis"

The question of diagnostic grouping has become clouded over the past decade. Where finding a single diagnosis was once the goal of assessment, the recognition of diagnostic comorbidity has become more commonplace. This has in turn led to the development of new combined treatment strategies. To that end, many of the chapters in this volume specifically consider the issue of comorbidity. Concern has focused mainly on the coexistence of substance abuse disorders and other psychiatric illnesses. Initial consideration was focused on whether the substance abuse or the mental illness was primary. We now accept that the disorders coexist and require combined treatment. We are, however, faced with the challenge of differentiating between organically generated conditions (e.g., a drug-induced psychosis) and those where a "functional" psychiatric illness and a substance abuse disorder both are present.

It is likely that this interest in dual diagnoses will expand in coming years and that new and more effective approaches to treatment will emerge. Presumably, greater attention will be drawn to other comorbid conditions, including traumatic brain injury/psychiatric disorder, Axis I/Axis II, and other amalgams.

Community Control and Involvement

Another great achievement of the community mental health movement has been the involvement of the community-at-large in planning and implementing mental health services. This was originally executed through the establishment of community mental health boards that served as boards of directors for community mental health centers. Many state and local governments set up parallel bodies with similar charges. These groups varied along the continuum of control from oversight or advisory bodies with little or no direct authority over service provision through formal boards of directors with direct supervisory control over a community mental health center's executive director.

Community involvement has evolved through many stages since its first renderings. One important effect of this is the high level of family and consumer involvement in community mental health care. Efforts such as those by the National Alliance for the Mentally Ill and the major consumer groups have been pivotal in redressing stigmatization of the mentally ill and improving funding for research about and treatment of mental illness. We look forward to the deepening of this involvement in the planning and operation of community-based systems of mental health care.

Psychiatric Leadership: Executive Director, Medical Director, or...

When community mental health centers first were established, most were directed by psychiatrists. In fact, regulations mandated that psychiatrists occupy executive director positions. Furthermore, this seemed a natural development, as most state hospital superintendents and state mental health directors were medical doctors. This regulation was overturned, and other mental health professionals and others assumed greater responsibility for patient care and administration. Since that time, psychiatrists have left administrative positions in community mental health settings to an alarming degree. By the mid-1980s, fewer than 5% of CMHCs had psychiatrists as directors. More disturbing, very few centers even had medical director positions. Psychiatrists' involvement in community settings was becoming severely fragmented, with the overall number of psychiatrists per CMHC going up but the total number of psychiatrist hours per CMHC dropping precipitously. Essentially, many psychiatrists used CMHCs as secondary practice sites, and CMHCs came to regard psychiatrists as dispensable. Factors cited for this exodus include inadequate training opportunities (Talbott 1991), poor salaries, and poor fit between authority and responsibility (Clark and Vaccaro 1987). Concomitantly, concerns developed regarding the deterioration in the quality of care provided in CMHCs (Freedman 1978; Arce and Vergare 1985; Perr 1986) and the apparent abandonment of their original mission, care of the seriously and chronically mentally ill patient (Group for the Adancement of Psychiatry 1983).

This trend has begun to change. The American Association of Community Psychiatrists and American Psychiatric Association have paid considerable attention to this matter and both have promulgated guidelines for psychiatrists practicing in community settings; these are reviewed by Young and Clark elsewhere in this volume. The role of the psychiatrist has undergone change as community mental health centers and public psychiatric programs have evolved. No longer can we assert our claim on positions of authority simply by virtue of our medical degrees. In the best situations, overall clinical and administrative leadership derives from competence in those areas. In the future, we should define appropriate leadership roles for ourselves and other professionals that ensure high quality clinical care.

Community psychiatry may well offer the prospective practitioner the greatest variety of experiences available within the field of psychiatry. There is variety in the ages of patients, spectrum and severity of illness, and cultural and socioeconomic groups served. There is variety in terms of treatment sites: outpatient clinics, emergency rooms, alternative acute care settings, partial hospital and inpatient programs, clubhouses and other rehabilitation programs, homes of patients and their family members, group homes, nursing homes, and prisons. Indeed, the CMHC is only one of a number of settings where one may practice community psychiatry. There is variety in terms of collaborators, including other clinicians (both within and outside the agency), members of the state or local departments of mental health, members of the judiciary, and members of local affiliates of groups such as the National Alliance for the Mentally Ill. The actual role of the community psychiatrist also is quite varied, including functions as a clinician, supervisor, administrator, teacher and researcher. Finally, in attending to patients' comprehensive biopsychosocial needs, there is variety in applied treatment modalities: somatic therapies; individual, couple, family, and group psychotherapy; behavioral strategies; and psychiatric rehabilitation interventions.

Community Psychiatric Interventions: Progress and Reform

Psychiatry in general, and community psychiatry more particularly, were often criticized as being too ideology-bound, and not sufficiently based in scientific theory and practice. To a large extent this has changed. The American Psychiatric Association's Diagnostic and Statistical Manuals have done much to advance the cause of rigorous diagnostic assessment. The greater reliance on outcomes research has led to the refinement of psychopharmacologic, psychotherapeutic, and psychosocial techniques and technologies. For example, Vaccaro and Young in their chapter detail psychopharmacologic treatments for individuals with schizophrenia that are now better targeted to specific symptom clusters and their relapse and remission (also see Stein et al. 1990), and Diamond speaks of better defined models of clinical case management. In other publications, authors have demonstrated the value of specific psychotherapeutic interventions for certain symptoms or disorders, the value of social skills training in the treatment of schizophrenia, and the efficacy of various forms of family interventions. We are now in a position to target more carefully the symptoms of psychiatric disorders for treatment. In a parallel manner, psychiatric rehabilitation has gained credibility as a unique area of practice.

Conclusions

In a special issue of the *Community Mental Health Journal* in 1987, entitled "Psychiatrists and CMHCs: A Recovering Relationship?" the question was asked, "Will CMHCs and CMHC psychiatrists survive, and what will be their relationships?" It would seem that this question has been modified, in that both parties have survived, and are poised at the threshold of a newly configured health care system in the United States. Given the prevalence of community mental health settings, and the consistency of their missions with the views put forward by health care reform architects, we will be presented with, and should seek out opportunities to be creative and further extend the initial mission of the community mental health movement: to provide quality mental health care for Americans in the communities in which they live, and in particular, to improve the lots of those with the most severe illnesses.

References

Arce AA, Vergare MJ: Psychiatrists and interprofessional role conflict in community mental health centers, in Community Mental Health Centers and Psychiatrists. Washington, DC: American Psychiatric Association and National Council of CMHCs, 1985

American Psychiatric Association: Diagnostic and Statistical Manual of Mental Disorders, 4th Edition. Washington, DC, American Psychiatric Association, 1994

Bellack L (ed): Handbook of Community Psychiatry and Community Mental Health. New York, Grune & Stratton, 1964

Clark GH, Vaccaro JV: Burnout among CMHC psychiatrists and the struggle to survive. Hosp Community Psychiatry 38:843–847, 1987

Freedman DX: Community mental health: slogan and a history of the mission, in Controversy in Psychiatry. Edited by Brady JP, Brodie HKH. Philadelphia, PA, WB Saunders, 1978

Group for the Advancement of Psychiatry: Community Psychiatry: A Reappraisal. New York, Mental Health Materials Center, 1983

Perr IN: New multi-tier system in psychiatry. Psychiatric Times 3:1, 1986

Stein LI, Diamond RJ, Factor RM: A systems approach to the care of persons with schizophrenia, in Handbook of Schizophrenia, Vol 5: Psychosocial Therapies. Edited by Herz MI, Keith SJ, Docherty JP. Amsterdam, The Netherlands, Elsevier, 1990

Talbott JA (ed): State university collaboration project, collected articles, Hosp Community Psychiatry 42:39–73, 1991

Torrey EF, Wolfe SM, Erdman K, et al: Care of the Seriously Mentally Ill: A Rating of State Programs, 3rd Edition. Washington, DC, Public Citizen Health Research Group and the National Alliance for the Mentally Ill, 1990

The Treatment Continuum

Chapter 3

Time-Efficient Therapy in Community Settings

Richard Chung, M.D.
Jerome V. Vaccaro, M.D.
Orlando J. Cartaya, M.D.

Outpatient care was one of the original five mandated services that community mental health centers (CMHCs) were expected to offer to citizens in their catchment areas. This initially occurred at a time when outpatient care was essentially unavailable to most citizens. This lack of available services was fueled by a variety of factors, including a dearth of providers, lack of consensus regarding the existence of illnesses other than chronic mental illnesses, a lack of information regarding effective treatments, and community stigmatization and poor understanding of mental illness.

For the most part, these conditions have changed dramatically. The number of mental health care providers has literally exploded, so that problems currently have more to do with role definition and boundary setting among professionals than with basic human resource availability. Fundamental advancements have greatly improved the precision with which diagnostic assessments can be undertaken. The current diagnostic classification system for mental disorders (DSM-IV) (American Psychiatric Association 1994) has led to greater reliability in the dialogue among professionals about mental illness and contributes to the progressive refinement of therapeutic interventions. Finally, the increasing sophistication of the general population (and resulting decrease in stigmatization) about mental illness has been spurred by family and consumer group advocacy and education, by the community mental health movement's successes, and by dissemination of information regarding the high prevalence of psychiatric disorders, their frequent biological substrates, and the efficacy of certain treatments.

In this chapter we highlight what we believe to be the principles for high-quality, efficient outpatient therapy with members of the general population who present for treatment. This includes the ways in which the current emphasis on managed care influences the provision of psychotherapy, the role that community psychiatrists may occupy in today's mental health care environment, and the necessary shifts in the way community psychiatrists think about psychotherapy. Because of space constraints, we do not review the many schools of psychotherapy or provide a guide to psychotherapy in community settings. The reader is referred to the listed references (Barten 1971; Budman 1988; Sifneos 1961) for such comprehensive or detailed readings. Similarly, we do not review the available research data in this area. Instead, we highlight ways to think about psychotherapy in the contemporary community mental health environment.

Currently there is an increasingly supportive environment for the growth of economically successful opportunities in community psychiatry and community mental health. Health care costs, specifically mental health care costs, have increased in recent years. Current plans to provide health care coverage to uninsured and indigent individuals in American society may carry significant increases in the allocation of resources for mental health services. This offers an opportunity to utilize the principles of community psychiatry in the design and practice of cost-effective mental health care services. Since their inception, community mental health systems have struggled with the problem of providing care to indigent populations in the face of economic constraints. As a result, the field of community psychiatry is noted for developing innovative, population-based changes conducive to the delivery of optimal care to the most people at the least cost.

Managed Care and Community Mental Health

Even as CMHCs in earlier decades were transforming mental health care delivery, their funding and success eventually were limited. At the same time, increasing health care costs in the private sector curtailed the availability of care. For example, it has been estimated that for every automobile made by a major American manufacturer, $600 in costs are attributed to health care utilization. The growth of managed care began with the use of benefit design to control access to care, and copayments to control utilization of care. This was followed by the use of preferred provider organizations or discounted networks of providers. The use of utilization review and current variants of utilization management and case management followed these developments.

The Scope of the Problem

One in three Americans will suffer a disabling mental illness at some time during their lives. Furthermore, one in five Americans suffers from mental illness at any given time (Robins et al. 1991). Although most of these individuals currently seek assistance from general health care providers and agencies, evidence suggests that the emergence of managed care has led to an appropriate increase in the use of mental health services by patients.

Currently the managed care industry has made use of such time-honored community mental health care principles as comprehensive continuums of care, interdisciplinary teams, and continuity of care. These principles have become the foundation for most mental health care delivery systems for private sector clients. The use of a manager who is responsible and accountable for resource utilization and quality of care, combined with careful underwriting analysis in a business environment, has led to successful cost control of mental health care services to large and varied populations of patients, including those on Medicare and Medicaid. Expertise in the management of resources, administration of claims and support activities, and response to customer service demands have led to the development of responsive, innovative, quality, and cost-effective care delivery systems to large populations of patients.

Managed care systems, through various reimbursement models, have allowed the "dollars to follow the patient" and have demonstrated success in cost control. Using managed care approaches and funding arrangements with stringent financial accountability, and marrying them to the innovations, flexibility, and population-based approaches of community mental health care, providers can be paid for the care they provide. For example, treatment plans can be approved for reimbursement, including such innovative combinations of services as 24-hour home care (with crisis stabilization beds for backup), and intensive outpatient treatment with a case manager to access a community drop-in center or psychosocial clubhouse. This kind of arrangement could be developed for especially difficult patients under managed care plans.

The Role of Community Psychiatry

The American Association of Community Psychiatrists estimates that there are between 6,000 and 12,000 psychiatrists practicing at least part time in the more than 2,000 community mental health care agencies throughout the country (Clark and Vaccaro 1987). These agencies have a history of providing a substantial proportion of total outpatient psychiatric care, particularly to indigent and underinsured populations. In many areas, services to these groups have undergone retrenchment owing to restricted public funding. This has led many community psychiatrists to reevaluate the focus and mode of the treatment they provide to this population.

The principles that have guided community mental health care through the course of its first 30 years of formal existence have been adopted by many and have even guided public policy groups as they contemplate mental health care reform. In fact, a reading of the managed care literature reveals that many principles of community psychiatry have been appropriated by those leading this movement. For example, continuity and comprehensiveness of services are hallmarks for systems that endeavor to reduce costs and provide clinically sound care. Most community mental health care systems have refined the use of alternatives to acute and long-term hospital care, another centerpiece for contemporary managed care strategies. Cost-efficiency has long been a central thematic chord in community psychiatry, as have concerns about enhancing accessibility and availability of mental health care services, all elements at the heart of managed mental health care. Other principles of community mental health care that prevail in managed care delivery systems include a reliance on optimal care in the least restrictive environment and in the least intrusive manner, and a model of care that values and rewards interdisciplinary efforts.

The Target Population

Patients who are the focus in this chapter are those who have a mental disorder that disrupts their lives in some way but is not usually considered to be a chronic mental illness. Their diagnoses range from acute depressive disorders to anxiety disorders, personality disorders, and others. We exclude in this chapter those patients whose identified need for treatment relates only to a substance abuse disorder (considered elsewhere in this volume), although many of the patients we discuss here will have comorbid substance abuse disorders.

For the most part, our emphasis in this chapter is on the resolution of functional impairment and focal psychiatric symptoms. Functional impairment usually consists of an inability to perform important social, occupational, or vocational tasks. The following case vignette illustrates the characteristics of this patient population and the types of therapy we discuss in this chapter.

> Bill is a 38-year-old construction worker who began seeing his family practitioner about 2 months ago for vague somatic complaints, for which his physician could find no cause. After several visits for these problems, Bill indicated that he had also noticed that he'd been less interested in his normal recreational and social activities and had actually found himself ruminating about death and dying. This concerned him greatly, as his brother had committed suicide when he was 28. Bill also noted a strong family history of depression. Bill said that at the time of his brother's death, he found his church priest to be extremely helpful, and since that time he had turned to his priest on many occasions for assistance. Bill's physician then referred him to his local CMHC for evaluation.
>
> Bill saw the psychiatrist at the CMHC, who elicited other signs and symptoms of major depression and learned that in addition to these symptoms, Bill's marital relationship had deteriorated over the preceding year. It was unclear whether his eventual separation from his wife had been the actual precipitant for the depressive episode, but this clearly played a role in the course of the depression. Bill's treatment consisted of a course of antidepressant medication (which resolved the major depressive symptoms in about a month), followed by four psychotherapy sessions whose focus was helping Bill and his wife repair their relationship and develop more effective communication and coping styles for the future. They were then referred to their church's family program, which consisted of regular group meetings and annual retreats.

The Approach to Outpatient Treatment

To provide clinically sound and economically viable services in the contemporary outpatient environment, there is clearly a paradigmatic shift that the individual psychiatrist or care provider must embrace. This attitudinal shift is probably more important than actually learning a different model of treatment or psychotherapy. Brief treatment approaches have been articulated for nearly all models of psychotherapy or treatment paradigms (Budman 1981; Budman and Gurman 1988; Malan 1976). The underlying assumption embodied in many of these models is that the intervention should help the patient return to a level of functioning that allows him or her to remain outside the hospital or to function at a level that does not require the formal intervention of a mental health care professional. Many of these models use the patient's community or social environment to facilitate and sustain changes that restore the functional capacities; many make use of a biopsychosocial assessment; and all make use of active, usually directive, interventions to promote change. In essence, these models share qualities of efficiency, an emphasis on being innovative, a systems orientation, and all stress rehabilitation as a primary goal.

A Paradigmatic Shift

The model in this approach to outpatient care is one that truly assumes the rehabilitative paradigm: cure is not the only acceptable goal. Instead, outcome is measured by the steps taken by the patient in his or her progress toward mutually identified, concrete goals such as the resumption of a productive, satisfying social or vocational role. The concept of cure tends to reflect a dichotomous state. If not "cured," the patient continues to be ill, and more treatment is required. There are few illnesses that fit this concept of "cure." In reality, medicine abounds with examples of brief, intermittent treatments for illnesses. For example, hypertension is rarely cured, but does require intermittent episodes of more intense treatment (e.g., weight reduction counseling or smoking cessation programs) or reevaluation of hypertensive pharmacotherapy. It also requires ongoing chronic maintenance treatment with medications and checkups on maintaining life-style changes.

Thus, part of the paradigmatic shift comes from the reconceptualization of "cure" from a dichotomous to a multifaceted definition, leading to a hierarchy of outcomes. "Cure" may be defined as 1) reversal of pathology, 2) the lack of residual symptoms, and 3) the prevention of recurrence. When considered in this fashion, psychiatry and mental health care interventions compare favorably with most medical or surgical interventions. For example, as noted earlier, hypertension may be well controlled with ongoing maintenance and brief, intermittent life-style change interventions that lead to enhanced prevention of future morbidity and mortality.

The treatment of depression is very similar. Depression, which is often a chronic illness, can be managed successfully with brief, intermittent medication management and brief, intermittent psychotherapy interventions in which coping skills can be learned to minimize future morbidity. In both situations, the patient may be able to return to satisfactory levels of functioning but may require ongoing chronic treatment and management. Both situations require patient-initiated and patient-maintained changes in behavior, such as dietary changes for many hypertensive patients; in the case of the patient with depression, there also may be required changes in social patterns, cognitive strategies, or physical exercise for improved functioning.

Structural Elements for Outpatient Community Psychiatry Practice

The implementation of efficacious treatment methods in the contemporary outpatient environment requires careful attention to time efficiency, continuity of care, the continuum of care, increased use of group therapy, and use of interdisciplinary perspectives. Thus, treatment approaches are modified to adapt to the constraints and goals of the *time-efficient* environment. This concern with time- and cost-efficiency is not new to community psychiatry or psychiatry in general. Many treatment or psychotherapy models addressed the issues of time and length of treatment long before the advent of managed care. Thus, the constraints of cost-effectiveness have only given time-efficient and brief therapies more relevance in the current cost-conscious health care environment.

To optimize time-efficient treatment and provide high-quality care, there must be easy access to a continuum of care and continuity of care. Once more, this concept is not alien to community psychiatry and the community mental health care movement. Since the mid-1960s, the concepts and practices of community psychiatry have been developed and actualized through the design and implementation of crisis treatment teams, crisis beds, partial care programs, and case management activities.

Attitudinal Elements

Along with the shift in paradigm and structural elements that are required for the successful outpatient treatment of the general population, there are significant therapist characteristics that contribute to successful practice. Innovation and flexibility are essential to the practice of efficient outpatient treatment. The psychiatrist should continually examine his or her practice to question whether interventions are effective or dogmatic, whether they are efficient or preferential, and whether the treatment is catalyzing growth or substituting for other relationships. This flexibility and innovative approach enhances the use of rehabilitative treatment approaches and emphasizes the progress of the patient through successive approximations and "levels of cure."

These attitudinal elements encourage the psychiatrist to move beyond traditional confines to practice creatively, using whatever resources and techniques prove effective in creating change. As a result, the psychiatrist is not "office bound." The use of family and significant others to foster behavioral change, the use of "exercises" in the patient's everyday life to practice change or to enhance the understanding of the effects of behavior on attitudes, and formal family or group interventions are all potential treatment methods available to or considered by the psychiatrist.

Time-Efficient Therapy

Similarly, treatment models or schools of therapy should be examined, but this does not necessarily require that the therapist be retrained. The community psychiatrist is more interested in time-efficient therapy than in a specific model or school of therapy. In essence, the goal is to maximize change efficiently and effectively. As there are limited empirical data to identify which aspects and components of therapy allow for rapid and effective change, the psychiatrist must be vigilant for opportunities to use less costly methods whenever clinically appropriate. This is a significant statement when we consider that much of what we do as clinicians is determined by preference and precedent rather than by empirically based information. For example, after many years of widespread use of fetal monitoring, this procedure has not been demonstrated as a uniformly significant advantage. However, it can change a physician's course of treatment or practice. The impact of small area analyses that generate differences in practice patterns—and, therefore, in outcome and cost—surely will influence the practice of psychiatry as practice guidelines evolve and similar analyses are undertaken.

The first session.   The self-examination of an individual psychiatrist's practice for efficiencies should begin with the first session. It is here that the patient will be socialized to the experience and conduct of psychotherapy and medical treatment. The patient will present with a set of expectations that are often not the same as the therapist's. For example, in a survey of more than 700 outpatients across the United States, patients were most often satisfied when helped with the specific problems that brought them to treatment. Few patients expect to be cured or to undergo extensive psychotherapy. In fact, they often expected what psychiatrists might consider a "medical practice model" approach. They believed that there was a "good enough" stage in treatment that allowed them to continue on with their lives.

Thus, the psychiatrist should articulate the basic assumptions about treatment as being solution oriented, pragmatic, and focused on defining goals of treatment that are measurable and attainable in a limited amount of time. The patient should be encouraged to see that there are levels of success in therapy which build on previous treatment successes. The expectation of 5–10 sessions versus unlimited sessions is communicated by how carefully and explicitly the goals of the treatment are targeted and how focused the treatment plan is. Thus, with more behavioral descriptions of the goals and more specific intervention plans, it is more likely the patient will expect that progress and time in the treatment will be carefully assessed.

Thus, when plateaus of progress occur, the therapist can introduce specific changes such as extending the interval of therapy or introducing periods of "practicing what has been learned" in therapy. These are then seen by the patient as steps to generalize change or to "road test" the improvements of treatment, rather than an abrupt termination of treatment or insurance-determined changes.

A time-efficient or brief, intermittent approach also allows the psychiatrist to communicate the developmental aspects of treatment. By emphasizing milestones in the interventions and a rehabilitative orientation, the expectation of continued growth outside of the psychiatrist's office is reinforced, and the availability of an intermittent or fading schedule of contact reassures the patient of a "safe harbor." This also provides for a pragmatic use of insurance limits. In fact, the psychiatrist can describe to a managed care entity a rational, clear, behavioral, and pragmatically based treatment plan that includes defined milestones for the assessment of progress.

The following vignette illustrates these points.

A 30-year-old male medical resident was found crying at the nurses' station. The supervising physician found that the resident was having marital problems and wanted a divorce. The resident had wanted to leave the marriage for almost 2 years and had thought that starting his residency in a new city would help the marriage by trying to "start fresh." The resident was referred to a psychiatrist and evaluated. There was no family history of depression or emotional disorders. The evaluation revealed a profile consistent with an adjustment disorder with mixed features.

The patient was extremely unhappy with his wife, who shared none of his interests and was socially and culturally unacceptable to his family. He recalls proposing to her because he was afraid of being alone, as he was transferring to another college farther away from her. She had threatened to stop seeing him because he would have been coming home only during breaks and vacations. He had decided to leave the marriage nearly 4 months previously, but he was afraid of hurting their two young children.

It became clear that the patient was reasonably certain of his decision and had made two attempts at marital therapy, but his wife discontinued the therapy.

The patient improved rapidly as he was treated in group therapy (six sessions) and began talking to others in the self-help group about his problems and fears and saw how others handled marital crises. As the patient became aware of decreased anxiety and depressive symptoms, the therapist pointed out to the patient that it was acceptable to stop therapy. At this point, the patient confirmed that he had not really wanted to come to therapy for the last two sessions. He was asked to keep in touch with the therapist and encouraged to call or return if necessary.

The patient eventually divorced, requested joint custody, and remarried some years later. He later reported that he has never regretted his decision and is currently happily married.

The patient could have been seen as a very dependent, unassertive man who demonstrated personality traits that led him to marry impulsively, suppress his rage, and compensate for his dependency through a marriage to a dominant wife. Instead, he was treated in a group, encouraged to make a decision, and received support from a self-help group. He has been successful and currently appears to be assertive in his personal relationships.

Targeted and focused assessments. Based on the characteristics of the approach that we have outlined, the assessment should be pragmatic, focused, and targeted. It is pragmatic in that it attempts to use the resources and strengths of the patient and his or her environment, which includes financial limitations. The assessment must be focused, returning the patient to a level of functioning that is and was satisfactory. This also means that the psychiatrist must be a catalyst in the patient's continued growth rather than a substitute for the relationships and institutions in the patient's life. Finally, the assessment must be targeted; specifically, it must remediate or change the cognitive, behavioral, or emotional excesses or deficits leading to and maintaining the patient's problematic situation.

One approach in developing a targeted and focused assessment is derived from crisis theory and adapted from Sheldon Kardener's article, "A Methodologic Approach to Crisis Therapy" (Kardener 1975). We outline and apply this approach for the purpose of highlighting several principles, with the understanding that other approaches also may be employed effectively. The basic assumptions of crisis theory allow for the identification and prioritization of the problems that bring a patient to treatment. Even more importantly, crisis theory emphasizes the central role of the "why now" element in the precipitation and alleviation of the patient's symptoms and resolution of the identified conflict or problem. The emphasis on the "why now," with a good understanding of the patient's relevant psychodynamic issues, allows for efficient and practical attention to a specific problem that will stabilize the patient and in many cases attains a level of resolution satisfactory to the patient. It also focuses attention on the specific behaviors and cognitions or attitudes that led to the precipitation of the problem or its exacerbation. This then facilitates psychoeducational interventions designed to prevent relapse or control future exacerbation.

> A 30-year-old man presented to the emergency department for admission to the drug abuse treatment ward. He sought treatment for alcohol, marijuana, and cocaine abuse. There was no evidence of physical dependency. He had been using for nearly 15 years, initially alcohol, then marijuana, and finally cocaine over the past 12–18 months. He had tried to stop two or three times in the past, but always dropped out of treatment. His wife also used marijuana and alcohol. He claimed to be fed up and wanted to get his life straight.
>
> The "why now" event turned out to be an argument with his wife over his being very late coming home. (He had stopped to get drugs from his source, who was also his former girlfriend.) His wife threatened to leave him if he did not stop drug and alcohol use. She went on to say that she wanted to stop using drugs and wanted him to stop seeing his girlfriend.
>
> He had hoped to prove to her that he had not been unfaithful and believed that by going in for treatment she would be convinced of his love. The history of prior treatment appeared to have a similar pattern, but this was not clear.
>
> The evaluation revealed no significant physical problems and no evidence of recent alcohol use. He was placed in a crisis bed for the night and returned for evaluation for the substance abuse treatment unit. His wife was called to assure her that he was seeking treatment and to explain the treatment recommendations. Because she was a critical part of the motivation and because he was self-employed, he was started on an intensive outpatient program (evening treatment program 4 days per week). As a condition, his wife was asked to be an active participant in his treatment and recovery.
>
> Her abuse and their trust in their relationship soon took on a major role in their participation. It was clear that neither saw their substance abuse as the critical factor in seeking help. They stayed in treatment, however, and maintained abstinence for several months before being lost to follow-up.

Kardener predicts that patients seek help when there is a perceived loss (imagined, potential, or real) of a strategic or significant support that has maintained the patient at some level of functioning. The patient seeks this help only after all other coping attempts have been made; the "loss" is the "final straw" that leads them to seek help. Kardener (1975) pointed out that a systematic evaluation of major functional areas of the patient's life could reveal the "why now" or the perceived "loss." Thus, the goal of the treatment plan would be to replace or reestablish this loss.

The psychiatrist must be especially skillful in understanding the "why now" and its relationship to the psychodynamics of the patient and, in turn, to the therapeutic relationship. The underlying or unstated expectations and assumptions of the patient can interfere with treatment in the remediation of the "why now." This is illustrated in the case of Bill earlier in this chapter.

Finally, it should be stated that a targeted and focused treatment plan is the heart of the practice of outpatient community psychiatry. The treatment plan should emphasize the restoration and stabilization of the patient using pragmatic interventions, catalyze growth or learning outside treatment, recognize the use of a continuum of care levels or community resources, and achieve attainable levels of functioning in a context of a rehabilitation philosophy of care rather than a unitary "curative" model. The treatment process identifies and targets the "why now" to focus the reparative work of therapy and treatment. The psychodynamic influences are recognized as modifiers of treatment process and outcomes; they are accounted for in the treatment goals and objectives.

Future Directions

The future for outpatient community mental health care is hopeful. Given the nation's preoccupation with health care reform, those individuals and agencies who can deliver effective and efficient quality health care will be sought-after as providers. Those CMHCs and others whose practices are consistent with an approach that stresses the treatment of populations using interventions that embody a continuum of care and continuity of care will be able to adapt and survive future changes in the outpatient landscape.

References

American Psychiatric Association: Diagnostic and Statistical Manual of Mental Disorders, 4th Edition. Washington, DC, American Psychiatric Association, 1994

Barten HH: Brief Therapies. New York, Behavioral Publications, 1971

Budman SH: Forms of Brief Therapy. New York, Guilford, 1981

Budman SH, Gurman AS: Theory and Practice of Brief Therapy. New York, Guilford, 1988

Clark GH, Vaccaro TV: Burnout among CMHC psychiatrists and the struggle to survive. Hosp Community Psychiatry 38:843–847, 1987

Kardener SH: A methodologic approach to crisis therapy. Am J Psychother 29:4–13, 1975

Malan DH: The Frontier of Brief Psychotherapy. New York, Plenum, 1976

Robins LN, Locke B, Regier DA: An overview of psychiatric disorders in America, in Psychiatric Disorders in America. Edited by Robins LN, Regier DA. New York, Macmillan, 1991

Sifneos PE: Dynamic psychotherapy in a psychiatric clinic, in Current Psychiatric Therapies. Edited by Masserman I. New York, Grune & Stratton, 1961

Talbot J: Unified mental health systems: utopia unrealized. New Dir Ment Health Serv 18:107–111, 1983

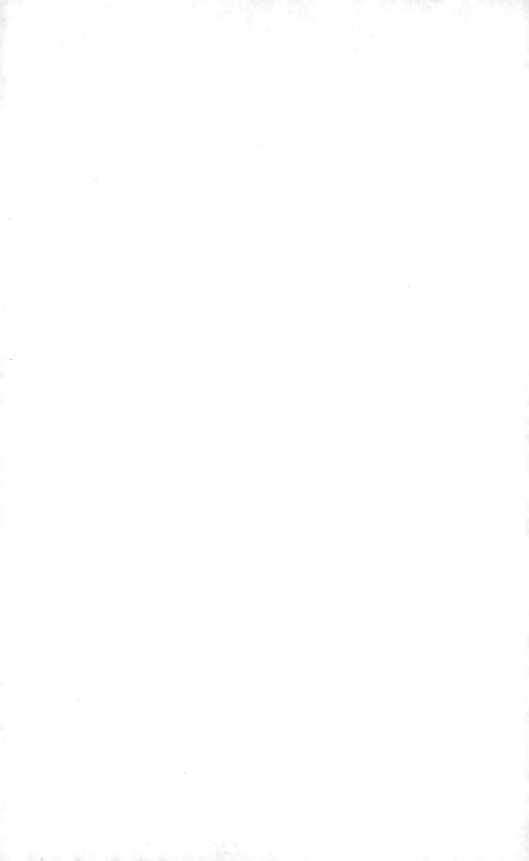

Chapter 4

Emergency Psychiatry and Crisis Resolution

Robert M. Factor, M.D., Ph.D.
Ronald J. Diamond, M.D.

C rises are an inherent part of the course of every chronic illness. This is particularly true of serious mental illness, where instability in a patient's life can be caused both by exacerbation of the illness and by disruptions in a patient's support system. Clinicians should expect these crises and be prepared to deal with them.

Unfortunately, emergency services that stress evaluation and disposition are not enough to help people with psychiatric illness lead stable lives in the community. Too often, psychiatric crises lead to psychiatric hospitalization that could have been averted were other interventions available. In this chapter we present an overview of effective clinical strategies, the goals of which are resolution of the crisis, reestablishment of the person's stability, and support of the person's ability to function at as high a level as possible.

Persons with serious mental illness often experience a crisis because their concrete needs are not being met. One person may need help obtaining and keeping a place to live, budgeting money, or having something enjoyable to do during the day. Another may need assistance getting treatment for a medical illness or ensuring that psychotropic medication is taken reliably. Most persons with serious mental illness can live in the community if they receive the supportive services that they need to complement the particular deficits caused by their illness (Stein et al. 1990). However, if appropriate support services are not available or not provided, persons with serious mental illness may run into difficulty in their apartment or home and risk eviction, run out of money, or fail to take medication. If a "best friend" leaves town, this may add to their social isolation. The increased stress caused by any one or more of these events can precipitate an increase in psychiatric symptoms and a psychiatric crisis. Although the presenting problem may be an increase in auditory hallucinations or bizarre behavior, the proximate cause may be the stress of running out of money or of an upcoming Social Security Income (SSI) evaluation.

The first step in effective crisis intervention should be to determine what combination of services the person will need to restabilize, resume, and maintain life in the community. Once this is clear, it is easier to be creative about how to provide these services. The issue is what treatment the patient needs. Traditional psychiatric emergency services often start with the question of whether to hospitalize. This involves a decision about where treatment will be performed, not what treatment is needed. Although hospitalization is sometimes necessary and may at times be lifesaving, the question of whether to hospitalize should never be the initial starting point for effective crisis intervention.

General Principles of Crisis Intervention

Plan First: Do Things One Step at a Time and Do Not Make Decisions Prematurely

In the midst of the turmoil of a crisis, it is often tempting to "do something." The police may want something done right away so that they can leave the emergency department, the patient may be yelling, and the family may be demanding some immediate intervention such as medication or hospitalization. At each stage it is important to determine what needs to be done at that moment and what does not. Initially the most important requirement is to ensure that everyone is physically safe. Later it is important to ensure that everyone has been heard and that all points of view have been considered. A treatment intervention, such as dispensing medication, should always follow an assessment and plan.

A large, angry, and disheveled man was brought into a psychiatric emergency service by the police after he frightened and then pushed a resident at the group home where his girlfriend was living. He was disorganized and described auditory hallucinations; both police and group home staff assumed that he would need hospitalization. Despite his disorganization, the crisis intervention staff could elicit the history that his long-term girlfriend had been refusing to go out with him and that he had gone to the group home where she lived and had gotten into a verbal argument with her there. Another resident had come into the living room in the midst of this argument and tried to intervene, but the patient pushed him away, whereupon the group home staff called the police. When everyone arrived at the emergency service, the scene was loud and confusing. After the patient was given a chance to calm down and be heard, it turned out that he had been living with psychotic symptoms for many years and had been regularly taking his prescribed antipsychotic medications. He was able to go back to his own apartment and agreed to stay away from the group home until he and his girlfriend could get some help to resolve their relationship.

Unfortunately, some of the pressure to "do something" prematurely often comes from psychiatrists, who are often too busy to do the kind of job that they would like. Although clinicians must face this reality, they must also resist the pressure to intervene before they have assessed what kind of intervention would make sense.

Do What Is Needed but No More

In the midst of a crisis, there is often pressure to do too much. Clinicians are asked to ensure that the patient eats regularly, takes medication as prescribed, and shows up for follow-up appointments. Most importantly, they are asked to guarantee that their patients will be safe, both to themselves and with others. Patients are often hospitalized because clinicians cannot guarantee that these needs will be met.

As psychiatrists, we must be selective in deciding what must be done and how much we can do. We do not have the resources to do everything for everyone. If we do too much, we risk creating dependence and interfering with the patient's self-esteem and autonomy. If we do not do enough, we allow someone who has already faced more than life's share of hardship to fall down again.

For example, if someone with a psychotic illness has stopped eating because he or she has no food, the psychiatrist must decide what kind of help to provide. Depending on the patient's clinical situation and the resources available in the community, a wide range of options can be considered. The patient could be hospitalized to ensure nutritional intake. Alternatively, the psychiatrist could arrange emergency housing for the patient where meals are provided, arrange for staff to go with the patient to obtain free food or food stamps, or provide the patient with information about how to obtain assistance. Hospitalization may be the safest option with respect to ensuring nutritional intake, but it may not be the best solution to help the patient learn new coping skills to obtain food in the community. The more the patient's needs can be met by his or her own internal resources and can be assisted by his or her own natural support system, the better it will be for the patient.

There is no absolute dose of intervention. The proper dose of intervention is "enough," as measured empirically by the outcome. Clinicians must also realize—especially when working in a public mental health system—that resources are limited. Giving more than is needed to some patients may mean that there may not be enough left to give to all patients in need.

> A patient was brought into the emergency department by his family because he was eating out of dumpsters, despite having access to other food. He was a reasonably built man who did not appear to have lost weight. In talking with him, he appeared proud that he knew when various restaurants put leftover food in their dumpsters and that he could fend for himself. While involving him in ongoing treatment posed a challenge, he was clearly safe; there was no reason to hospitalize him, despite his family's request, and no way to guarantee that anyone could prevent him from eating from dumpsters in the immediate future.

Clinicians' concern to avoid doing too much leads them to prefer outpatient treatment whenever the particular combination of services a person needs can be provided in the community. Unfortunately, in many areas, community-based resources are extremely limited. Community-based crisis resolution programs and continuing-care programs may not exist, and staff may lack the training needed to work in community-based settings (Factor et al. 1988). However, even when community-based options are limited, it may be possible to put together effective crisis intervention plans that do not require hospitalization, if alternatives are actively sought. A crisis can sometimes be resolved during the initial contact with the crisis service, but more often the resolution requires closely integrated follow-up.

Consider the Needs of the Entire Support System

The needs of the patient's entire social system are critical. Often family, friends, housemates, emergency department staff, landlords, employers, and police all have their own views of the problem and their own needs that must be met. In the earlier example of the man who ate out of dumpsters, the patient's behavior had not changed in some time, but the family felt that they had to do something immediately once they learned about it.

A decision to support a patient in the community may be an appropriate way to deal with the patient's crisis, but it may do little to help the family with their sense of responsibility, the landlord with his or her disturbing tenant, or the police who must wait in the emergency room as follow-up arrangements are made. If the clinician understands the needs of all the people connected with the crisis, it will be easier to come up with a solution that all parties can accept. Often the extended support system can play an important role in an intervention strategy. To orchestrate this, the clinician must understand the crisis from everyone's point of view, including each person's ideas about what would constitute a good solution, what is acceptable, and what is possible.

Basic Strategies for Working in Crisis Situations

Be active. Be willing to be directive and to make decisions. A crisis situation is inherently chaotic. People are in turmoil, and the anxiety level of all participants is usually very high. The anxiety of both the patient and of others involved will often decrease if the clinician takes charge and provides some structure. Actively collecting information, directing questions, making sure that only one person talks at a time, and ensuring that everyone has a say are all ways to reestablish order. The clinician must have considerable skill to stay above the fray and avoid getting into arguments that would interfere with his or her ability to provide a safe, organized holding environment.

Be willing to take calculated risks. By their very nature, crises are unstable. While a crisis carries with it certain risks, it also allows for positive changes and gives the clinician several temporary prerogatives. For example, during a crisis the clinician may get permission to telephone the patient's family, even if this had previously been resisted. In certain situations, if there is a risk of life-threatening behavior, it may be ethically and legally justified to contact family or other significant persons, despite the patient's objection (Applebaum and Gutheil 1991); this may establish a relationship that had not been possible earlier. At times, the crisis can be used to make unusual demands on others (e.g., to participate in family meetings, ask friends to take someone in on a temporary basis). People also may be willing to drop longstanding psychological defenses because of the emergency.

Try to appear calm and in control regardless of the situation. Clinicians serve as a model for those in crisis. If the clinician is calm and communicates that a reasonable resolution of the crisis is possible, the other people involved in the crisis will tend to calm down and participate in finding a solution. At times patients may behave in ways that frighten others, including the clinician. It is often very useful to tell the patient that he or she is frightening others. At the same time, it is important to maintain a calm voice and a sense of being in control even as the information is communicated. If the clinician appears to be overwhelmed by the patient's threat, the patient may lose more control. This is not to say that the clinician should pretend to know everything or control everything. Clinicians can actively seek help from the patient as well as other participants, and they can share the limits of what they know and can accomplish. The clinician does have the obligation, however, not to be drawn into the chaos of the crisis situation.

Be sure to have your own support system. When dealing with a potentially violent patient, it is often important to have security personnel readily available. If the patient is actively threatening, it might be necessary to have police or security in the room during the assessment (Factor 1991). Although the clinician must always respect confidentiality, he or she must feel safe and secure in order to focus on the psychiatric issues, without having to worry unduly about immediate personal safety.

When working with a patient who manifests a significant risk of violence to self or others, it may be extremely helpful if colleagues, other consultants, family members, and others in the patient's support network can be present either in person or by telephone (Factor 1991). This leads to better problem solving and helps ensure that the clinician does not overlook possible solutions. Equally importantly, the clinician can share the burden of responsibility inherent in making high-risk decisions. Although hospitalizing a patient who is chronically suicidal may decrease the short-term risk of suicide, it may increase the long-term risk. Hospitalization may interfere with the patient's ability to learn new ways to cope outside the hospital with chronic suicidal feelings. Hospitalization may also decrease self-esteem. As with any treatment decision, the participants in the decision (including the patient and family) must balance all potential benefits and risks.

It is also important for clinicians to involve their own support system when dealing with patients who are particularly demanding or who tend to "burn out" staff. Some patients make clinicians feel that anything they do is wrong and that every attempt made to be useful only makes the situation worse. Patients with personality disorders with dramatic features (including borderline personality disorder) who are difficult to work with often use misery as a way to try to get what they need and relate to others as if "my misery is your command" (Benjamin 1993, p. 121). Realizing this can help clinicians avoid becoming overwhelmed and trapped. In a crisis, emergency staff should involve other clinicians who already know the patient in formulating a joint treatment plan (Nehls and Diamond 1993). Clinicians in a crisis service should support one another with specific decisions and generally help each other acknowledge the good work they do with challenging patients.

Know your own goals for each intervention. Usually the primary goal is the clinical one of doing what is best for the patient. At other times, however, the goal might be more programmatic. For example, the outpatient clinician may request that a patient be hospitalized for a few days to give the outpatient staff a brief respite, or an emergency service that usually can find alternatives to hospitalization may have to lower its threshold and admit more patients to a hospital if its workload is exceptionally high. Although clinicians all like to think that they are always doing things entirely in their patients' best interests, it is important to acknowledge that providing respite for staff is also a valid consideration.

There can be a variety of programmatic and political influences on a clinician's decision making. For example, patients are often admitted to one hospital rather than another for administrative or financial reasons, which may at times conflict with the unit that would be clinically best for the patient. Similarly, a patient who has bothered a well-known politician will be dealt with differently from the patient who has bothered someone less well known. In all of these cases, if clinicians take a moment to clarify the pressures influencing the clinical decisions, they will likely make a better decision and be more comfortable with it.

Separate the crisis from other kinds of life problems. Crisis, by definition, refers to a change in the patient's ongoing behavior, function, or support system. A patient whose wife has just left him and who is feeling suicidal for the first time is in crisis. A patient who is chronically suicidal and whose wife has been on the verge of leaving throughout their marriage may have a severe life problem and may even end up killing himself, but he is not in crisis. Crisis does not refer to the severity of the problem or even the risk of lethality. A problem is a crisis when it represents something new or different in a person's life, rather than part of an ongoing pattern. People who live lives of "chronic chaos" often present to emergency departments as though they are in a crisis, often feeling suicidal or out of control (Bassuk and Gerson 1980). It is important to assess whether what they describe is part of an ongoing life struggle, or whether some fundamental change has occurred in their lives.

The intervention for a true crisis will be very different from the intervention for similar behavior that is part of an ongoing life problem. In a true crisis, the problem is of recent onset or is the result of recent change, and a rapid intervention is likely to be of benefit. If the patient has a chronic problem, a brief crisis-oriented intervention is unlikely to achieve more than momentary relief and may make the ongoing problem worse. People whose lives are chronically in a state of chaos and crisis, who often have disabling personality disorders in addition to any Axis I diagnosis, present extremely difficult problems. Intervention in these cases should be guided by a treatment plan that is informed by the patient's character and a knowledge, if possible, of what does and does not work. Clinicians should respond to the "chronic state of crisis" and not treat each crisis as a unique event. Such treatment plans work best when they are written collaboratively by the consumer, ongoing treaters, and crisis staff (Nehls and Diamond 1993).

For example, if a person presents to an emergency department with extreme anxiety over some recent event, after a medical and psychological assessment, it might be very appropriate to provide a few doses of an anxiolytic medication. If a person presented with the same complaint but with a history of chronic anxiety going back for many years with many medication trials and many physician visits, treatment in the emergency department might be inappropriate, no matter how distressed the patient.

Crises represent changes in someone's normal state of being; they are temporary, no matter how severe. Although the time course may be highly variable, it is often helpful to consider the crisis as evolving over time, starting with an initial period of precrisis during which tension increases, reaches a peak during the crisis period, and then resolves (Bartolucci and Drayer 1973; Rapoport 1962).

> A man with chronic schizophrenia was living in his own apartment with support from an assertive, continuous care team. Despite very close monitoring of his medications, he began to decompensate, shouting in his apartment and leaving on the burners of his stove because of paranoid delusions that his noisy neighbors would harm him. The clinical goals were to ensure his safety, to help him feel less frightened, to help him restabilize as quickly as possible, and to allow him to continue living in his apartment building. Based on his past history, the team believed he would restabilize quickly following a temporary increase in his antipsychotic medication and a change in his living situation away from his neighbors. He was very frightened of hospitals, but there were significant risks in leaving him in the community. If he caused a fire, he not only might harm himself or another, but could jeopardize the opportunity of all persons with mental illness to get good housing in that community. After some negotiation, he agreed to go into the hospital for 3 days until he was less paranoid, and then stay 1 week in a motel where he could be monitored by the continuous care team several times a day. This allowed him to remain away from the neighbors until he stabilized and was no longer frightened of them. The team also worked with the landlord to deal with the overall noise level in the building. At each step along the way, the members of the team consulted with and supported each other in assessing the risks and benefits and in carrying out the plan.

Initial Approach to the Crisis Situation

Listen to the story of the crisis from the various people involved. Taking a careful step-by-step history of what happened first and what happened next can often be useful, both in obtaining critical information and in helping those present to organize their thoughts and decrease their sense of chaos. As they feel heard and understood, the process of telling the story can help everyone involved to calm down and feel less out of control. Ask yourself, "For whom is this a crisis?" Establish the interpersonal context. How does this crisis fit into the person's life? What other crises has the person had, and how were they handled? Is this similar to or different from previous crises? What are the person's strengths and usual coping mechanisms? What support system does the person have?

The patient and family may want to focus only on the immediate event that precipitated the crisis and then jump to some solution. People in the midst of crisis often feel as though nothing can possibly help. Knowing what has been useful in the past and helping to develop ways for the patient to use the same strategy can increase the patient's sense of mastery. As part of the history, the clinician can collect information about solutions that have already been attempted. For example, the clinician might learn that in an effort to calm down, the patient had already taken some extra medication or tried to talk with friends. If the clinician then were simply to suggest that the patient try these very same actions, in all likelihood this would not be very productive; it might only make all parties feel that they had not been heard and the clinician was not going to be of any use.

It is important to start by promising that everyone will have the chance to be heard and to make sure that everyone has had their say before deciding on a solution. The various points of view will often present a more complete picture than will that of any one participant. Even a psychotic patient who feels that neighbors are trying to harm him has important information, both about how he is feeling and about details of the interaction between him and his neighbors that led to the crisis. If people feel heard and their views are seriously considered, they are much more likely to be willing to participate in a treatment plan, even if it is not exactly the one that they would have preferred.

Assess risk. Pay particular attention to information about dangerous behavior and the risk of such behavior in the future, either to self or to others. It is important to get as much detailed information about the risk as possible. For example, if someone is described as being dangerous, it is important to know specifically why this label was assigned and by whom. Has the patient verbally threatened someone in the past? Has the patient actually assaulted someone? If so, was the assaulted person known to the patient, or a stranger walking down the street? Were weapons ever involved, and are weapons available now? Was previous dangerous behavior associated with being intoxicated or stopping psychotropic medication? A particularly relevant issue in working with a potentially dangerous person is any history of aggressive behavior toward authority figures or treatment staff. Is anything happening now that suggests that the person may behave in a dangerous fashion (Factor 1991)?

There is an emotional burden in working with patients who have significant risk of dangerous behavior. There is always a possibility that someone may be hurt or even die. The decision to hospitalize a suicidal patient does not prevent risk: the loss of self-esteem connected with hospitalization can increase the long-term risk of suicide in some patients, and even hospitalization does not completely eliminate the short-term risk. It is important to share this burden with other experienced clinicians, especially in high-risk situations. As discussed earlier, this can minimize blind spots and errors and decrease the emotional burden of making difficult decisions.

Involve the patient as much as possible. Patients in the midst of a crisis feel out of control. They may be angry, especially if they have been brought to a crisis service or emergency department against their will. Often the expectation of the patient, the family, the police, or others involved is that the clinician will do something to this patient and "fix" him or her, perhaps even in short order. From the opening introductions through the history taking and the formulation of the plan, it is important to try to convert this expectation to a more collaborative one of working together toward goals shared by the patient, the family, and the clinician. This is easy when the patient wants "my voices to go away" or wants "to feel less frightened." It can be far more difficult if the patient's description of the problem is very different from that of the clinician or the family.

For example, a psychotic patient may feel that his behavior is entirely justified, even after he is brought into an emergency department by police after yelling at neighbors. At first, the only goal shared by the clinician and the patient may be to arrange things so that the police can safely exit. Accomplishing this may decrease an immediate source of stress. This goal may not completely reflect the problem, but it is at least a starting point for the clinician and patient to work together toward additional common goals.

Even when psychotic, patients can often use a number of effective coping mechanisms once everyone is working toward a common goal. In the example above, the patient may know that if he talks to friends, calls the crisis telephone line, or just spends a few days away from his apartment, he could control his anger better. Once all parties can agree on some common goal (even if seemingly minor), the patient may play a much larger role in finding ways to achieve it. Alternatively, once the goal is clear, the patient may be more willing to accept help. The above patient might be more willing to accept antipsychotic medication once he views the medication as causing the police to leave him alone, albeit by helping him control his psychosis and his anger.

Involve as many collateral sources as possible. Often people outside the treatment network have important information about the problem, about what has worked in the past, and about options that might currently be available. Such people also have needs and concerns that must be addressed if a crisis treatment plan is to be successful. The clinician must carefully balance treatment needs with the patient's own wishes, right to privacy, and confidentiality (Diamond and Wikler 1985). When contacting others, stay in a problem-solving role. It is easy to make incorrect assumptions that an outside clinician is incompetent or, conversely, is more competent than you. At times, it feels as if the patient and the clinician are both "stuck" and that no resolution of the problem is possible. A very useful dictum is, "If you are stuck, expand the field." Think creatively about others you can involve, either in person or by telephone.

Be flexible and creative with the telephone. Whenever possible, have conversations with the patient present. Speakerphones are an inexpensive way to involve a group in a consultation. At times the most appropriate person is someone from the patient's support system, such as a family member or friend. At other times the patient's outpatient therapist or case manager must get involved before a resolution is possible. In still other cases, the clinician in the crisis service should contact a consultant to talk through options with a trusted colleague less directly involved in the situation. When working in the field and away from fixed telephones, a cellular telephone can also provide a very useful communication link with other crisis staff, consultants, or members of a support network.

Evaluate and maximize cooperation from both patient and others. Try to find out what each person wants, from his or her own perspective. As the saying goes, "You can't please all the people all the time . . . ," but people will cooperate much better if they feel they are getting at least something that they want. For example, in dealing with a patient who is ambivalent or reluctant to take medications, begin by trying to understand from the patient's perspective why he or she does not want to take medications. Then try to find even a small reason why he or she might want to take medications. Also explore the perspectives of the family, the landlord, and others involved.

A patient with schizophrenia did not want to take medications because of troubling side effects, manifested by a mild tremor and a feeling that "my head has a vise on it and is shut down." Yet he would readily acknowledge that while on medications, he could play chess better and could function well at a part-time job and earn a small amount of extra money, both of which were very important to him. He was more willing to take medications when he was reminded of the advantages that were important to him, not just the advantages perceived by others, albeit accurately, that he was safer, more organized, and "looked better."

Formulate a Differential Diagnosis

Consider medical illnesses (for examples, see Hyman and Tesar [1994]). If you do not look for a medical illness you will not find one. It is important to continue considering the possibility of organic illness even after the patient has been cleared medically by an emergency department physician. Psychiatric patients, especially those with severe and persistent illness, may get less than a complete evaluation and treatment from some nonpsychiatric physicians or may have medical problems falsely attributed to their psychiatric condition (Weissberg 1979). Areas for special consideration include drug intoxication or withdrawal states; delirium; and neurological, endocrinological, and infectious disorders, among others.

For the psychotic patient in whom a medical illness has been excluded, the clinician should make a differential diagnosis of psychosis (for examples, see Hyman and Tesar [1994]). Is this an acute episode or part of a chronic illness? What is the context in which the person became psychotic? A DSM-IV (American Psychiatric Association 1994) differential diagnosis is useful insofar as it changes immediate treatment. Other factors concerning history, symptoms, and psychosocial function are often more important in both crisis and long-term treatment planning (Stein et al. 1990).

Develop a Crisis Treatment Plan

Consider the necessary information—medical, social, psychological, and historical—that is needed but not yet acquired. Identify gaps in information so that such information is not overlooked as the treatment plan is developed. Rank the patient's needs, and use this to gather the information needed. Some information will have to be collected before a crisis treatment plan can be developed, but all the information does not have to be obtained at the start; note other information for you or someone else to collect later, once the immediate crisis has resolved.

Determine what this patient needs *now*. It often helps to break down the person's needs into the following basic categories:

- *Housing.* Does this person need a place to live? What kind? For the duration of the crisis or permanently?
- *Protection.* How much protection does this person need to prevent harming himself or herself or others, and for how long? How much observation or supervision, and what kinds of assistance, does this person need to live safely?
- *Structure.* How much structure does this person need to help organize his or her life at this time?

Other needs that may also have to be considered include social supports, medical treatment, or family issues. The clinician can then consider how these needs can be met: Where can one obtain emergency housing or a place where a patient can be observed over the next few days?

Once the needs of the patient have been clearly established, it becomes easier to consider the range of settings in both the community and the hospital that provide the appropriate degree of protection, observation, supervision, and structure. The central question is, "What does the patient need, and where can he or she get it?" rather than "Does this patient need admission to a hospital?" It is important that clinicians involved in crisis intervention know as many options as possible and stay informed about community resources. For example, when housing and monitoring are needed but not at the level present in a hospital, then a motel or a crisis home, with frequent visits from a crisis resolution team (Arce and Vergare 1985), might be a better option. At times friends or family may be able to provide enough supervision to offer a safe and effective alternative to the hospital.

At times hospitalization will be necessary. Before hospitalizing any patient, the clinician should be able to state what he or she hopes to accomplish with hospital admission in the specific crisis. Specific goals might include the following:

- To ensure safety when no less-restrictive methods will work
- To observe the patient especially closely or to evaluate medical conditions (being clear about what you are trying to find)

- To stabilize the patient on medications that cannot be safely administered outside the hospital (being clear about why, such as the need for close observation in order to titrate dosage or observe for medical complications)
- To give family, caregivers, or treaters a respite

It is also important to estimate the length of the hospitalization and discuss this with the patient. Goals and length of stay, of course, are always subject to modification later.

At the time of admission, the clinician should also develop clear criteria for discharge. For example, if a patient has had chronic delusions, it makes little sense to have the absence of delusions as a criterion for discharge; requiring that the patient be behaviorally stable and able to care for himself or herself is a much more reasonable criterion. Developing clear criteria is most difficult when the patient has been admitted for longstanding threats of suicide or assault. Unless the purpose of the hospitalization is clearly defined from the beginning, it will be difficult to decide when hospitalization is no longer needed.

> A man with chronic schizophrenia and longstanding threats to assault others was hospitalized after his parents, with whom he lived, evicted him. He had never actually hurt any one, but the crisis team was concerned that the eviction would increase his risk of violence. The purpose of the hospitalization was clearly defined from the beginning: to provide a safe place for him to work through issues with his family, and to give him and the community treatment system a safe period of time to find permanent housing. After 80 days, he was discharged to his own apartment with close follow-up from the continuous care team, still mumbling threats but back to his baseline behavior.

Determine the role of medication. Decide as clearly as possible the purpose of any proposed medication. In the midst of a crisis, there is often considerable pressure to prescribe a medication, as this helps everyone involved feel that something is being done. In reality, antidepressant and sometimes antipsychotic medications require from days to weeks to realize their specific effects, and any immediate response in the emergency department is either from the sedating effects or from nonpharmacological (although very important) symbolic effects of such drugs.

There are certainly crisis situations in which the use of psychotropic medication can be extremely useful. It is important to identify specific target symptoms and consider how long it will be before the medication is likely to be effective. Target symptoms allow both clinicians and patients to monitor the effectiveness of medication and to change or discontinue ineffective medication.

In addition to deciding what medications to use, it is important to consider how medication will be dispensed. The clinician can give an initial dose of a medication to an ambivalent patient while he or she is still in the emergency department. For some patients, acceptance of the medication at that time may help promote future medication use, as such acceptance represents a symbolic gesture of good faith toward the clinician. A patient is more likely to continue taking a medication once it has been started. Patients who are unwilling to take an initial dose in the emergency department under staff observation are unlikely to take medication on their own in the immediate future. For some patients it may be necessary to arrange for medication to be dispensed daily or several times a week to ensure that the patient is taking the medication and to minimize risk of overdose.

In all cases, decide what medication to use, in what dose, for what specific purpose, and how it is to be dispensed and monitored. Share this information with the patient and others in the network, as appropriate.

Many clinicians are not comfortable prescribing medications for patients in a crisis outside the supervision of a hospital. Generally such reservations center around the need for medical evaluation (including laboratory testing) and ongoing monitoring for desired and adverse effects. However, if the clinician thinks specifically of what is needed in both of these areas, there may well be others in addition to the psychiatrist (e.g., nonpsychiatric physicians, other mental health professionals, or others in the patient's network) who can provide safe monitoring in an outpatient setting. Information, education, and support from the psychiatrist may all help to increase the number of people willing to help monitor medication use.

Medications have symbolic and interpersonal effects that may be as important as their pharmacological effects. For example, a patient may take a pill as "proof" that he or she is "really ill." Medications may be seen as something that are given to a patient or something that a patient can use to take control over his or her illness. The more the clinician understands the phenomenology of the patient, the more effectively he or she will be able to intervene.

During a crisis, prescriptions can be given in small amounts and without refills. This does more than reduce the danger of overdose and allow more accurate monitoring of how much medication is being used. It also communicates to the patient that the physician (or other members of the team) wants to see him or her again soon to evaluate the effects of the medication and will be willing to make changes in dosage or in the medications themselves, depending on the experiences of the patient and the observations of the clinicians. A patient may pick up medications at the mental health center, or staff may deliver medications daily to the patient's home, depending in part on how frequently the physician wants to monitor medication effectiveness, side effects, or compliance.

Finally, cost is an important factor in the use of medication. Once the decision has been made to prescribe medication for a specific indication, cost should be one of several factors in the choice of the particular medication regimen. The clinician must also ensure that a patient can afford the medication that is prescribed or, alternatively, make other arrangements, such as providing medications from samples or stock purchased by the mental health center.

Long-Term Planning

Long-term planning should begin during the initial crisis response or before admission if the patient needs to enter the hospital. From the initial contact, the clinician should begin thinking about what the person will likely need at the end of the crisis or on discharge from the hospital. What kind of permanent housing is the person likely to need? What kinds of medical treatment or help with daily structure or finances will be needed? Is this person likely to need help with socialization or to need specialized kinds of social and psychological support? Are vocational services likely to be useful? Will this person need a case manager? These longer-term needs can often be predicted at the initial contact and should be considered in the initial crisis treatment plan.

It is also important to anticipate the difficulties that treaters might expect following resolution of the crisis, and try to prepare for them. This applies to discharge from a hospital, from a crisis home, from the emergency department, or from the care of a crisis team. For example, patients may fail to show up for appointments. Rather than just labeling the patient "unmotivated" and "treatment resistant," we can try to find out with as much specificity as possible what the patient wants (Diamond and Factor 1994). Consider whether outreach will be necessary, and if so, if it will be available.

Similarly, it is important to develop strategies for patients who are likely to refuse to take psychotropic medications (Diamond 1983, 1985). For patients whose crisis was associated with stopping medication, the clinician should ask the patient why he or she decided to stop taking the medication. Did the medications actually help the patient accomplish his or her own goals, as opposed to the treaters' goals? Did the patient experience side effects? Did taking medications touch off issues of control between the patient and treaters, family, or others? The clinician should attempt to negotiate with the patient. At times the only way to get a patient to take medication is involuntarily, through legal coercion. If so, the clinician must decide if medication is such an important part of treatment that seeking legal authority is worth its cost and whether such authority is likely to work legally and practically.

Pass control and information from the crisis team to the continuing care team. During the postcrisis phase, problems may develop in the support system. For example, a patient may upset or frighten neighbors in an apartment building or act in a bizarre manner with family, friends, or employers. The continuing care team, perhaps with assistance from the crisis team, must be available to provide contact, support, and consultation to the patient's support system so that all persons involved can deal with the patient's behavior more appropriately. A small investment supporting the patient's support system often pays off handsomely in the long run to resolve present and ongoing crises with less input from professionals. The crisis service can thus provide a critical role in keeping the long-term care system functioning smoothly (Stein 1992a).

Once a plan is in place, monitor it to see how it is progressing. Do not just "let it go." Make sure that there is a mechanism that is responsive to ongoing crises and stress. Consider what individual or team is going to be the crisis manager. This important job involves many responsibilities to ensure that 1) the plan is carried out; 2) information about how the plan is working and how the patient and support system are doing is appropriately collected, kept up to date, and passed along to treaters and the support system; 3) meetings are scheduled as necessary; 4) the treatment plan is coordinated and revised as necessary; 5) appropriate reevaluations and referrals are done; and 6) the patient does not "get lost" in the system. The crisis manager must monitor the efficacy of the entire plan. Monitoring and revision can be hourly, daily, weekly, monthly, or at whatever time intervals are appropriate. In this way, treaters can intervene early if things decompensate.

Asses for early signs of decompensation. The continuing-care team and others who will be in the patient's support network should know the early signs of decompensation, what to be concerned about, what not be to concerned about, what interventions they can try that usually work to reduce behavior that causes problems, and how they can get help from crisis personnel when they need it. As with other elements of treatment planning, the details should be specific to the patient and his or her support network.

After the crisis has stabilized and resolved, develop a long-term treatment plan that will maintain the patient in treatment. It is important to reassess the patient once the crisis has resolved, both from the perspective of DSM-IV and from the perspective of the patient characteristics that influence the selection of a service delivery system. These include the willingness to come in for services, medication compliance, the need for structured daily activities, the ability to monitor oneself, the frequency and severity of crises, the need for professional psychological support, and the need for case management services (Stein et al. 1990). As in other phases of treatment, the clinician should make sure the patient does not "get lost" in the transition from crisis to ongoing treatment. If the crisis manager is different from the manager of ongoing treatment, the former should not relinquish responsibility until the patient is well connected with the latter, not immediately after a referral has been made on paper.

The Mentally Ill, Substance-Abusing Patient

Persons with mental illness who also abuse substances present special problems for the psychiatric crisis service. These patients are often brought into the crisis service against their will, acutely intoxicated, and when they are least amenable to treatment. Their disorganization or risk of life-threatening behavior often necessitates an involuntary hospitalization that appears to accomplish little other than temporary drug or alcohol detoxification. From the perspective of the patients, these recurrent hospitalizations increasingly serve to alienate them from the treatment system that they perceive accurately as controlling and coercive. Attempts to develop a collaborative relationship may be futile with someone who is acutely intoxicated, and the risk of violence may be increased during a lengthy interview.

It is important for the clinicians at the crisis service to recognize their limitations and not attempt more than they can realistically accomplish. The immediate need is often safe detoxification in a facility that can contain the patient's behavior and monitor the patient's medical status. As long as the patient is intoxicated, it does not matter whether this occurs in a hospital, a detoxification unit, or some alternative facility. Psychiatric evaluation and treatment begin after acute detoxification is complete. Patients with both substance abuse and mental illness can be effectively treated in community support programs that pay attention to both of the patient's problems, but this requires an ongoing and coordinated treatment approach that cannot easily be orchestrated by a crisis service (Drake et al. 1991).

The Mentally Ill Person Who Commits Minor Crimes

Persons with mental illness who commit minor crimes, once or repetitively, also present special problems for the psychiatric crisis service. These persons are often bounced back and forth between the mental health and criminal justice systems without fitting well into either (Teplin and Pruett 1992). Special difficulties almost always arise whenever someone with a major mental illness is arrested. However, individuals differ greatly in terms of the relationship between their illness and any criminal behavior, and in the amount of responsibility that they should bear.

Some patients commit minor crimes because of the direct effects of their psychotic thinking. Examples include a patient with schizophrenia who broke a shop window because his thinking and behavior were so disorganized that he was unaware of the effects of his actions; a patient with schizophrenia and command hallucinations who engaged in shoplifting because a voice told her that the merchandise she took belonged to her; and the patient with florid mania who got into a fight with police after they stopped him from driving backward around the block in what he believed was a way to make the United States independent of foreign oil. Persons such as these are clearly not responsible for their actions and need treatment within the mental health system rather than incarceration. Our experience is that police and district attorneys are more than willing to let the mental health system assume responsibility for these persons, as long as the system is also responsive to the need of the police to stop the illegal and socially disruptive behavior in a timely manner.

More commonly, patients with serious mental illness commit minor crimes as part of their life-style or become psychotic because of a competent choice they made when not psychotic. Examples include a patient with schizophrenia who repeatedly engaged in shoplifting because he spent all of his money on drugs; a patient with schizophrenia who repeatedly broke some store windows while drunk; a patient with bipolar disorder who forged some checks while manic after discontinuing lithium for the fourth time, despite many discussions with and warnings to the patient (while the patient was euthymic) about the possible consequences of discontinuing lithium; or a patient with a severe mixed personality disorder with narcissistic and histrionic features who repeatedly engaged in shoplifting as one of a variety of attempts to test whether a good friend really cared about him and would get him off this time on the criminal charge. These persons have a major mental illness but should be held responsible for their own behavior while also receiving appropriate mental health treatment. This means that the criminal justice system should deal with the criminal part of the behavior while the mental health system continues to provide support and treatment, whether the person is in jail, on probation, or in the process of hearings and legal decision making.

These patients are best managed by a cooperative effort between the criminal justice system (police, attorneys, courts, and jails) and the mental health system (Stein and Diamond 1985). Although such an integrative approach involving both the criminal justice and mental health systems is difficult to implement in many communities, when it can be accomplished, there is a significant benefit for all concerned. Cooperation can allow the staff of each system to do their particular jobs well, rather than feeling "used" by someone else. It can help optimize the use of limited resources, and it can minimize the chances of a patient falling between systems. Most importantly, a cooperative approach can help patients receive needed mental health treatment while also being held responsible for their behavior when this is appropriate. Clinicians should presume that most of their patients are competent most of the time and, like anyone else, have a citizen's responsibility to face the consequences of their competent actions.

In a crisis situation, this cooperation requires that the crisis service be able and willing to respond rapidly to a request for help by police and have a range of immediate and follow-up options that can be used. Staff working in the crisis service must work with police as professional colleagues who have their own skills, priorities, and jobs to do. Before any of this can occur, there must be a significant investment in providing education and support to patients, patients' families, and criminal justice professionals about the appropriate role for both the mental health and criminal justice systems. Involvement by the mental health system in the form of support for the patient, and for the criminal justice system in working with the patient, should occur throughout the entire judicial process. The involvement of the criminal justice system is not a substitute for treatment by the mental health system, nor should arrest or incarceration be used simply because mental health treatment is unavailable.

A corollary of the principle that these patients should be held responsible for competent actions is that they are entitled to the same rights accorded all citizens. Mental health professionals in particular should guard against any stigmatization of persons with mental illness. In this context, people with mental illness should not be treated more harshly by the criminal justice system simply because their behavior is different or bizarre. For example, someone with schizophrenia should not be arrested for vagrancy unless the vagrancy laws are applied similarly to everyone, and bail should be set for someone with mental illness using the same standards used for anyone else.

Providing Services at Times of Natural or Human-Caused Disasters

Disasters include a wide range of events. Floods, hurricanes, tornadoes, and urban violence may affect large numbers of people in a community. House fires, traumatic accidents, violent crimes, or other causes of sudden injury or death may affect a single person or family. Disasters may be natural or human-caused. Those affected may be suffering distress from the psychological trauma of the event itself. They may be suffering losses of family or friends or of a home or other property. They may also be suffering physical injury. Clinicians may be called on to treat victims, affected family and friends, witnesses, and caregivers.

The early development of the practice of crisis intervention was strongly influenced by Lindemann's classic paper on the survivors of the Coconut Grove fire in Boston in 1942, and his finding that appropriate crisis intervention could decrease later psychological sequelae (Lindemann 1944). Based on this and subsequent research, effective ways have evolved for working with people who have experienced overwhelming events. People go through four typical phases following a disaster (or any significant loss), although reactions vary depending on the individual's character and style, cultural background, personal history of loss, and social network and on the particular nature of the disaster and losses suffered. The first phase may involve some degree of warning or anticipation of the event. At the time of the event and the immediate aftermath, the person experiences shock and disbelief and relative psychological numbness, which may last hours to many days. Next follows a period when the shock wears off, and the person experiences the loss maximally and grieves it. Ideally, after what may be many months, the person enters a period of resolution, with acceptance of and adaptation to the loss and return to more typical functioning (Raphael 1986).

Each phase can raise potential issues for the disaster victim that are important for the crisis worker to identify and utilize in the intervention. A person might feel that he or she ignored a potential warning of the disaster or did not take sufficient action to avoid it. During the disaster itself, the person may have responded effectively or with a considerable degree of help-lessness. A person may be able to mobilize psychological resources such as prayer or hope during the immediate aftermath or may be overwhelmed and paralyzed. An individual may experience degrees of helplessness from the effects of the trauma, as well as pain from the human and physical losses sustained. Survivors may feel considerable guilt. The clinician should tailor interventions to the characteristics of the person and the issues involved. Appropriate interventions help the victim cope with the psychological ef-fects of the disaster and decrease the likelihood of long-lasting posttrau-matic symptoms.

Some general strategies that are helpful in working with individuals in-clude allowing victims to express their grief; providing information to vic-tims, who may be confused and in psychological shock about what has happened to them and to others; offering medications if appropriate; and arranging for follow-up care for individuals or groups if appropriate. Above all, clinicians should recognize that a variety of reactions on the part of vic-tims may be adaptive and should try to maintain a sympathetic and flexible attitude toward victims. People need the opportunity to utilize supportive services without being labeled inappropriately as having psychopathology. As with any crisis, people may be psychologically more accessible at the time of the crisis than later, so that it is best to make initial contact with those affected as soon as possible after the disaster.

One group intervention that can be particularly useful for victims, wit-nesses, and other persons affected by an acute disaster is a debriefing ses-sion (Rubin 1990). Sessions can start with each person retelling his or her story or role. As each person's story is shared within the group, members begin to organize the events and to understand what has happened and con-tinues to happen to them. They have the opportunity to feel some sense of mastery over the traumatic experience and that they are going to be able to live with it. Sessions also help to restore members' lost confidence in the safety of their environment.

Debriefing can also be useful for professional caregivers, including health professionals, police, firefighters, and other disaster workers. In addition to the above, sessions can also include a discussion of interpersonal issues among members of the team, of treatment plans, or of revisions in the policies and procedures for handling such situations. Sessions can help members restore lost confidence in their efficacy, preserve their ability to cope with stress, and work as an effective team.

Providing disaster-related services on a large scale can be very difficult unless some planning has been done ahead of time. A disaster plan should identify key individuals, as well as programs and agencies that have trained personnel in place who would be able to devote themselves to working with victims. The plan should also include a way of mobilizing these services rapidly and with minimal effort, such as through "telephone trees." Individual contacts and debriefing sessions should be led by trained personnel. It is also useful to have on hand printed material that includes the stages of adaptation to loss, common symptoms that people may expect to experience, reassurance about what does and does not need further treatment, and information on what to expect, along with referral resources for medical, psychological, social, economic, and legal help. Information specific to the particular disaster can be added to previously prepared handouts, which is much easier than preparing all material freshly at the time of the disaster.

Changing the System

On a system level, mental health professionals should work administratively and politically to improve (or create) a system of services that cares for seriously ill people as well as possible, using information and techniques that are presently established but often not employed for a variety of reasons (Factor et al. 1988; Stein et al. 1990). The variety of services needed may not be not available in the community in which the crisis occurs. This may be because staff lack some specific skills or sufficient time to manage some clients, or because the caseloads are too big or too heterogeneous in relation to the service needs of patients. The solution for the most needy patients may lie in multidisciplinary continuous care teams specializing in working with subpopulations of seriously mentally ill individuals (Stein 1992b).

Conclusion

Mobile crisis intervention services and psychiatric emergency departments are important parts of the mental health service system. Many patients come to these crisis services struggling to live their lives while burdened with a serious psychiatric illness. Others come overwhelmed by an acute stress, with little evidence of preexisting psychiatric problems. Many patients come to these crisis services in a true crisis, with sudden disruptions in their lives that overwhelm their ability to cope. Others live in chronic states of crisis, with ongoing life problems that fill their lives with chaos. In each case, the clinician's job is to listen to the patient's story, help to organize the crisis, and help the patient restabilize his or her life to function as well as possible. Crisis workers often attempt to do this with too many patients who need their help and too little time to do all that they would like. Crisis workers are often forced to make decisions with too little information and to deal with situations that include the risk of violence to others or suicide.

Despite all of these problems, there is no area of psychiatry where one can make so great a difference in a patient's life in so short a period of time. One important element of the job must include helping people to be safe. Beyond this, however, an intervention can sometimes transform the crisis into an opportunity to learn a new way to cope. The crisis can be the time when family can get reinvolved or when a patient decides to restart needed medication. A period of crisis might be the best time to make a human connection with someone who desperately needs help but has been unwilling to seek treatment. Treatment that begins on an involuntary basis may evolve into treatment that becomes more collaborative and voluntary, as patients achieve goals that make palpable improvements in the quality of their lives. This may happen quickly, or it may take significant amounts of time, and the crisis may be only the beginning. In each case, clinicians should see their job as an opportunity not only to assess and perform triage, but also to help patients to resolve the crisis and carry on with their lives.

References

American Psychiatric Association: Diagnostic and Statistical Manual of Mental Disorders, 4th Edition. Washington, DC, American Psychiatric Association, 1994

Applebaum PS, Gutheil TG: Clinical Handbook of Psychiatry and the Law, 2nd Edition. Baltimore, MD, Williams & Wilkins, 1991

Arce AA, Vergare M: An overview of community residences as alternatives to hospitalization. Psychiatr Clin North Am 8:423–436, 1985

Bartolucci G, Drayer CS: An overview of crisis intervention in the emergency rooms of general hospitals. Am J Psychiatry 130:953–960, 1973

Bassuk E, Gerson S: Chronic crisis patients: a discrete clinical group. Am J Psychiatry 137:1513–1517, 1980

Benjamin LS: Interpersonal Diagnosis and Treatment of Personality Disorders. New York, Guilford, 1993

Diamond RJ: Enhancing medication use in schizophrenic patients. J Clin Psychiatry 44:6(section 2):7–14, 1983

Diamond RJ: Drugs and the quality of life: the patient's point of view. J Clin Psychiatry 46:5(section 2):29–35, 1985

Diamond RJ, Factor RM: Treatment-resistant patients or a treatment-resistant system? (editorial) Hosp Community Psychiatry 45:197, 1994

Diamond RJ, Wikler DI: Ethical problems in community treatment of the chronically mentally ill. Directions for Mental Health Services 26:85–93, 1985

Drake RE, McLaughlin P, Pepper B, et al: Dual diagnosis of major mental illness and substance disorder: an overview. New Dir Ment Health Serv 50:3–12, 1991

Factor RM: Managing the violent patient in the emergency department. Emergency Care Quarterly 7:82–93, 1991

Factor RM, Stein LI, Diamond RJ: A model community psychiatry curriculum for psychiatric residents. Community Ment Health J 24:310–327, 1988

Hyman SE, Tesar GE (eds): Manual of Psychiatric Emergencies, 3rd Edition. Boston, MA, Little, Brown, 1994

Lindemann E: Symptomatology and management of acute grief. Am J Psychiatry 101:141–148, 1944

Nehls N, Diamond RJ: Developing a systems approach to caring for persons with borderline personality disorder. Community Ment Health J 29: 161–172, 1993

Raphael B: When Disaster Strikes: How Individuals and Communities Cope With Catastrophe. New York, Basic Books, 1986

Rapoport L: The state of crisis: some theoretical considerations. Soc Serv Rev 36:211–217, 1962

Rubin JG: Critical incident stress debriefing: helping the helpers. J Emerg Nurs 16:255–258, 1990

Stein LI: Crisis stabilization services for persons with psychotic illnesses, in Emergency Psychiatry Today. Edited by van Luyn JB. Amsterdam, The Netherlands, Elsevier Science Publishers, 1992a, pp 25–28

Stein LI: On the abolishment of the case manager. Health Affairs 11:172–177, 1992b

Stein LI, Diamond RJ: The chronic mentally ill and the criminal justice system: when to call the police. Hosp Community Psychiatry 36:271–274, 1985

Stein LI, Diamond RJ, Factor RM: A system approach to the care of persons with schizophrenia, in Handbook of Schizophrenia, Vol 4: Psychosocial Treatment of Schizophrenia. Edited by Herz MI, Keith JJ, Docherty

JP. Amsterdam, The Netherlands, Elsevier Science Publishers, 1990, pp 213–246

Teplin LA, Pruett NS: Police as streetcorner psychiatrist: managing the mentally ill. Int J Law Psychiatry 15:139–156, 1992

Weissberg MP: Emergency room medical clearance: an educational problem. Am J Psychiatry 136:787–790, 1979

Chapter 5

Psychiatric Rehabilitation in Community Settings

Jerome V. Vaccaro, M.D.
Deborah B. Pitts, M.B.A, O.T.R.

P sychiatric rehabilitation has assumed new prominence as attention is given to the long-term community adaptation of individuals with mental illness. In most areas, psychiatric rehabilitation programs have developed independently from community mental health programs. In fact, many rehabilitation practitioners articulate the view that this separation is desirable. The focus of conventional treatment settings is on early intervention and effective treatment of psychiatric symptoms. Although this is clearly important and necessary to address, psychiatric rehabilitation emphasizes continuous treatment of lifelong disorders, targeted at ameliorating symptoms; preventing or reducing relapses; and improving patients' performance in social, vocational, educational, and familial roles. In addition, the practice of psychiatric rehabilitation stresses empowerment of the mentally disabled person to be actively involved in treatment decisions and to achieve satisfactory life quality (Anthony et al. 1992; Kuchnel et al. 1990; Liberman 1988).

In this chapter we provide an overview of contemporary issues in psychiatric rehabilitation, highlight a number of specific technologies, and suggest roles for the psychiatrist in the practice of psychiatric rehabilitation.

Conceptual Issues

Psychiatric rehabilitation may be seen as a set of methods and techniques that can accelerate social and symptomatic recoveries among seriously mentally ill individuals. The conceptual model that is currently used to explain our understanding of the process of rehabilitation has been called the *stress-vulnerability-protective factors model* of psychiatric impairment, disability, and handicap (Liberman et al. 1995). Its main features are an assumption that individuals with mental illness possess some biological or behavioral diathesis that results in the production of psychiatric symptoms when the effect of stressors overwhelms the individual's coping strategies and competencies.

Psychiatrists speak of an individual's *impairments,* such as the psychotic symptoms, affective abnormalities, cognitive deficits, and other psychiatric symptoms and signs. These impairments may then result in *disabilities,* or restrictions, in various functional life domains such as vocational performance, recreational pursuits, family and social relationships, and self-care. A *handicap* is said to exist when these disabilities place the individual at a disadvantage to others in his or her environment, including roles such as worker, student, citizen, and family member. The focus of rehabilitative interventions, then, is to enhance protective factors. Examples of such protective factors are psychopharmacological interventions that reduce symptoms with minimal side effects, the individual's coping skills and competencies, and social supports such as safe and secure housing.

Functional Assessment

As with any intervention, careful initial and ongoing assessments improve efficacy and ensure that timely and appropriate care is offered. Of particular importance to ensure success are an individual's self-identified goals and desired life roles. Too frequently, psychiatrists plan and offer services with little or no attention to these issues. Not surprisingly, poor compliance results when goals are not clear or if the individual feels that treatment and rehabilitative services are irrelevant to or conflict with his or her needs. Clinicians should conceptually separate the evaluation process into two overlapping but distinct procedures: functional and symptom assessments.

Goal Setting

Goal setting is usually the pivotal event in the process of functional assessment and psychiatric rehabilitation. Interventions that are offered cannot be or appear to be inconsistent with the individual's perceived needs and goals. This stage of rehabilitation planning is also the most difficult to accomplish, as many clinicians do not feel comfortable discussing life goals with their patients. Commonly cited concerns are that individuals will identify unreasonable or unrealistic goals or that setting goals may be a demoralizing process for seriously impaired individuals. In fact we have found this not to be the case; instead, the goal-setting process energizes treatment and rehabilitation, bringing the individual, psychiatrist, and rehabilitation team into a closer working alliance. Goals most commonly identified include improving family relations, maintaining housing, obtaining employment or pursuing occupational objectives, and establishing social networks.

Once goals are established, the individual is engaged in identifying his or her own adaptive skills, deficits, and resources. When asked about obstacles that might block progress, individuals often identify psychiatric symptoms, illicit drug use, side effects from prescribed medications, inadequate social and independent living skills, alienation from families, and lack of money and housing. Adaptive skills such as coping with mental illness, interpersonal negotiation skills, development of family bonds, and friendship skills can be identified and reinforced. The following case vignette illustrates this process.

K.A. was a 26-year-old man who had been diagnosed as having paranoid schizophrenia. Once his psychotic symptoms were controlled with antipsychotic medications, he engaged in a rehabilitation planning effort with an occupational therapist who was a member of a community mental health center treatment team. When first asked to identify his goals, he said he wanted to enter college and complete his bachelor's degree. He had not been in school for 6 years and said he wanted to matriculate as a full-time student in a prestigious school in engineering. On further exploration, it was learned that K.A. had felt happiest when he was in school, and he now thought this would be the best way to realize his goal of being "happy and independent."

Once this goal of becoming independent and more pleased with himself was identified, he was helped by his therapist to set as a long-term goal resumption of his schooling at a local community college that had a supported education program. He then began to work with his therapist to target skills and deficits in the areas of time management, organization of scheduled activities, and self-assertion. He saw these as essential to prepare for his goal of entering school. He had been an organized person with good study habits prior to developing his illness, so these were seen as potential assets. His basic conversational skills were more than adequate, but he needed training in speaking up to meet his needs in the classroom, with teachers and with peers. He had the prerequisite resources to engage in the recommended training sessions—namely, time, an automobile for transportation, and the availability of social skills training services in his local community support program. Six months later, after benefiting from structured and systematic skills training, he returned to school.

Functional assessments can be performed with observational, interview, or self-report instruments—focusing on the performance of the individual in self-care, social, family, recreational, vocational, and financial domains. Instruments selected for use in clinical practice should be congruent with the purposes and logistics of the assessment; thus, time sample behavioral observations are useful in residential settings, whereas interview and self-report formats are more suitable for outpatient settings.

Social Skills Training

Social skills training interventions are characterized by behavioral techniques or learning activities that enable individuals to acquire skills in areas required to meet the interpersonal, self-care, and coping demands of community living. A typical skills training session is conducted educationally as a class with 1 or 2 cotherapists and 5 to 10 participants. Sessions are conducted for 45–90 minutes, depending on the individuals' level of concentration and symptom control, and meet 1 to 5 times a week. Because most mentally disabled individuals have pervasive deficits in social functioning, skills training should become a central element in their long-term rehabilitation.

In conducting social skills training, therapists engage seriously mentally ill individuals in goal setting and motivational enhancement. They are given an understanding of how the skills to be learned can help them achieve their own personalized needs and desires. For example, in generating motivation to participate in a conversation skills group, they are given illustrations of how good conversation skills can enhance friendships, dating, and job success. It is important to note that social skills training is an active, highly interactive, and directive experience. Thus, therapists actively teach skills to patients, ensure that these skills are learned adequately (e.g., through the use of role play), and induce generalization (e.g., through the use of homework assignments).

Social skills training can be conducted in the context of individual, family, or group therapy. Goals can be individualized to fit the functional and symptomatic needs of each person or can follow a prescriptive format in which preset goals are pursued that have general relevance for a large proportion of a target population. For example, clinics may offer individualized social skills training through therapists or clinical case managers and group social skills training in the form of goal-directed courses (e.g., classes on medication or symptom management, community living skills, conversation skills, or self-care skills).

Full discussion of methods employed to implement social skills training programs is beyond the scope of this chapter. However, it is useful to note that several centers (e.g., the University of California, Los Angeles, Clinical Research Center for Schizophrenia and Psychiatric Rehabilitation; Boston University's Center for Psychiatric Rehabilitation; and the center at the Albert Einstein College of Medicine program) (Anthony et al. 1990; Liberman 1992a; Liberman et al. 1989) have packaged social skills training programs (e.g., as modules or classes) that are available to clinicians.

Family Psychoeducation

Success in treatment and rehabilitation can be enhanced by involving the family as well as the mentally ill relative in a collective enterprise of 1) education about the designated person's particular mental disorder and ways to obtain professional and community services for him or her, 2) training in communication skills, and 3) use of communication skills in systematic application of problem solving. The family comprises an important part of the natural support system and living environment—even those with chronic mental illness living apart from their relatives maintain significant contact with them and is a powerful force in the recovery process.

With many international replications of the findings that family stress, as reflected in the "high expressed emotion" attitudes of criticism and emotional overinvolvement toward the mentally ill relative, is the most powerful predictor of relapse in schizophrenia and affective disorders, several modes of family intervention have been designed and empirically validated for their ability to equip relatives with coping skills and thereby change the emotional climate of the family and reduce the incidence of relapses and rehospitalizations (Falloon et al. 1984). From the vantage point of the stress-vulnerability-protective factors model of serious mental illness, families are viewed as struggling with the stress produced by the positive and negative symptoms and disability of their severely mentally ill relatives. In an interactive process, the stress load produces demoralization, tension, and emotional and financial burdens on the family and can precipitate relapse in the index patient who has fragile coping capacity and significant psychobiological vulnerability to stress.

Disavowing the now anachronistic and antitherapeutic theories of the past that implicated family interaction in the etiology of schizophrenia, clinicians engage relatives as essential allies in the treatment process. Family members' needs for coping skills and social support are recognized, given their serving as the primary caregivers of an individual with a chronic and disabling mental disorder. After an initial period of assessment with individual members of the family unit, the family alone or in combination with the individual begins a psychoeducational process aimed at translating in lay terms what is known scientifically and professionally about the person's mental disorder. Topics might include information about positive and negative symptoms, effects of psychotropic medications, and treatment options in psychiatric rehabilitation. Factual material is typically presented during the first half of an education session, followed by a guided discussion in which families are helped to personalize their learning with comments or questions regarding their own experiences. Sometimes the mentally ill relative attends these meetings and is invited to explain various points about symptoms and treatments in terms of their own experiences. In many areas of the United States, self-help groups such as affiliates of the National Alliance of Mentally Ill or local mental health associations have shared the education function.

To produce durable clinical effects, family interventions must go beyond education, and train family members in necessary coping skills, including basic communication and problem solving. Families are better able to address recurring difficulties associated with their family member's symptoms and disabilities when these skills are added to their behavioral repertoires. Skills training strategies similar to those reviewed previously in this chapter are used to help individual families learn to interact in more constructive and goal-oriented ways. These family interventions may be offered to individual families or to groups of families. In fact, evidence suggests that multiple-family group interventions may have some benefits over single-family interventions (McFarlane 1990). The following case vignette illustrates the effects of family interventions such as those described here.

Most of the members of the Aiello family have been concerned about Jim's smoking in his room at night. His parents, Gilda and Eugene, were particularly worried that Jim might fall asleep smoking in bed and start a fire. Using the problem-solving steps they learned in the family skills training sessions, the parents decided to call a meeting to discuss the matter. The Aiello family rotated leadership of the meeting each session, and this time it was Jim's sister, Andrea's, turn to review the steps.

Although Jim first saw the problem as his parents' nagging him about his smoking habits, with gentle pressure from Gilda and Andrea, Jim soon agreed with the others that he had a problem with smoking in his room at night. Andrea then encouraged everyone to generate solutions to the problem. Gilda said that Jim should be encouraged to learn new ways to stop smoking and thought he should be rewarded with $1 for each day he went without smoking in his room. Eugene did not like this idea, because he thought this would only "coddle" his son. Andrea reminded Eugene that the family should evaluate the solutions only after several had been generated and challenged him instead to come up with a solution. Eugene said that they should take away Jim's smoking privileges altogether.

After listing six solutions, the group reviewed the pros and cons of each alternative. Family members were then asked to vote on the worth of each solution. Four of the five agreed that finding Jim another place to smoke at night would be a good alternative. To implement the solution, Andrea volunteered to help Jim walk through the house after the meeting to find a safe and quiet place for him to smoke between 8:00 and 10:00 P.M. They agreed that the basement family room would be just such a place. The plan was to start the next night, and a week later the group was to reconvene and discuss progress.

The following week it was Eugene's turn to lead the family meeting. Under his guidance, the group discussed whether the frequency of Jim's bedroom smoking had decreased. Jim reported that he had smoked in his room at night only once the preceding week, about which everyone was happy. Gilda, however, said she now found watching television in the family room a bit unpleasant at night because of Jim's smoke. Because the original target of bedroom smoking had decreased markedly, the family decided to wait a week before deciding whether and how to tackle the smoke problem in the family room.

Cognitive Remediation

In addition to cognitive models of skills training, treatment researchers have designed techniques that target the various cognitive deficits presumed to mediate the symptoms and social dysfunctions of severe mental illness

(Liberman and Green 1992). Proponents of cognitive remediation view these cognitive functions and their brain substrates as plastic and amenable to direct rehabilitative interventions. Although some biologically focused psychiatrists might counter that the cognitive deficits of schizophrenia represent an irreversible and enduring form of dementia and hence cannot be mitigated by rehabilitation, evidence is gradually accumulating to justify clinical research in this area. For example, studies have documented the predictive relationship between information-processing deficits (e.g., such as vigilance and short-term memory) and the ability of individuals with schizophrenia to learn psychosocial skills.

Allen et al. (1992) formulated a theory of cognitive disability that conceptualizes a hierarchy of cognitive functioning in which the individual is increasingly able to incorporate sensory information from the environment and therefore function more adaptively in social and task environments. This theory, when applied to the clinical setting, can 1) assist the biomedical practitioner in measuring and monitoring response to psychiatric medications, and 2) assist the rehabilitation practitioner in knowing when the introduction of cognitive remediation or skills training technology will have the optimal effect. It is beyond the scope of this chapter to examine cognitive remediation interventions in detail, but readers are encouraged to seek information regarding this new and promising area through the references (e.g., Liberman 1992b).

Supportive Environments

In addition to the various skills training initiatives described, comprehensive psychiatric rehabilitation programs must provide individuals with opportunities for engaging in personally meaningful and relevant daily routines and opportunities for safe and supportive living environments (Fairweather et al. 1969). Organized as an integrated network, each residential, vocational, social, and educational rehabilitation environment has increasing skill requirements and decreasing amounts of support.

Psychosocial Rehabilitation Clubhouses

One of the fastest growing approaches for this aspect of rehabilitation is the psychosocial rehabilitation movement, with Fountain House in New York City as its prototype and inspiration. Fountain House was organized in the late 1940s when patients released from state hospitals met regularly as a social club to satisfy their needs for acceptance, destigmatization, activities, and emotional support. At "clubhouse" programs, now disseminated throughout the United States, staff and patients work side by side in common activities such as meal preparation, cleaning, office work, editing a newsletter, recreation, and self-governance. The basic goals of stabilizing persons with mental illness in a normalizing environment with reduced needs for mental hospitalization are achieved through peer support, participation in meaningful and gainful tasks, and active involvement in planning one's own rehabilitation program.

Central to the psychosocial rehabilitation philosophy is the belief that persons with psychiatric disorders have a fundamental right to work and a home, and that these basic needs, when satisfied, generate self-esteem and a positive identity necessary for community adjustment. Thus, psychosocial clubhouses have invested time and money in developing transitional employment and housing programs. In transitional employment, after a period spent acquiring prevocational skills such as punctuality and neatness in the clubhouse, members are placed in jobs in normal places of business. Ranging from large corporations to small firms, these jobs are entry-level positions requiring minimal training or skills. The clubhouse staff guarantees that the job will be performed reliably, even if staff members must fill in occasionally for an absent clubhouse member. These transitional jobs are opportunities for club members to work temporarily and under supervision in preparation for full-time, gainful employment. The popularity and growth of psychosocial rehabilitation programs are reflected by their services being reimbursed by Medicaid, Medicare, and state departments of rehabilitation; by their certification by accreditation agencies; and by the vitality of the International Association of Psychosocial Rehabilitation Services, an organization spawned by the clubhouse network.

Supported Employment

The federally sponsored supported employment initiative springs from the understanding that individuals with psychiatric disabilities require ongoing services, such as training in the skills necessary to maintain employment, once they secure competitive employment. It deemphasizes the importance of what has been labeled "prevocational" training, advocating instead a "place-train" approach. Individuals are placed in employment settings and then offered the training necessary to maintain their positions. In its fully applied form, individuals are offered services indefinitely, with "job coaches" visiting them at their workplaces to help them learn and retain the technical, interpersonal, and problem-solving skills they need to sustain employment.

For example, the job coach assesses an individual's stamina, emergent psychopathology, medication side effects, and interpersonal relations directly on the job site. In league with the other members of the community support mental health team, the job coach or case manager ensures that interventions are delivered to strengthen stamina, prevent relapses, control side effects, and improve social skills. In mastering the technical aspects of a job, the job coach carries out a task analysis of the requisite work, and breaks down the training process into component, incremental steps. Job coaching for persons with mental illness demands crisis intervention and liaison with psychiatrists providing medication to promote the individuals' tenure on the job.

Supported Education

As in the supported employment approach, the effort in supported education is to provide the social and structural supports needed by individuals with psychiatric disabilities to be successful in their efforts to pursue higher education. Through the collaborative efforts of educational institutions and community mental health or rehabilitation agencies, a variety of accommodations are made to ensure the individual's success in the educational environment. Accommodations include tutorials and alternative presentations of educational material congruent with learning styles or cognitive disabilities experienced by many persons with psychiatric disabilities.

Supported Housing

Residential environments that may be included in the network include halfway houses, group homes, and supervised apartments. The range of supported housing alternatives available in a given community should reflect the values as well as the functional abilities of the individuals they are intended to serve. Through the integration of interpersonal supports and targeted independent living skills training, these environments afford individuals the opportunity to live with the least amount of professional supervision.

The Role of the Psychiatrist

Most psychosocial or psychiatric rehabilitation settings lack significant involvement of psychiatrists, and psychiatric leadership in these settings is minimal. This is reflected in the relative shortage of curricular exposure to rehabilitation during residency training and the limited presence of psychiatric rehabilitation experts in departments of psychiatry. If psychiatrists are to be accepted in rehabilitation settings and guide the efforts of those in such settings to any meaningful extent, greater attention must be paid to their roles here. For one thing, psychiatrists must better educate themselves about the content of rehabilitation programs and be thoroughly familiar with their interventions. They should also become familiar with research findings in the field and accept the validity of rehabilitative efforts. The foregoing sections in this chapter are meant to be a primer in this regard.

Second, psychiatrists must be full collaborators on rehabilitation teams, supporting and enhancing the work of their rehabilitation practitioner colleagues. The following example illustrates this point.

> Joan is a 27-year-old woman who is a member of a psychosocial clubhouse, where it is noticed that her behavior is disruptive and prevents her from fully engaging in her own rehabilitation. It is further noted that her behavioral problems are the result of her psychotic and disorganized thinking. She tells her rehabilitation counselor that she has been diagnosed as having schizophrenia for 5 years and has taken antipsychotic medications in the past, with thioridazine being the most helpful. Joan and the rehabilitation counselor agree that she should see the psychiatrist at the local community mental health center for an evaluation.
>
> When Joan sees the psychiatrist for her initial evaluation, she presents none of the psychotic thinking or behavioral problems noted. After some discussion, Joan and the psychiatrist agree that the psychiatrist should call her counselor and discuss the referral. During the conversation, the psychiatrist learns of her past history of and present difficulties caused by psychotic symptoms. This leads to a discussion with the psychiatrist in which Joan tells him that she presented a "rosy picture" because she feared she would be overmedicated to the point of incapacity, limiting her ability to engage in meaningful activities at the clubhouse. With this in mind, she and her psychiatrist agree to a trial of low-dose thioridazine with frequent, brief follow-up visits.

In addition to collecting (and placing value on) information from the rehabilitation counselor, the psychiatrist in this example developed a contract with his patient so that he, the patient, and the counselor could carefully and collaboratively monitor the patient's responses to the medication. The psychiatrist valued the patient's initiative in her own rehabilitation and remained vigilant about the toxic effects medications sometimes have on rehabilitation. Thus, psychopharmacotherapeutic interventions must be consistent with and supportive of rehabilitation practice.

Finally, the psychiatrist practicing in rehabilitation settings can lead only through demonstrated competence. This can be as the general psychiatrist who is familiar with and respective of rehabilitation interventions, or as the psychiatrist who is thoroughly familiar with rehabilitation practice and who can deliver specific rehabilitative interventions. For example, a psychiatrist who has been trained in psychiatric rehabilitation may lead social skills training groups, educate patients and their families, and teach rehabilitation practice to other practitioners.

References

Allen CK, Earhart CA, Blue T: Occupational Therapy Treatment Goals for the Physically and Cognitively Disabled. Rockville, MD, American Occupational Therapy Association, 1992

Anthony WA, Blanch A: Research on community support services: what have we learned? Psychosocial Rehabilitation Journal 12:55–81, 1989

Anthony WA, Cohen M, Farkas M: Psychiatric Rehabilitation. Boston, MA, Center for Psychiatric Rehabilitation, Boston University, Sargent College of Allied Health Professions, 1990

Fairweather GW, Sanders DH, Maynard H, et al: Community Life for the Mentally Ill: An Alternative to Institutional Care. Chicago, IL, Aldine, 1969

Falloon IRH, Boyd JL, McGill G: Family Care of Schizophrenia. New York, Guilford, 1984

Kuehnel TG, Liberman RP, Rose G, et al: Resource Book for Psychiatric Rehabilitation. Baltimore, MD, Williams & Wilkins, 1990

Liberman RP (ed): Psychiatric Rehabilitation of Chronic Mental Patients. Washington, DC, American Psychiatric Press, 1988

Liberman RP (ed): Effective Psychiatric Rehabilitation. New Directions for Mental Health Services, No 53. San Francisco, CA, Jossey-Bass, 1992a

Liberman RP (ed): Handbook of Psychiatric Rehabilitation. New York, Macmillan, 1992b

Liberman RP, DeRisi WJ, Mueser KT: Social Skills Training for Psychiatric Patients. Elmsford, NY, Pergamon, 1989

Liberman RP, Green MF: Whither cognitive-behavior therapy for schizophrenia. Schizophr Bull 18:27-35, 1992

Liberman RP, Vaccaro JV, Corrigan PW: Psychiatric rehabilitation, in Comprehensive Textbook of Psychiatry, 6th Edition. Edited by Kaplan HI, Sadock BJ. Baltimore, MD, Williams & Wilkins, 1995, pp 2696–2717

McFarlane WR: Multiple family groups in the treatment of schizophrenia, in Handbook of Schizophrenia. Edited by Nasrallah HA. New York, Elsevier, 1990, pp 167–189

Paul GL, Lentz R: Psychosocial Treatment of Chronic Mental Patients. Cambridge, MA, Harvard University Press, 1977

Chapter 6

Alternative Acute Treatment Settings

Richard Warner, M.B., D.P.M.
Charlotte Wolleson, M.A.

I n this chapter we describe in some detail a community-based program for the treatment of acute psychiatric disorders—namely, Cedar House, in Boulder, Colorado—and present brief descriptions of a number of other acute nonhospital treatment programs in the United States and abroad. These facilities cover a broad range of settings: locked and open-door, voluntary and involuntary, public and private, nontraditional, and strictly medical settings. Each of these programs can be found described in depth, along with details of staffing, management and cost, in *Alternatives to the Hospital for Acute Psychiatric Treatment* (Warner 1995a).

Why Develop Alternatives?

Domestic settings for the treatment of acutely disturbed, mentally ill adult patients offer a number of benefits. They provide care that is much cheaper than hospital treatment, less coercive, and less alienating. Despite these ad-

This chapter is adapted from Warner R (ed.): *Alternatives to the Hospital for Acute Psychiatric Treatment.* Washington, DC, American Psychiatric Press, 1995. Used with permission.

vantages, there are fewer such treatment settings in the United States than might be expected, given the number of patients who can benefit.

Why are there not more such programs? Current health insurance mechanisms do not support their use. Managed care providers are becoming aware, however, that nonhospital programs offer substantial cost-benefit advantages. In Boulder, Colorado, for example, health maintenance organizations (HMOs) contract with the community mental health center for emergency psychiatric and inpatient services, in part because the range of inpatient options offered by the center includes Cedar House, the hospital alternative described later, which costs a fraction of psychiatric hospital care. Where Medicaid capitation schemes for the provision of health care are being introduced—for instance, in Utah and Colorado—we can expect to see hospital-alternative settings, with their opportunities for cost savings, become used more frequently in preference to conventional care.

Going beyond cost savings, it is important to recognize that these settings produce a different result. People receiving services in a noninstitutional setting are called on to use their own inner resources. They must exercise a degree of self-control and accept responsibility for their actions and for the preservation of their living environment. Consequently, patients retain more of their self-respect, their skills, and their sense of mastery. The domestic and noncoercive nature of most of the alternatives described in this chapter makes human contact with the person in crisis easier than it is in the hospital.

Philosophical Origins

There are common origins for many of the alternative settings for the treatment of acute mental disorders. Some (e.g., Paul Polak's crisis home program, described later) have links to the postwar therapeutic community movement, of which British psychiatrist Maxwell Jones was a major force (Jones 1968). Others, such as Soteria, have their roots in the experimental treatment environments of Laing and his associates in the Philadelphia Association in London in the 1960s (Barnes and Berke 1972; Sedgwick 1982). Crisis intervention facilities in the Netherlands were developed in response to the concept of primary prevention of emotional disorder, espoused by Gerald Caplan in his 1963 book, *The Principles of Preventive Psychiatry.*

The thread runs back through these revolutionary postwar developments in social psychiatry to an even earlier source: the successful elements of early 19th century moral management. There are common themes—active ingredients—in these alternative treatment programs and in the models to which they are linked, from this century and the last, that tell us something about the human needs of patients and the nature of the illnesses being treated (Jones 1972; Warner 1994). Currently, as in the moral treatment era, effective psychosocial treatment settings tend to be small, family style, and normalizing. They are open-door programs, genuinely in the community, and allow the user to stay in touch with friends, relatives, work, and social life. They are flexible and noncoercive and are often based more on peer relationships than hierarchical power structures. They involve patients in running their own environment and use whatever work capacity patients have to offer. The pace of treatment is not as fast as a hospital, and the units generally try to provide a quiet form of genuine "asylum."

Cedar House, Boulder, Colorado

Cedar House is a large home on a busy residential street in Boulder, Colorado. It was established in the late 1970s as a program of a comprehensive community mental health center to control ballooning hospital expenses. Inpatient treatment at Cedar House costs one-fourth of the daily rate in local psychiatric hospital wards, and it has proved its worth in other ways. Patients and staff like the facility because it is less confining, coercive, and alienating. As a result, patients make an effort to comply with house rules, and severely disturbed patients seem to behave less aggressively than they would in hospital. The program is fairly small, and although it is domestic in style, it is assertively medical in treatment orientation.

Staffed, like an acute psychiatric hospital ward, with nurses, a psychiatrist, and mental health workers, Cedar House functions as an alternative to the hospital for the acutely disturbed patients of the Mental Health Center of Boulder County. Like a hospital, it offers all the usual psychiatric diagnostic and treatment services (except electroconvulsive therapy). Routine medical evaluations are performed on the premises: patients requiring advanced medical and neurological investigation, including those with acute or chronic organic brain disorders, are evaluated by consulting physicians and in local hospital departments. Unlike a hospital, it is homelike, unlocked, and noncoercive.

As far as possible, Cedar House has the appearance of a middle-class home, not a hospital. Residents and staff may bring their pets with them to the house. A bird may be heard singing in one of the bedrooms, and a dog may be curled up on the sofa. On winter nights, a fire burns in the hearth. Staff and patients interact casually and share household duties. Residents come and go fairly freely (some attend work while in treatment), once they have negotiated passes with the therapist. Staff must encourage patients to comply willingly with treatment and house rules: no one can be strapped down, locked in, or medicated by force. Many patients, nevertheless, are treated involuntarily at Cedar House under the provisions of the state mental illness statute; they accept the restrictions because the alternative is hospital treatment, which virtually none of them prefer.

Patients

Patients who cannot be treated in the house are those who are violent or threatening, those who are so loud and agitated that they would make the house intolerable for other residents, and those who are so confused that they cannot follow staff direction. The house cannot handle individuals who repeatedly walk away or patients who are likely to elope and who, as a result, would be likely to harm themselves seriously. Patients who have direct access to guns and present some risk of using them are not admitted. In practice, just about everybody with a psychotic depression, most people with an acute episode of schizophrenia, and many people with mania can be treated in the facility. Some people with adjustment disorders or personality disorders are considered appropriate for admission. Many patients have a dual diagnosis of mental illness with substance abuse. Very few patients—fewer than 10%—need to be transferred to the hospital. Cedar House has not entirely replaced locked hospital care, but it provides nearly two-thirds of the acute inpatient treatment for the mental health center's patients and could provide an even greater proportion if more beds of this type were available.

Issues that definitely do not, by themselves, preclude admission to Cedar House include the following:

- Severe psychosis
- Concurrent medical problems
- Organic brain abnormality
- Suicidal ideas or gestures
- Age (any age above 16 is acceptable; people older than 65 are commonly admitted)
- Social class (although it sometimes takes a while for new upper-middle-class patients and their families to perceive advantages that Cedar House may have over a private hospital setting)
- Ability to pay for treatment (those who have good hospital insurance are no more likely to be admitted to the hospital and those with no insur-

ance are not rejected from Cedar House—care is provided under the center's usual sliding scale)
- Unpleasant disposition
- Illnesses such as *Phthirus pubis* infection ("crabs"), infectious hepatitis, acquired immunodeficiency syndrome (AIDS), or any contagious conditions that can be controlled by standard infectious precautions

Treatment

A number of the people treated in Cedar House would be subject to coercive measures, such as restraints and seclusion, if they were admitted to a hospital where such approaches are available and routinely used. The avoidance of coercion is an important benefit of the residential program—important in maintaining the mentally ill person's sense of self-esteem and self-control. As the moral treatment advocates of the early 19th century discovered, treating people with respect in a home-like and normalizing environment leads them to exercise "moral restraint" or self-control over their impulses.

The normalizing treatment style has many of the features of the therapeutic community approach. Residents take a hand in the day-to-day operations of the household. Every patient has a daily chore, and one resident—the chore leader—supervises the work of others. Higher functioning residents assist in aspects of treatment and may, for example, escort more disturbed patients on trips outside the house when needed. Although the engagement of patients in the management of the household and in the treatment process is empowering, the extent of patient government is limited. This is because the average length of patient stay is brief, and it is necessary for staff to exercise close control over admissions and discharges in order to make room available at all times for new admissions.

Cedar House is busy. Patients are admitted at any hour of the day or night, as in a hospital. All new patients go through a formal admission procedure and are seen by a psychiatrist within 24 hours. There are usually about 20 to 25 admissions a month. The need to create bed vacancies for the next emergency admission places pressure on staff and patients alike to limit length of stay to a brief period. Most patients stay 1 or 2 weeks, but some stay much longer. The occasional person who stays months is generally a high-risk patient, sometimes potentially dangerous, sometimes medically unstable, who proves difficult to place in the community, even with extensive supports and elaborate treatment.

An essential initial step in the treatment of those entering Cedar House is the evaluation of the patient's social system. What has happened to bring the person in at this point in time? What are his or her financial circumstances, living arrangements, and work situation? Have there been recent changes? Are there family tensions? Has the person relapsed more since establishing the current living arrangements? From the answers to such questions, a short- and long-term treatment plan is developed that will, it is hoped, not only lead to the patient's immediate improvement, but also reduce the chances of relapse after discharge. The goal for all patients is to leave Cedar House for suitable living conditions and coordinated treatment designed to prevent the revolving-door syndrome and provide a decent quality of life. Virtually no one who leaves is expected to stay at a homeless shelter.

An advantage of intensive residential treatment over hospital care is that the lower cost allows treatment to proceed at a more leisurely pace. More time can be spent observing the features and course of the patient's illness, selecting and adjusting medications, eliminating side effects, and evaluating benefits of treatment. Selected patients suffering from psychoses with a good prognosis can be treated without recourse to antipsychotic drugs.

Benzodiazepines are used extensively at Cedar House as a supplement, or sometimes as an alternative, to the antipsychotic drugs. Moderate doses of benzodiazepines, such as diazepam (Valium) or lorazepam (Ativan), have been found to be more effective than neuroleptic agents in calming acutely agitated and psychotic patients and have proven invaluable in the early phases of treatment in Cedar House's open-door setting. Newly admitted patients with psychotic relapse are routinely treated with modest maintenance doses of neuroleptic medication combined with flexible, as-needed doses of a benzodiazepine.

Safety is an important issue for patients and staff, and every effort is made to ensure that no one is allowed to become aggressive. Crisis intervention techniques are used to deescalate arguments or acute upsets, and staff members listen carefully to any patient who reports that another resident may be becoming dangerous. Agitated patients may be offered medication or hospitalized if necessary. Everyone is expected to treat everyone else with respect. Patients are generally supportive of one another and, along with staff, are culture carriers for nonviolence and safety. Staff members work as a team, and each has the opportunity and responsibility to give input into treatment planning along with the therapist and the patient.

Staffing

Residential treatment of this intensity requires a staffing pattern similar to that of a hospital. A mental health worker (psychiatric aide) and a nurse are on duty at all times. On weekdays, two experienced therapists with psychology or social work degrees provide services to the residents; they offer psychotherapy, family therapy, and help with practical issues such as obtaining disability benefits, and they make arrangements for the patient's move back to the community. A half-time consumer case manager aide—a person who has experienced serious mental illness and has been trained in the principles of case management (Sherman and Porter 1991)—also assists residents with practical issues of accommodation and entitlements. A psychiatrist is present for 3 hours a day and is available by telephone around the clock. A team leader directs the program, and a secretarial assistant manages the office work; building repairs; and purchasing of supplies, food, and furnishings. Students and volunteers are used in a variety of ways.

A part-time cook prepares the meals with help from the mental health worker. In the early days of Cedar House, the residents did much of the cooking, but complaints were so plentiful that this is now rare. A cleaning person comes in a few times a week. Many of the acutely disturbed patients are too dysfunctional to assist much in the upkeep of the house, cooking, or repairs, and the staff are too busy doing other things. The house is cleaner, the food is of better quality, and things work better if these extras are squeezed into the budget.

Cedar House is staffed by people with diverse backgrounds who are experienced in the care of severely mentally ill patients. At least two staff members—one of them a nurse—are in the house at all times. At night the nurse sleeps, but is available if needed. Employees must have high professional standards, be bright and flexible, and be able to handle crisis situations and work under stress. They must be positive, friendly, and good with co-workers; they must enjoy working with the patient population and treat them with respect and dignity.

Management Issues

It has turned out to be important that Cedar House was set up in a neighborhood that is partly commercial. Within a few blocks are many community resources that patients use, such as grocery stores, a post office, a coffee shop, a hospital emergency department, a park, and a recreation center. The neighbors have shown little concern over the years about the presence of Cedar House. Early on it was necessary to erect a privacy fence around the property, and measures are taken to keep the noise down, especially at night, but for the most part, there have been few complaints.

The staffing of Cedar House imposes relatively high fixed costs that cannot be reduced without significantly altering the nature of the program. The therapeutic design would be improved if there were fewer than 15 acutely disturbed patients in residence, but this can be achieved only by driving up the per capita daily cost or by reducing staffing to a level that would restrict the severity of the patients who can be treated.

At $160 a day, Cedar House costs one-fourth as much as a private hospital. Only a small proportion of the actual costs, however, are covered by reimbursement from the patient or insurance companies. The program is not considered a hospital, and thus most insurance companies do not reimburse the treatment at an inpatient rate: Medicaid pays for the treatment at the long-term partial care rate. Some HMOs, however, appreciate that Cedar House is a bargain compared with hospital care and reimburse at the full rate. As capitated Medicaid mental health reimbursement mechanisms are established in Colorado, mental health agencies will find inexpensive nonhospital settings such as Cedar House far more attractive than traditional hospital units. Until then, the reason that Cedar House is financially viable is that it offers a treatment alternative for medically indigent patients.

The high fixed costs of Cedar House would be hard to justify for a mental health agency with a catchment area much below 200,000. With this proviso, the Cedar House model is appropriate for both rural and urban settings. The Colorado Division of Mental Health has replicated the Cedar House design in the northern part of the state and on the western slope of the Rockies as closer-to-home alternatives to state hospital admission for those in far-flung rural areas.

The Range of Alternatives

Venture, Vancouver, British Columbia

Venture, an acute treatment facility in Vancouver, British Columbia, is similar in several important ways to Cedar House (Sladen-Dew et al. 1995). It is an open-door household with an informal, relaxed atmosphere, yet offering close supervision. Residents are encouraged to do household chores and may leave to run errands and take care of business matters. The facility is under the same administration as the Greater Vancouver Mental Health Service and provides good continuity of care to the community care teams; psychiatrists and staff of the community programs come to Venture to provide treatment for the acutely ill patients. Venture admits about 350 patients a year, about half of all the inpatient admissions for the Vancouver mental health system. The average length of stay is 8 days. Close to three-fourths of the people admitted to Venture suffer from a psychosis.

At 20 beds, Venture is larger than Cedar House. The administrators of the program recognize that the increase in cost-efficiency with the larger size comes at the expense of the environmental benefits associated with a more home-like, small-scale setting. Staff find it difficult to keep track of all the patients in the larger setting, and some patients report that the facility is too busy, crowded, and noisy. "In hindsight," the administrators comment, "we would have given serious consideration to building two 10-bed facilities and to adopting a slightly higher staffing ratio" (Sladen-Dew et al. 1995).

Crossing Place, Washington, DC

Crossing Place is an independent acute treatment program taking referrals for a range of seriously disturbed patients from the public mental health system and operating out of a house on a busy street near the center of Washington, DC (Bourgeois 1995). More than half of the patients treated by the program in 1992 were suffering from schizophrenia, and nearly 60% were black. The household, which is small (eight residents) and home-like, uses a therapeutic community approach and emphasizes the human element in acute treatment. Staff and patients are involved in decision making, and an effort is made to determine the social factors that trigger acute episodes of illness. The treatment program takes a supportive and educational approach, using skills training; expressive therapies; and group, individual, and family psychotherapy.

Progress Foundation, San Francisco, California

The Progress Foundation in San Francisco, California, has established a series of four acute treatment facilities that are small, normalizing, human-scale establishments. The size of the households ranges from 7 to 10 residents, with 2 to 4 staff on duty at all times. Staff are picked as much for their life experience and their talent in working with others as for their specific professional training. Patients are involved in decision making, and each facility adapts itself to meet the needs of the patient.

The administrator of the program, Steve Fields, emphasizes that these are not mini-hospitals: In some ways, these facilities are the antithesis of standard treatment institutions and achieve results that hospitals cannot. There are inherent risks in running an informal program that does not respond to problems with a predetermined protocol, but this risk taking, Fields argues, is a key issue in making treatment effective. Every proposed new rule or procedure, he suggests, should be subjected to an "environmental impact study" to assess potentially adverse effects on rehabilitation goals and to ensure that the program does not gradually change into an institutional environment in the community (Fields 1995).

Northwest Evaluation and
Treatment Center, Seattle, Washington

This alternative to a psychiatric hospital was established as an evaluation and treatment unit for acutely disturbed, involuntary psychiatric patients from a large urban area. The facility is distinctly different from the other programs described in this chapter; it is similar in many ways to a traditional psychiatric hospital unit but is not licensed as one and is not as expensive as a hospital ward (Table 6–1). It is a large (32 patients), locked, nondomestic facility with ambulance entrances and large elevators to accommodate patients strapped to gurneys. Four psychiatrists are on staff to conduct psychiatric evaluations for the court and to provide treatment. Out of concern that the facility will not be viewed as a real hospital, the staff go to lengths to emphasize the medical nature of the program. It has three secure rooms and clearly defined institutional operating procedures; patients progress through a four-level system of privileges based on staff assessment. As a locked facility, the program is not integrated into the community: patients cannot leave the unit to conduct business. They are not involved in the operation of the treatment environment; instead they are involved in recreational, art, and movement therapy (Ferguson and Dowd 1995). The program is included here to illustrate the breadth of possibilities encompassed by the term *hospital alternative*.

Crisis Intervention Centers, The Netherlands

Crisis intervention centers were originally developed in the Netherlands in response to the theoretical approach outlined by Caplan in *Principles of Preventive Psychiatry* (1963). The original goal of providing preventive intervention to previously healthy people under severe stress did not prove as feasible as was hoped, but the crisis centers demonstrated their value in other ways, developing into short-term treatment units for more chronically disturbed individuals. At some of the centers, for instance, about one-fourth of the users suffer from a psychosis. However, the centers continue to function as a resource for less disturbed persons under acute stress. Many of those admitted have no diagnosable mental disorder, and a large number of admissions are for psychosocial problems such as domestic abuse.

Seven of these short-term residential facilities are in operation in the Netherlands in Groningen, The Hague, Rotterdam, and other cities. Although more expensive than hospital treatment, these facilities have become important components of the Dutch mental health system, offering asylum to a surprisingly broad range of people (Schudel 1995).

Table 6–1. Daily patient treatment cost in 12 hospital alternative programs

	Cost/patient/ day	Cost as % of private hospital cost	Cost as % of state hospital cost
Cedar House Boulder, CO	$160	25	57
Venture Vancouver, BC, Canada	160	36	54
Crossing Place Washington, DC	156	17	35
Progress Foundation San Francisco, CA	215–230	33	66
Northwest Evaluation Seattle, WA	249	31	83
Crisis Intervention Centers The Netherlands	300–365	200	200
Soteria Project San Francisco, CA	125	18	39
Soteria Berne Berne, Switzerland	300	75	100
Windhorse Northampton, MA	169–238	25	80
Clustered Apartments Santa Clara County, CA	12–27	N/A	N/A
Family Sponsor Homes Denver, CO	150 (1980s)	33	60
Crisis Homes Madison, WI	80	12	20

Soteria, San Francisco Bay Area, California

Soteria is a descendent of Kingsley Hall, a novel nonmedical community for people suffering from psychosis that was developed in London in the 1960s by radical British psychiatrists R. D. Laing and David Cooper (Barnes and Berke 1972; Sedgwick 1982). Soteria and its sister program, Emanon, were small, supportive households established in California in the 1970s to provide care for people with first-break schizophrenia, using minimal amounts of antipsychotic medication. The houses accommodated two staff members and six resident patients. Staff members, usually young people with no professional mental health training, stayed at the facility for 48-hour shifts and developed close nurturing relationships with the residents. A controlled investigation, funded by the National Institute of Mental Health and conducted by Loren Mosher, demonstrated that psychosocial care in this type of therapeutic milieu produced results that were equivalent to or better than standard hospital and outpatient treatment—at no greater cost and without reliance on usual doses of neuroleptic medication (Mosher and Menn 1978; Mosher 1995).

Soteria Berne, Berne, Switzerland

Soteria Berne, a Swiss therapeutic household for the treatment of early schizophrenia, borrows many ideas from the Soteria Project. Like the California-based program, the household in Berne aims to manage the illness in a small, quiet, and relaxing environment using neuroleptic medication in low doses and only in unusual circumstances. The 12-room house accommodates six to eight patients and two nurses. The program sets out to establish supportive bonds between the patient and only a few carefully selected people; to collaborate closely with relatives; and, as the patient moves toward discharge, to provide education about the illness, realistic expectations for future functioning, and recognition of prodromal symptoms.

As in the earlier Soteria Project, the outcome of treatment in this domestic setting, with very restricted use of antipsychotic medication, is equal to that with standard hospital and outpatient care (Ciompi et al. 1992). An important lesson of both the Swiss and American Soteria Projects is that remission often occurs in early schizophrenia without the use of neuroleptic medication if patients are managed in a supportive and human-scale environment.

Windhorse, Northampton, Massachussetts

The Windhorse Program is as noninstitutional as the treatment of acute psychosis can be. The approach was developed by psychiatrist Ed Podvoll and the faculty and graduates of the East-West Psychology Program of the Naropa Institute, a Buddhist college in Boulder, Colorado (Podvoll 1990). In this program, the patient lives in his or her own home and is helped by a team of people who join the patient in a variety of daily activities. Some may be live-in housemates, whereas others may join the patient to play basketball or chess, to go for hikes, or to talk about politics or spiritual issues. Throughout, there is an underlying sense of the benefit of human contact, the value in being with the patient rather than doing things to him or her, and an emphasis on patience and empathy. An attempt is made to keep the use of antipsychotic medication to a minimum in the hope that the healing nature of the environment will change the course of the patient's illness (Fortuna 1995).

Clustered Apartments, Santa Clara County, California

An innovative series of programs, conceived and established by James Mandiberg and his associates at a large mental health agency centered in San Jose, California, has created living communities of mentally ill persons based on mutual support and interdependence. Communities have been established at three sites: an urban community of 68 people, a suburban program for 73 persons, and a rural site for 90. These communities of clustered apartments are set up to be assertively nonclinical in style. Staff are encouraged to abandon traditional roles and to instead become community organizers. Their role is to help patients establish a network of mutual support as an alternative to dependency on the treatment system.

Can such strengthened communities develop ways to support their members so that hospital admission for acute psychiatric distress becomes less necessary? As the project has taken shape, each of the communities has developed in different ways, and each has devised mechanisms to avoid the hospitalization of community members. In one program, for example, the community members have reserved a housing unit as a crisis apartment and use it to provide respite care to members who were acutely disturbed. Residents in this program are trained to provide help to community members in acute psychotic distress and stay with the disturbed person through the crisis. Another of the programs has developed a less structured approach, providing neighbor-based crisis support to individuals in their own apartments (Mandiberg 1995).

Family Sponsor Homes, Southwest Denver, Colorado

During the 1970s and 1980s, Paul Polak and his associates at Southwest Denver Mental Health Center in Colorado established and operated a revolutionary system of family sponsor homes for the care of acutely disturbed psychiatric patients. This program consisted of a number of private homes where patients were helped through their crises by carefully screened and selected families. Mobile teams of psychiatrists, nurses, and other professionals provided treatment to the patients placed in the sponsor homes: rapid tranquilization was sometimes used in the management of acutely psychotic patients. The program proved to be suitable for the large majority of the agency's acute admissions and helped reduce the daily use of hospital beds to 1 per 100,000 of the catchment area population (Polak et al. 1995).

Southwest Denver Mental Health Center no longer exists as an independent agency, and the system of family sponsor homes is no longer in operation. The system, however, became a model for other agencies, including the mental health center in Madison, Wisconsin.

Crisis Homes, Madison, Wisconsin

A network of family crisis homes based on the Southwest Denver model is currently in operation at Dane County Mental Health Center in Madison. Ten family homes provide care to a wide variety of people in crisis, most of whom would otherwise be in the hospital: nearly three-fourths of these patients suffer from acute psychotic illness, and others are acutely suicidal. About 40% of the patients entering the program are admitted from the community as an alternative to hospital care, 40% are patients in transition out of the hospital, and 20% are people whose clinical condition is not severe enough to require hospital care but who have housing problems or social crises. The average length of stay is only 3 days.

Violence committed by people admitted to the crisis home is almost never a problem, partly because of careful selection of appropriate patients and partly because patients feel privileged to be invited into another person's home—they try to behave with the courtesy of house guests. For this reason, people with difficult personality disorders seem to behave better in the crisis home than they would in a hospital ward (Bennett 1995).

Because fixed costs are low (see Table 6–1), the crisis home model can be established with quite a small number of treatment beds (four to six) without significant loss of cost-efficiency. For rural communities, the model has the advantage that the crisis homes can be widely dispersed, not centrally located like a hospital, making it possible to provide intensive treatment close to the patient's home. To be effective, the treatment agency must sustain a high level of commitment to the success of the program. Each foster-care family requires a substantial amount of support from a consistently available professional, and the patients placed in the home must have intensive psychiatric treatment from a mobile team of professionals available 24 hours a day.

Management Issues

One may wonder whether the human-scale programs described in this chapter—nearly all of them unlocked, domestic and informal in style—can address the needs of the difficult-to-treat patients who form a core constituency for community mental health care systems. Can they handle those who are violent or facing criminal charges, those who actively resist treatment, those with AIDS or other medical problems, and those who prefer to live on the streets or who combine substance abuse with mental illness? A review of Table 6–2, which presents information about each of the programs previously described, reveals that North American programs that are integrated with or contract with a broader community treatment system clearly do not exclude such patients.

In most of these programs, individuals who have been convicted of misdemeanors and, often, those who have been convicted of a felony are routinely accepted into treatment. In some instances, as at Cedar House in Boulder, Colorado, offenders are transferred directly into treatment from jail after evaluation by an outreach team. Similarly, mentally ill homeless persons are located by outreach workers at the local shelter and admitted to treatment at the alternative facility, involuntarily if necessary. A large proportion of the patients of Crossing Place in Washington, DC, are homeless: an outreach team invites homeless mentally ill people to visit the house, and sometimes after many attempts, some agree to stay (Bourgeois 1995).

Agitation, disruptiveness, threatening behavior, or imminent risk of violence or self-harm are not usually grounds for exclusion. In Madison, Wisconsin, agitated patients and people who are imminently suicidal may be placed in private family homes (Bennett 1995), as they were in the similar family sponsor home program in Southwest Denver when it was in operation (Polak et al. 1995). All of the alternative programs that are affiliated with a mental health system accept AIDS patients, and a few admit patients with significant medical problems that require nursing care (e.g., patients with brittle diabetes or leg ulcers requiring daily dressing, patients on oxygen, and those with indwelling urinary catheters). These programs also often accept patients in acute organic confusional states in order to pursue the diagnosis of the medical cause of the condition.

Lack of cooperation with treatment does not exclude patients from an alternative treatment setting. Virtually all of the programs accept people who are at risk of walking away from treatment, and where the state statute allows, most accept patients who are detained under involuntary treatment orders. Northwest Evaluation and Treatment Center in Seattle, Washington, a locked setting that admits only involuntary patients, treats many patients who are not welcome at local private hospitals (Ferguson and Dowd 1995).

Case examples provided by the hospital alternatives illustrate the severity of illness of the patients. At Crossing Place, a psychotic woman was admitted because she was bizarre and aggressive and had recently attacked a police officer (Bourgeois 1995). A catatonic patient at Cedar House was

Table 6–2.   Characteristics of 12 hospital alternative programs

	Cedar House Boulder, CO	Venture Vancouver, BC, Canada	Crossing Place Washington, DC	Progress Foundation San Francisco, CA	Northwest Evaluation Seattle, WA
Inpatient capacity	15	20	8	8–10 per house	32
Carry outpatients?	6	Evaluations	Sometimes	No	No
Associated with community mental health system					
As an integral part	Yes	Yes	No	Yes	Yes
By contractual agreement	—	—	Yes	—	—
Does program accept patients with					
Serious imminent suicide risk?	Sometimes	No	Yes	Yes	Yes
Serious non-imminent suicide risk?	Yes	Yes	Yes	Yes	Yes
Nonserious suicide attempts/ threats?	Yes	Yes	Yes	Sometimes	Yes
Agitation and disruptiveness?	Sometimes	Sometimes	Yes	Yes	Yes
Imminent risk of violence?	No	No	Sometimes	Yes	Yes
Current threatening/ menacing behavior?	Rarely	No	Yes	Yes	Yes
Obnoxious inter-personal behavior?	Yes	Yes	Yes	Yes	Yes
Organic confusional states?	Yes	No	Yes	Usually	Yes

Crisis Intervention Centers The Netherlands	Soteria Project San Francisco, CA	Soteria Berne Berne, Switzerland	Windhorse Northampton, MA	Clustered Apartments Santa Clara County, CA	Family Sponsor Homes Denver, CO	Crisis Homes Madison, WI
10–12	6	8	1 per house	60–75 per program	2/home in 3 homes	1/home in 6 homes
1–10	Drop-in	Informal	Yes	N/A	No	Informal only
Yes	No	No	No	Yes	Yes	Yes
—	No	Yes	No	—	—	—
Sometimes	Yes	Yes	No	Yes	Yes	Yes
Sometimes	Yes	Yes	Sometimes	Yes	Yes	Yes
Yes	Yes	Yes	Yes	Yes	No	Yes
No	Yes	Sometimes	Sometimes	Yes	Usually	Yes
No	Yes	Sometimes	No	Sometimes	No	No
No	Yes	Usually	Sometimes	Sometimes	Sometimes	No
Sometimes	Yes	Usually	Yes	Usually	Yes	Sometimes
No	No	No	Sometimes	No	Usually	Usually

(continued)

Table 6–2.   Characteristics of 12 hospital alternative programs (*continued*)

	Cedar House Boulder, CO	Venture Vancouver, BC, Canada	Crossing Place Washington, DC	Progress Foundation San Francisco, CA	Northwest Evaluation Seattle, WA
Does program accept patients with					
Significant medical problems (such as brittle diabetes, indwelling urinary catheter, etc.)?	Yes	Yes	No	No	No
Acquired immunodeficiency syndrome?	Yes	Yes	Yes	Yes	Yes
Significant substance abuse problems?	Yes	Yes	Yes	Yes	Yes
Risk of drug/alcohol withdrawal reaction?	Sometimes	No	Sometimes	Yes	Yes
Current drug/ alcohol intoxication?	No	No	Sometimes	Usually	Yes
Involuntary treatment order/civil commitment?	Yes	No	No	No	Yes
Current misdemeanor criminal proceedings?	Yes	Yes	Yes	Yes	Yes
Current felony criminal proceedings?	Yes	No	Sometimes	Yes	No
Risk of escape/ walking away from treatment?	Sometimes	Yes	Yes	Yes	Yes

near mute, almost immobile, and scarcely ate or drank (Warner and Wollesen 1995). In the Windhorse program, a patient muttered and snarled to himself continually and had periods of agitation and destructiveness (Fortuna 1995). Comparative research has documented the high degree of pathologic abnormality at one of these alternatives. A sample of patients at Cedar House was

Crisis Intervention Centers The Netherlands	Soteria Project San Francisco, CA	Soteria Berne Berne, Switzerland	Windhorse Northampton, MA	Clustered Apartments Santa Clara County, CA	Family Sponsor Homes Denver, CO	Crisis Homes Madison, WI
No	No	No	Sometimes	No	Sometimes	Usually
Sometimes	N/A	No	No	Yes	N/A	Yes
No	Yes	No	Usually	Sometimes	Usually	Usually
No	No	Sometimes	No	No	No	Sometimes
No	No	No	No	Sometimes	No	No
No	No	No	Sometimes	No	Yes	Yes
Sometimes	Yes	Sometimes	Yes	Yes	Yes	Yes
No	No	Sometimes	Yes	No	Usually	Sometimes
Yes	Yes	Yes	Sometimes	No	Yes	Yes

shown, on a standardized measure, to be significantly more disturbed than long-term patients on the ward of a district general hospital in Manchester, England. Cedar House patients had higher levels of both positive symptoms of psychosis and affective symptoms. Despite the greater severity of illness, the quality of life (measured by a standard quality-of-life profile) of the

Cedar House residents was significantly greater than that of the hospitalized patients (Warner and Huxley 1993).

Patient Selection

The selection of appropriate patients for the alternative settings is usually made by the crisis staff and psychiatrist of the mental health system after consultation with the staff of the acute facility. In the Madison crisis home program, the program coordinator determines who will be admitted, but the crisis home family and the patient have veto power (Bennett 1995). In most instances (at Crossing Place, Venture, and Cedar House, for example), the facility staff, with the backup of the house director when necessary, have the final decision about whether an admission is appropriate.

Progress Foundation in San Francisco has a virtual "no refusal" policy for its acute alternative houses. Psychiatric emergency staff at San Francisco General Hospital act as gatekeepers and select appropriate patients for admission. The patient is interviewed at the emergency department by a liaison from the Progress Foundation, who makes a referral to one of the houses. The patient is automatically accepted unless, on arrival at the house, the patient's symptoms have escalated, and inpatient care has become necessary (Fields 1995).

Patient Management

The broad acceptance of patients who would prove difficult even for a locked hospital unit poses the question, "How are such patients managed?" What do staff do, for example, when one of the patients in residential treatment comes back to the facility intoxicated with alcohol? In many instances, as at Crossing Place in Washington, DC, or Venture in Vancouver, British Columbia, such a patient is initially handled in a low-key way, if possible, and isolated (or sent to bed) until he or she is thinking more clearly. At Cedar House and at Venture, if the patient is grossly intoxicated or obnoxious, he or she may be transferred to a local detoxification facility until sober and later returned to the treatment facility (Bourgeois 1995; Sladen-Dew et al. 1995; Warner and Wollesen 1995). At the Progress Foundation in San Francisco, repeated substance use is dealt with in an individualized way, Steve Fields, the director, reports.

For some, the treatment plan includes working with them in spite of the use of substances. Others may have reached a point where they have a "no drinking or using" clause in their admission agreement. In those cases, the patient might be discharged to a program for patients with substance abuse problems. The disposition—to be hospitalized, to be discharged to another program, or to remain in the acute residential treatment program—depends upon the relative psychiatric stability of the patient (Warner 1995b).

Similarly, the response to patients who become assaultive or destructive is often determined by clinical and diagnostic considerations, although the first concern in all of the settings is to ensure the safety of the patient and other residents and staff. At Venture in Vancouver, British Columbia, for example, if a resident in an acute psychotic state assaults someone, he or she would probably be transferred to the hospital; the response to nonserious property damage might be to give the patient extra medication and allow him or her to stay in the facility. If a patient with a personality disorder were to assault someone, he or she would probably be discharged. At Venture, Crossing Place, or Cedar House, an attempt would be made to bill the patient for damaged property, and at some facilities, criminal charges may be made against those who are assaultive or destructive, especially if the patient is not acutely psychotic (Bourgeois 1995; Sladen-Dew et al. 1995; Warner and Wollesen 1995).

In noninstitutional settings where restraints and seclusion are not used, it is important to minimize a disturbed patient's agitation as soon as possible to prevent disruption of the environment and to ensure the safety of the patient and others. On admission to Cedar House, psychotic patients are likely to be offered benzodiazepines as needed to reduce agitation and psychotic symptoms. Agitated patients often require extra staff support and supervision to calm them and to ensure that they are not intrusive with other patients and do not walk away from the facility. Firm direction of the patient may be required, but head-to-head confrontation is avoided. A staff member or volunteer may take the patient for a walk to the park or involve him or her in some other activity to help reduce tension and restlessness.

It is not uncommon for a resident in an acute care setting, especially one with a personality disorder, to make a nondangerous self-harm gesture (e.g., making a superficial cut on the arm or wrist). At most of these alternative settings (e.g., at Soteria and Windhorse), staff members respond to gestures of this type by sitting and talking to the patient about what led to the behavior and by encouraging him or her to come to the staff in the future before making such gestures (Fortuna 1995; Mosher 1995). Some of the facilities, such as Crossing Place and Cedar House, emphasize that the response should be understated and should not reinforce the behavior by providing more attention than is strictly necessary to ensure the patient's safety and to provide medical care (Bourgeois 1995; Warner and Wollesen 1995). At none of the programs, except the crisis home program in Madison, Wisconsin, would such behavior lead to the patient being discharged or transferred. Even in the Madison program, however, such patients are almost always given a second chance to return to the crisis home (Bennett 1995).

Follow-Up Care

Most of the programs described previously are integral components of a broad community care system or have a close contractual relationship with one. They ensure continuity of care for patients through multiteam meetings and by making discharge planning an integral part of the residential treatment plan. At Cedar House, weekly meetings between psychiatrists and managers of the intensive outpatient, hospital, and hospital-alternative programs review the progress and community treatment needs of all patients receiving acute care. At Venture, similar multiservice meetings are held to review the treatment of patients who are difficult to manage.

Some programs allow outpatient contact with the acute care facility to continue after discharge. At Venture, daily drop-in for former patients is encouraged to allow reassessment if they are not doing well. Ex-residents of the crisis home programs in Madison and Denver often visit the family care sponsors on an informal basis just to stay in touch. Previous residents of Soteria Berne maintain contact with the treatment community while attending other agencies for outpatient care. At Crossing Place, previous residents may visit on "drop-in night"; others visit and come for dinner at different times. At Cedar House, some patients may continue to attend the house after discharge to receive extra supervision or medication monitoring, other outpatients may drop in for support or meals as an interim measure to prevent admission, and many welcome the opportunity to return as outpatients for Thanksgiving and Christmas dinner (Bennett 1995; Bourgeois 1995; Ciompi et al. 1992; Polak et al. 1995; Warner and Wollesen 1995).

Benefits

The flexibility of these alternative settings permits them to respond to the human needs of their clientele. Patients who would otherwise be in an institutional setting can retain their autonomy and links to the community. People who have used the crisis home programs in Madison, Wisconsin, and Denver, Colorado, feel less stigmatized by the experience than by hospital care, because treatment takes place in a normalizing environment where there is contact only with mentally healthy people (Bennett 1995; Polak et al. 1995). Patients at Cedar House, Progress Foundation, Crossing Place, and elsewhere maintain many of their social skills as a result of the expectation that they will continue to deal with many of their usual social responsibilities (Bourgeois 1995; Fields 1995; Warner and Wollesen 1995). Windhorse, which treats people in their own homes, goes farthest in empowering the patient in this respect: The patient has a sense of ownership of the household and responsibility for household management (Fortuna 1995). Virtually all of the users of domestic-style alternative facilities—more than 90% of Progress Foundation patients (Fields 1995), for example—say that they prefer the experience to a hospital.

The unusually supportive and personalized care in the nontraditional programs—at Soteria, Soteria Berne, and Windhorse—means that psychotic patients can be treated with lower doses of neuroleptic medication than is usual in standard inpatient care (Ciompi et al. 1992; Fortuna 1995; Mosher 1995). At Soteria Berne, the doses of antipsychotic medication used are about one-fourth of those employed at hospitals in the area (Ciompi et al. 1992). The lower cost of alternative settings means that the pace of treatment is less hectic than in a hospital: more time can be spent in evaluating patients before beginning drug therapy, patients need not be rushed into making a decision about medications, and dosages can be increased gradually.

For the mental health system, hospital alternatives offer several advantages. They permit scarce hospital beds to be reserved for very severely disturbed patients who require intensive care. If the alternative program is an integral component of the community agency, access for clients in need of inpatient care is assured and is not dependent on hospital protocols, quality of inpatient care is under the direct control of the community agency, and good continuity of care is much more readily accomplished. Hospital alternatives expand the range of options for the care of patients in crisis. The Crisis Centers in the Netherlands provide immediate care for patients with a host of psychosocial problems that would not warrant or benefit from hospital admission (Schudel 1995). For patients with severe personality disorders who may lose self-control in a hospital, a normalizing alternative placement may be much more clinically appropriate.

Cost

An important advantage of hospital alternatives is their low cost. As Table 6–1 shows, the programs that are integral to or in a close working relationship with a community care system are much cheaper than hospital care. These programs cost about one-fourth of the expense of local private hospital care, on average, and never more than one-third: they cost a little more than half of the expense of state hospital care, on average. Their small size explains much of the savings. Unlike hospitals, they do not require expensive dedicated service elements such as pharmacies, security personnel, laboratories, or emergency departments. Such services are often obtained by the alternative facility from an equivalent in the community. For example, at Cedar House the local police department provides the same function as hospital security personnel, when required, and laboratory services and medical investigations are obtained by contracts with community agencies and hospital outpatient departments.

The staffing flexibility of community agencies, the use of multidisciplinary teams, and the delegation of responsibility also permit considerable cost savings. In hospitals, protocols imposed by accreditation requirements and liability concerns lead to increased staffing requirements. For example, in many good private hospitals, a reasonable caseload for a full-time psychiatrist might be 10 inpatients. At a community alternative program, however, a psychiatrist can provide good care for this number of patients in half the time by delegating to well-trained mental health professionals many of the daily evaluation and treatment tasks—namely, individual and family psychotherapy, clinical information gathering, and disposition planning.

Risks and Risk Management

Many may feel that informal, open-door inpatient treatment facilities present greater risks in the care of severely disturbed patients. This need not be the case, however. Clearly, open-door facilities require careful selection of patients, day-by-day observation of the residents' changing condition, and expert supervision of treatment plans to ensure safety. The setting may be informal in style, but staff can never be casual in their efforts to observe and protect their patients. Patients are not admitted if they are at risk of walking away and if walking away is likely to lead to a serious problem. A patient who is so psychotic and agitated that he or she may run out into traffic is likely to be placed in the hospital. A resident who becomes so confused or autistic that he or she cannot follow staff direction will require additional staffing for continuous observation or transfer into a safer setting.

Program supervision is a key to risk management in these settings. Experienced professionals must have daily input into the treatment plans. At some of the more medically oriented treatment facilities, such as Venture and Cedar House, psychiatrists may be an important part of this daily supervision; at the more nontraditional programs such as Windhorse and Soteria, psychiatrists are less closely involved, but supervision by experienced professionals is equally close and detailed. The open-door environment calls for a high level of staff skill and attention. More responsibility for risk prevention is delegated to staff and, to a degree, to patients—giving patients the message that they are responsible for themselves.

Given this degree of care and professionalism in program operation, the level of risk does not appear to be higher for these programs. Over 16 years of operation, serving 10,000 acutely disturbed individuals, the Progress Foundation in San Francisco, has experienced fewer than a dozen violent episodes (Fields 1995). In the Madison, Wisconsin, program, no patient has ever assaulted a crisis home provider, although property damage and theft have occurred on occasions (Bennett 1995). At Cedar House, aggression and assault are less common than in the hospital. Patients sometimes walk away from treatment at Cedar House and must be brought back by family members or the police; elopement with resulting bad outcome, however, has been very rare. Over nearly two decades of operation, occurrences of this type, or similar critical incidents such as serious suicide attempts on the premises, have been no more frequent than among the mental health center's patients placed in the hospital (Warner and Wollesen 1995).

Many professionals argue, moreover, that the greatest risk for seriously mentally ill patients is not when they are in inpatient treatment but after discharge, when they may evade outpatient care and become severely disturbed again. If this is the case, lower cost, less alienating alternative facilities that are closely integrated with the outpatient system may reduce risk to users in the long run by allowing a longer period of inpatient treatment, by developing a better allegiance with the patient, and by leading to the formulation of a successful community treatment plan. Those who work in community mental health care understand that short-term concerns about liability and risk must be weighed against long-term benefits for the patient and overall quality of life. Nowhere is this more evident than in the choice of alternatives to hospital treatment.

References

Barnes M, Berke J: Mary Barnes: Two Accounts of a Journey Through Madness. New York, Harcourt Brace Jovanovich, 1972

Bennett R: The Crisis Home Program of Dane County, in Alternatives to Hospital for Acute Psychiatric Treatment. Edited by Warner R. Washington, DC, American Psychiatric Press, 1995, pp 227–235

Bourgeois P: Crossing Place, Washington, DC: Working with people in acute crisis, in Alternatives to Hospital for Acute Psychiatric Treatment. Edited by Warner R. Washington, DC, American Psychiatric Press, 1995, pp 37–54

Caplan G: Principles of Preventive Psychiatry. New York, Basic Books, 1963

Ciompi L, Dauwalder H-P, Maier C, et al: The pilot project "Soteria Berne": clinical experiences and results. Br J Psychiatry 161(suppl 18):145–153, 1992

Ferguson WD, Dowd D: Northwest Evaluation and Treatment Center, Seattle: alternative to hospital for involuntarily detained patients, in Alternatives to Hospital for Acute Psychiatric Treatment. Edited by Warner R. Washington, DC, American Psychiatric Press, 1995, pp 77–92

Fields S: The Progress Foundation, San Francisco: Principles of acute residential treatment, in Alternatives to Hospital for Acute Psychiatric Treatment. Edited by Warner R. Washington, DC, American Psychiatric Press, 1995, pp 57–76

Fortuna JM: The Windhorse program for recovery, in Alternatives to Hospital for Acute Psychiatric Treatment. Edited by Warner R. Washington, DC, American Psychiatric Press, 1995, pp 171–189

Jones K: A History of Mental Health Services. London, England, Routledge & Kegan Paul, 1972

Jones M: Social Psychiatry in Practice. Baltimore, MD, Penguin, 1968

Mandiberg J: Can interdependent mutual support function as an alternative to hospitalization? The Santa Clara County Clustered Apartment Project, in Alternatives to Hospital for Acute Psychiatric Treatment. Edited by Warner R. Washington, DC, American Psychiatric Press, 1995, pp 193–210

Mosher LR: The Soteria Project: the first generation American alternatives to psychiatric hospitalization, in Alternatives to Hospital for Acute Psychiatric Treatment. Edited by Warner R. Washington, DC, American Psychiatric Press, 1995, pp 111–129

Mosher LR, Menn AZ: Community residential treatment for schizophrenia: two-year follow-up. Hosp Community Psychiatry 29:715–723, 1978

Podvoll EM: The Seduction of Madness: Revolutionary Insights Into the World of Psychosis and a Compassionate Approach to Recovery at Home. New York, Harper Collins, 1990

Polak PR, Kirby MW, Deitchman WS: Treating acutely ill psychotic patients in private homes, in Alternatives to Hospital for Acute Psychiatric Treatment. Edited by Warner R. Washington, DC, American Psychiatric Press, 1995, pp 213–223

Schudel WJ: Acute hospital alternatives in the Netherlands: Crisis intervention centers, in Alternatives to Hospital for Acute Psychiatric Treatment. Edited by Warner R. Washington, DC, American Psychiatric Press, 1995, pp 95–108

Sedgwick P: Psycho Politics. New York, Harper & Row, 1982

Sherman PS, Porter R: Mental health consumers as case management aides. Hosp Community Psychiatry 42:494–498, 1991

Sladen-Dew N, Young AM, Parfitt H, et al: Short-term acute psychiatric treatment in the community: the Vancouver experience, in Alternatives to Hospital for Acute Psychiatric Treatment. Edited by Warner R. Washington, DC, American Psychiatric Press, 1995

Warner R: Recovery From Schizophrenia, 2nd Edition. London, England: Routledge, 1994

Warner R (ed): Alternatives to Hospital for Acute Psychiatric Treatment. Washington, DC, American Psychiatric Press, 1995a

Warner R: From patient management to risk management, in Alternatives to the Hospital for Acute Psychiatric Treatment. Edited by Warner R. Washington, DC, American Psychiatric Press, 1995b, pp 237–248

Warner R, Huxley P: Psychopathology and quality of life among mentally ill patients in the community: British and U.S. samples compared. Br J Psychiatry 163:505–509, 1993

Warner R, Wollesen C: Cedar House: a noncoercive hospital alternative in Boulder, Colorado, in Alternatives to the Hospital for Acute Psychiatric Treatment. Edited by Warner R. Washington, DC, American Psychiatric Press, 1995

Chapter 7

Inpatient Psychiatry

Kathleen Daly, M.D., M.P.H.
Martin Kaufman, M.D.
Gordon H. Clark, Jr., M.D., M.Div.

I mprovements in the reliability of diagnosis, pharmacological treatments, and focused psychotherapeutic interventions have placed greater emphasis on community-based support systems, especially in the treatment of seriously and chronically mentally ill patients (Bachrach 1983). Less restrictive community-based treatment settings became a possibility with developments over the second half of this century—namely, increased effectiveness of pharmacological treatments, concerns for patients' rights, and economic pressures (Hodge 1979). This trend has created a need for staff trained in a multitude of supportive services and has diminished the importance of hospital-based treatment (Thompson et al. 1990). Greater emphasis has also been focused on the important role of family and social support networks in providing an environment in which patients can maximize their potential.

An unavoidable influence has been that of shrinking financial support for mental health care, both in terms of public dollars and through the increasing use of managed care contracts in the private sector. The pressure to use less expensive outpatient services will affect patients, whose treatment options may be fewer and whose lengths of stay may be shortened and often determined by third-party payers rather than the clinicians responsible for their care. It is likely that those most in need of care will experience the greatest constraint, brought about by past abuses. Those taking care of patients in a system of care that relies on Medicare reimbursement must approach treatment with an eye toward conserving the patient's hospital days over his or her entire lifetime, as the number of days a seriously mentally ill individual can be hospitalized under Medicare is restricted to 190 per lifetime.

In light of these changes, there is a need to create a role for inpatient psychiatry within the broader concept of a system of mental health care. In this chapter we will review the following aspects of inpatient psychiatry: guiding principles of inpatient treatment; maintenance of a secure treatment setting; configuration of and participation in treatment teams; and assessment, treatment, and discharge planning.

Guiding Principles of Inpatient Treatment

Least Restrictive Alternative

The overall goal of providing the least restrictive treatment environment should be maintained. Clear criteria for admission must be established by members of the treatment team. Only when evaluation or treatment within the hospital would alleviate restrictions or provide a safer environment should inpatient treatment be considered.

Indications for inpatient treatment.   Patients who require hospitalization have needs that usually fall into one of three broad categories: protection, intensive evaluation or treatment, and restructuring of their outpatient support network (Stein and Test 1980). In 1969, California enacted a civil commitment statute, the Lanterman-Petris-Short Act, that set the standard followed by every state over the ensuing decade. Patients who are suicidal, homicidal, or unable to provide for their basic needs in the presence of mental illness and refusal of treatment can be involuntarily hospitalized (Lamb and Mills 1986). Virtually all states have statutes that permit outpatient commitment, but there is little uniformity in interpretation of these laws, with the result being that most states equate involuntary commitment with hospitalization (Keilitz and Hall 1985). Often patients who are suicidal recognize their need for protection and agree to inpatient treatment.

Hospitalization can benefit patients who require extensive diagnostic tests that cannot be accomplished as an outpatient, or in cases where observation of behavior such as sleep patterns will aid in understanding and treating illness. Comorbid medical conditions that dictate close observation to initiate psychotropic medication often require the level of care that hospitalization provides. Comorbid substance abuse may require inpatient observation to adequately monitor for withdrawal symptoms. A course of electroconvulsive therapy usually requires hospitalization because of the need for general anesthesia and the observation required during the post-treatment period of transient memory impairment. Finally, a failure in the support system (e.g., family or board and care) may precipitate a crisis that warrants hospitalization.

Patients' Rights

On admission to an inpatient setting, many patients may be uncertain about their civil rights. Their low self-esteem and sense of powerlessness adds to the misinformation most laypersons have about psychiatric hospitalization. It is important that staff attend to this need and help patients understand their legal rights, particularly because many have court-appointed guardians and in fact do have limitations on their civil rights (Wolpe et al. 1991).

Maintenance of a Secure Environment

Concerns for patient safety are often the primary reason for admission to an inpatient unit. Staff cannot provide for patients' safety unless they feel safe. Procedures to ensure staff safety must be addressed with the same vigor as are policies and procedures for patient safety. Safety concerns by the staff should be addressed regularly in an open and supportive manner. Ongoing attention must be given to the potential for self-injury from the physical environment, as well as to maximizing the potential for safety and security by attending to the milieu.

Brief Hospitalization

Rather than a long-lasting and life-changing event, hospitalization must be viewed as a brief interlude providing an important and safe treatment alternative, not as an exclusive and independent source of treatment. Inpatient treatment exists on a continuum of care, particularly in the context of a chronically mentally ill patient's life and treatment. Longer stays in which a patient was evaluated within the sometimes protected, sometimes regressive milieu and that provided far-reaching recommendations for all aspects of a patient's social and treatment environment are no longer financially feasible, responsible, or the best therapeutic alternative (Test and Stein 1978). Hospitalization must be brief, limited in perspective, and specifically focused on treatment goals. Although economic pressures may have stimulated this trend, it is clinically preferable, as prolonged hospitalization creates barriers to the support of family and friends in the community and has greater stigma associated with it.

Continuity of Care

It is assumed that continuity of care is better than disjointed, uncoordinated, or stop-gap treatment (Test 1992). A single treatment team providing care in and out of the hospital would be the best way to ensure continuity, but this ideal is rarely realized. More often, separate teams work independently, and therefore, it is essential that working relationships between inpatient and outpatient treatment teams be established. Designated team members from each setting can work together to integrate the expectations of the outpatient team with the reality of the inpatient team's capacity and strengths, thus establishing reasonable treatment goals, length of stay, and discharge plans; avoiding splitting of the two teams; and clearly delineating responsibility, such as who will be the therapist while the patient is in hospital and who will provide case management services. In addition, the outpatient team has the opportunity to receive consultation about the longer course of treatment, including alternative treatment settings.

Discharge Planning

Discharge planning should begin on admission to ensure that follow-up services are in place when the patient moves from inpatient to outpatient treatment. Sources of care should be identified and included in the treatment process as early as possible. This often depends on an accurate assessment of length of stay, as openings in placement settings may dictate the site of aftercare. Family or other members of the social support network should be included as early as possible, as they will likely play a crucial role in supporting plans for care after discharge.

Patient Evaluation

Hospitalization is often precipitated by a need for a comprehensive evaluation, which should include biological, psychological, social, and rehabilitative perspectives. An interdisciplinary approach is preferable, but it is important not to limit the strengths of team members by restricting their input to that of their training. Just as the strengths of our patients may not be reflected in their diagnoses, the experience team members bring to the treatment process may not be reflected by their degrees. All team members should be encouraged to share their expertise in formulating an assessment of patient needs. Training in different areas may provide various treatment interventions for a particular patient need. Interdisciplinary teams combine various perspectives to better understand patients' needs, whereas a multidisciplinary process implies the presence of different specialists without integration of their efforts and perspectives (Zablocki 1991).

Patient Participation

In addition to the members of the outpatient team, it is important for the patient and family or social support network to have a meaningful role in treatment planning. This can be accomplished by discussions before and after team meetings to plan treatment. Ideally patients and significant others can be invited to team meetings where treatment options are discussed. Attention to legal and ethical issues concerning communication with family members and others is essential.

Case Management Services

Careful attention to linkages with community services, the outpatient therapist, and other programs in which the patient may be involved can provide valuable information to aid in evaluation and treatment. Day treatment centers, group home managers, and the van driver who provides transportation contribute valuable insight into a patient's behavior that can predict the likelihood that a particular approach will succeed. A case manager can provide essential linkage between inpatient and outpatient teams and facilitate discharge planning.

Program Design

The inpatient program should be designed to support the specific goals of the unit but be sufficiently flexible to accommodate the individual needs of each patient. A treatment program typically provides the following elements:

1. A community meeting to establish and maintain a respectful, secure, and therapeutic milieu.
2. Educational groups run by trained staff to discuss medications and side effect management, coping skills, social skills, problem solving, assertiveness training, abstinence from illicit drugs, diet, or other topics.
3. Therapeutic groups tailored to the target population, such as eating disorders, problems encountered by elderly individuals, or posttraumatic stress disorder. Group leaders must be cognizant of the brief duration of treatment and the impact of turnover as patients are admitted and discharged from the hospital.
4. Supportive and educational groups for members of the family and social support network.
5. Individual, marital, family, or social support network therapy should be done in cooperation with outpatient therapists and focused on issues consistent with inpatient treatment goals.

6. Therapeutic structured activities directed by recreational, rehabilitative, occupational, art, dance, physical, and drama therapists.
7. Special groups such as Alcoholics Anonymous or Narcotics Anonymous, when patients have substance abuse problems and such activities support the goals of treatment.
8. Staff meetings to facilitate discussion of issues that enhance patient care.
9. Discharge planning meetings that include a liaison from or to the outpatient team.

Maintenance of a Secure Treatment Setting

Some patients come to a psychiatric unit in search of security. For some the need is for protection from others in cases of spouse abuse, elder abuse, or child abuse. For others the need is for protection against their own impulses, whether directed at themselves or others. Inpatient staff must think of and ensure security. The staff must be well trained and empathic as they attend to patients' security needs. Procedures for patient and room searches should be delineated, and training in thorough but sensitive searches of patients and their belongings should be reviewed frequently.

The rate of occurrence of violent events in institutional settings has increased (Davis 1991). When violence occurs, it is crucial that the staff effectively work as a team in seclusion and restraint of the patient and emergent administration of medication (Tardiff 1988). Procedures for seclusion and restraint must be clear, and guidelines should be reviewed frequently to minimize injury to staff and patients. Additional staff support must be available through an established in-hospital code when there is a crisis involving violence.

Local law enforcement may be of assistance, and it is important to maintain a good working relationship with the police and to offer training to community agencies that occasionally interact with psychiatric patients. Being prepared to respond in a violent situation by making a quick assessment and employing appropriate techniques and medications allows for the safe treatment of all patients on an inpatient unit.

The psychiatrist must carefully consider the etiology of any violent outburst in order to guide medication use.

Investigators have overcome methodological difficulties to demonstrate the correlation between crowding on a psychiatric unit and aggressive behavior (Planstierna et al. 1991). It is important to observe a newly admitted patient continuously, as violence is more likely to occur early in the course of hospitalization. Persistent observation beyond 72 hours is probably deleterious for both patients and staff (Davis 1991). Past history of violence is a better predictor of violent behavior than diagnosis (Janofsky et al. 1988; Monahan 1984; Noble and Rodger 1989). Indications of violence potential are often recognized in retrospect but are rarely helpful in advance, and thus staff always feel taken by surprise. When an act of violence occurs and has been witnessed by other patients, a community meeting to discuss the event is an effective means of restoring trust in the staff's ability to protect and contain patients' behavior, alleviate unnecessary guilt, and restore a respectful, empathic working relationship between patients and staff. A willingness to listen, to strive toward achieving a nonjudgmental attitude, and to foster open communication are most likely to identify the full range of security issues and bring them into the treatment process.

Efforts to educate and orient the patient to the rules and social mores of the unit may help in the adjustment to an unfamiliar environment. Allowing patients as much autonomy as possible may minimize the authoritarian quality of the psychiatric unit. Independent decisions about nonessential aspects of care, such as the time to shower, dietary choices, or style of dress, should be encouraged whenever possible. A brief community meeting to review unit issues, answer questions regarding rules and function of the unit, and provide information to patients about expected admissions and discharges should be held every morning to minimize the anxiety associated with unknown and unexpected occurrences.

Configuration of and Participation in Treatment Teams

Treatment teams are as varied and individual as their component members. Differences can be defined by discipline, specialty training, interests, function, or role. Teams that include multiple disciplines function in several different ways. It is important that an established team agree on the model of interaction it uses. Disagreement about how the team should function will cripple its effectiveness. To operate effectively, a treatment team must be well organized and managed, aware of its own functioning, and capable of changing as new treatment strategies become available or new members bring different skills to the team. Ongoing efforts at education of members about the expertise, treatment approach and philosophy, and roles of team members are integral to effective team functioning.

Zablocki (1991) described the traditional model of a multidisciplinary team as one in which health professionals from diverse disciplinary backgrounds perform within a prescribed role according to specialty training. Interactions with other members are consultations or an exchange of information about planning or treatment, but little work is done in cooperation with team members outside of one's discipline. Members of each discipline assess and treat a patient according to their expertise. Although there may be some overlap with other disciplines, little cooperation in assessment or treatment beyond exchange of information is required of team members. Individual team members are more important than the team. The highest ranking professional (usually a psychiatrist on inpatient units) is usually the team leader, and little note is made of the team process or functioning (Zablocki 1991).

Zablocki also distinguished an interdisciplinary treatment approach in which expertise and interest guide participation. Team members share information to arrive at a common understanding of the needs and goals that will be addressed in treatment. There is less independent action on the part of the members and a greater emphasis placed on the team's importance. More collaboration and trust are required for this model to work effectively, but less individual responsibility is attributed. The team takes credit and accepts responsibility for successes and failures. A case manager or treatment coordinator can be from any discipline and is often a different team member in each case. Communication, role negotiation, and other skills are practiced, and responsibility for team effectiveness is shared by all members (Zablocki 1991). The function and role of an individual is not dictated by specialty training.

Team Composition

The disciplines represented on a treatment team vary according to the specialty focus of the unit. It would be important to include a dietitian and a behavioral therapist on an eating disorders unit, whereas a geriatrician or geriatrics nurse practitioner would be a necessary member of the team on a geriatrics unit. Seriously mentally ill individuals benefit from rehabilitative specialists with expertise in social skills training. Homeless patients require more intensive social services intervention. The following disciplines are represented on most teams: psychiatry, psychology, social work, nursing, occupational therapy, rehabilitative therapy, and activities therapy. In addition to these disciplines, several functional roles for which there is no specific training are vital to team functioning; these include case manager, unit coordinator, and community liaison. The role of case manager is important in coordinating all aspects of an individual's care. A unit coordinator plays a vital role in maintaining the functional capacity of the unit but is rarely asked to participate in team meetings. The community liaison can be a role taken on by the unit coordinator or the case manager and is imperative for attaining the goal of continuity of care.

Authority and Responsibility

As the task of patient care becomes more complex, the psychiatrist's role changes from team member as consultant to manager (Pepper 1991). Although a treatment team may function without traditional divisions of authority and responsibility, the unit director must take administrative responsibility for the care provided and therefore has ultimate authority. A conceptual approach that is useful in understanding these complex relationships is one in which responsibility falls into one of three categories: exclusive, ultimate, and shared. An example of *exclusive* responsibility is the role of the psychiatrist as physician in charge in an emergency situation when there is not any opportunity for discussion about decisions. In the case of decisions where collaboration among team members is essential, such as determining privileges, *ultimate* responsibility remains with the physician who writes the order. *Shared* responsibility describes most team problem solving in which solutions are arrived at by consensus. It is necessary to remain flexible in a changing health care environment where there are increasing economic pressures on hospitals, concerns about liability, changing organizational structures, changing institutional roles for state hospitals and inpatient units, and changing roles within specialties (Pepper 1991). The increasing trend toward treatment within a community setting has diminished the role of institutions for those in need of long-term care and shifted such treatment toward outpatient management punctuated by brief inpatient hospitalization for exacerbation of a chronic illness. There are increased burdens on the inpatient staff for greater communication with the outpatient team to ensure continuity of care. Again, the focus on a team member as liaison becomes imperative.

Case Management

The role of case coordinator or case manager has become increasingly important as shorter hospital stays and broader community involvement have become the norm for treatment. The professional discipline of the case manager is less important than the interest in working creatively to maximize inpatient interventions and outpatient treatment resources. Rarely are seriously ill individuals treated by a single person or agency. Issues such as transportation and coordination of scheduling become an important aspect of care. The functions of a case manager vary according to individual treatment needs, and the term is used in myriad of ways (Fiorentine and Grusky 1990). In an outpatient setting, the case manager is often a care provider who helps an individual perform the tasks of daily living that most healthy individuals take for granted: for example, making appointments, arranging transportation, paying the rent and utility bills, and meal planning or preparation. For many, the case manger becomes a substitute for a family member. In the context of inpatient care, a case manager is the coordinator of care, linking the patient to community services and working closely with an outpatient case manager to identify and respond to needs, particularly those that are being met within the hospital and that will be difficult for the patient to accomplish independently as an outpatient.

Patient Participation

Patients' participation in the treatment planning process is necessary to establish goals that are attainable and to ensure patient agreement and cooperation. In some cases patients may choose to be present at team meetings where their treatment is discussed. This usually requires very little alteration in discussion to accommodate a patient's presence and can have a therapeutic benefit in cases where splitting of team members is occurring. In other cases the focus and goals of treatment are discussed with the patient individually, and a team member acts as a liaison between the patient and the team. Ideally, the patient will review and sign the documented treatment plan.

Family or Social Network Participation

Family and other social network members are crucial in engaging patients' cooperation. It is essential that the patient consent to the participation of people outside the treatment team (just as the patient consented to treatment by the team), but whenever possible, members of the social support network should be included. An opportunity is afforded for staff to obtain additional history, observe interactions, support, and educate an important member of the outpatient team when family or others are involved. The need for family therapy can be assessed. Elaborate plans for treatment that do not include the cooperation of the support system risk sabotage or abandonment.

Unit Coordinator

The unit coordinator is vital to maintaining the integration of a system of services. As competition for patients increases, hospitals are becoming more aware of the need to work closely with referring agencies to attract business. Working with outside service providers has not been valued and has rarely been paid for, but the focus is changing, and more attention is being paid to the interface among residential homes, day programs, and outpatient care providers. As the inpatient treatment team becomes more integrated into the broader system of community care and expands its communication with outside agencies, the unit coordinator becomes a more important team member in negotiating the boundary between inpatient and aftercare. Efforts to involve outside therapists or case managers must be supported. When distance or schedules dictate that inpatient and outpatient care be discontinuous, conference calls can be used to coordinate the efforts of different care providers. Although they aid in communication, fax machines must be used with caution, as it is impossible to guarantee confidentiality of the information that is transmitted.

Assessment, Treatment, and Discharge Planning

The focus of this section is to highlight the opportunities for enhancing the assessment-treatment-discharge planning continuum when an inpatient hospitalization is integrated in a comprehensive mental health services system. This concept is less of an administrative reality than a practical one. The programs commonly found within such a system include group homes; board and care programs; shared or supervised apartments; day treatment or drop-in centers; rehabilitative or work reentry programs; and community mental health centers where case management, medication management, and group and individual therapy often take place. Various degrees of independence from the mental health structure and staff are represented in these different settings. All have in common the opportunity to observe an individual and evaluate stressors, coping mechanisms, transference, countertransference, and social relations. It is critical that adequate and timely communication be maintained between inpatient and outpatient sources of care. It is important to remember that patients come to the hospital at their worst functional levels, and their initial presentation will improve at least to the level of earlier functioning. Although frustrating, an assessment is not stagnant but dynamic, and must evolve as the patient improves. It must be assumed that a patient will be able to resume at least his or her prior level of functioning and independence.

Functional Assessment

Functional assessment focuses on answering how the individual is getting along in different settings: work skills; social and interpersonal skills; independent living skills; and all concrete issues of daily living, including the ability to access medical, social, rehabilitative, and legal resources. Although the goal of functional assessment is to identify needs, the emphasis is placed on identifying strengths and capabilities in the face of disability.

Social Assessment

Family relationships, housing needs, financial concerns, and the need for legal services are among patients' social considerations. A comprehensive evaluation must be flexible, as a patient's social needs often change through the course of hospitalization as an exacerbation or its precipitant resolves.

Medical Assessment

The presence and significance of medical conditions among psychiatric patients has been well documented (Lieberman and Coburn 1986) but often neglected by medical and emergency personnel (D'Ercole et al. 1991). This underscores the importance of a systematic review of physical health problems and the availability of consultation to ensure that adequate treatment is provided.

Psychiatric Assessment

The psychiatric evaluation uses a medical model to organize the details of the developmental, past personal, family, medical psychiatric, and present illness histories, as well as a comprehensive mental status examination to establish the psychiatric diagnosis and guide pharmacological management. The etiologies of most psychiatric illnesses are an interplay among biological, psychological, and social or environmental factors. Inpatient admission is often precipitated by a crisis or exacerbation that occurs in response to some change in this complex interplay. It is the intent of the biopsychosocial paradigm to conceptualize and respond to clinical issues in as broad a manner as possible so that more effective treatment can improve a patient's quality of life. It is important that any changes in medication be carefully reviewed with the outpatient psychiatrist, as his or her experience with a particular patient may be invaluable regarding issues of response, compliance, and side effects.

Mental Health System Assessment

The importance of collaborative efforts with the outpatient system of care has been stressed, but hospitalization provides the opportunity to reevaluate the appropriateness of care in the outpatient setting. For those patients whose social, recreational, housing, occupational, and treatment activities include other patients and staff, interpersonal difficulties will occur in relation to that community. If those relationships can be brought into focus during inpatient treatment, problems identified, and corrective measures suggested, then a therapeutic benefit may result. Issues of medication noncompliance, transference, countertransference, intrapatient rivalries, jealousies, intimacy fears, anxieties, psychotic decompensation, and existential dilemmas exist within the various social, treatment, living, and work situations. These issues serve as important reminders to staff of the need to maintain a humanistic view of patients in an era in which mental health care is becoming increasingly focused on biology and economics.

Inpatient Psychotherapy

The emphasis of inpatient treatment has shifted from Maxwell Jones' therapeutic community and long-term, insight-oriented inpatient therapy to more concrete, problem-solving approaches (Santter et al. 1991). Brief hospitalization allows a treatment team to identify problems and offer ideas about solutions. All group, family, couples, and individual work should be focused on restoring function rather than on uncovering new issues. Observations that occur during work with a patient can certainly help those who will be working with the patient on a longer term basis, but "breakthroughs" are likely to precipitate a crisis and prolong hospital stay.

Discharge Planning

A good understanding of the patient's living situation prior to admission will aid the process of discharge planning and expedite a return to the community and a less restrictive environment as soon as possible. After evaluation and prognosis are established in the inpatient setting, the team will be in a better position to determine whether the prior accommodations were meeting the patient's needs.

Collaboration With Community Agencies

Often the length of stay in the hospital is mandated by insurance providers or by concerns about using limited numbers of days. Collaboration with community agencies and coordination of care after discharge will help reduce the length of stay, reduce recidivism, and foster the successful return to the community.

Summary

Our intent in this chapter has been to emphasize the importance of inpatient care as one aspect of community-based care and the need to locate inpatient units in communities where they can support the work of outpatient clinicians. The brief and intermittent nature of inpatient treatment underscores the importance of establishing a comprehensive system of care outside the hospital that includes day treatment, social environments, therapeutic housing, and rehabilitative work settings. In the past, inpatient treatment had the luxury of long stays and was the focus around which all other treatment revolved. The reverse is now the case, at least within the realm of community psychiatry. It has been stressed that to create a secure environment, staff and patients must all feel safe. Treatment team configuration and models were discussed, outlining the differences between multidisciplinary and interdisciplinary teams. The need to maintain linkages with the community-based system of care is vital to the smooth transition between inpatient and outpatient treatment. Such linkages are so vital to ensure continuity of care, particularly in the treatment of seriously mentally ill, that they justify expenditures for a designated staff person and technological support. Because length of inpatient stay is usually short, diagnostic assessments and treatment strategies must be focused but not compromised by purely economic considerations. Perhaps most importantly, as the focus of treatment for the seriously mentally ill patient evolves in the community, requiring a special relationship between the inpatient unit and less restrictive outpatient services, there is an increasing need for well-trained, adequately compensated day center and residential group home staff, case management personnel, and, finally, some form of compensation for family or social support network members who provide invaluable informal care.

References

Bachrach LL: An overview of deinstitutionalization. New Dir Ment Health Serv 17:5–14, 1983

Davis S: Violence by psychiatric inpatients: a review. Hosp Community Psychiatry 42:585–590, 1991

D'Ercole A, Skodol A, Struening E, et al: Diagnosis of physical illness in psychiatric patients using Axis III and a standardized medical history. Hosp Community Psychiatry 42:395–400, 1991

Fiorentine R, Grusky O: When case managers manage the seriously mentally ill: a role contingency approach. Soc Serv Rev March:79–93, 1990

Hodge MJ: Social forces, ideology, and the domain of mental health services. Psychiatr Q 51(4):280–293 1979

Janofsky JS, Spears S, Neubauer DN: Psychiatrists' accuracy in predicting violent behavior on an inpatient unit. Hosp Community Psychiatry 39:1090–1094, 1988

Keilitz I, Hall T: State statutes governing involuntary outpatient civil commitment. Mental and Physical Disability Law Reporter 9:378–397, 1985

Lamb HR, Mills MJ: Needed changes in laws and procedure for the chronically mentally ill. Hosp Community Psychiatry 37:475–480, 1986

Lieberman AA, Coburn AF: The health of the chronically mentally ill: a review of the literature. Community Ment Health J 22:104–116, 1986

Monahan J: The prediction of violent behavior: toward a second generation of theory and policy. Am J Psychiatry 141:10–15, 1984

Noble P, Rodger S: Violence by psychiatric inpatients. Br J Psychiatry 155:384–390, 1989

Pepper B: Power and governance issues in the general hospital (letter). Hosp Community Psychiatry 42:1169, 1991

Planstierna T, Huitfeldt B, Wistedt B: The relationship of crowding and aggressive behavior on a psychiatric intensive care unit. Hosp Community Psychiatry 42:1237–1240, 1991

Santter F, Heaney C, O'Neil P: A problem-solving approach to group psychotherapy in the inpatient milieu. Hosp Community Psychiatry 42:732–735, 1991

Stein LI, Test MA: Alternative to mental hospital treatment, I: conceptual model, treatment program, and clinical evaluation. Arch Gen Psychiatry 37:392–397, 1980

Tardiff K: Management of the violent patient in an emergency situation. Psychiatr Clin North Am 11(4):539–549, 1988

Test MA: The Training in Community Living Model: delivering treatment and rehabilitation services through a continuous treatment team, in Handbook of Psychiatric Rehabilitation. Edited by Liberman RP. New York, Macmillan, 1992, pp 153–170

Test MA, Stein LI: The clinical rationale for community treatment: a review of the literature, in Alternatives to Mental Hospital Treatment. Edited by Stein LI, Test MA. New York, Plenum, 1978, pp 3–22

Thompson KS, Griffith EE, Leaf PJ: A historical review of the Madison model of community care. Hosp Community Psychiatry 41:625–634, 1990

Wolpe P, Schwarz D, Sanford B: Psychiatric inpatients' knowledge of their rights. Hosp Community Psychiatry 42:1168–1169, 1991

Zablocki CJ: A Guide for Interdisciplinary Resident Care Planning in the Nursing Home Care Unit, 2nd Edition. Milwaukee, WI, VAMC, April 1991

Section III
Target Populations

Chapter 8

Child and Adolescent Psychiatry in the Community

M. Steven Sager, M.D.

Perhaps the best known community child psychiatrist is Lucy from the *Peanuts* cartoon strip. She sits outside, offering other *Peanuts* child characters community-based psychiatric care at affordable rates (only five cents). Similarly, community child and adolescent psychiatrists continue to offer individual psychiatric care, but the role has expanded to include many other services, such as school and other consultative work, psychotropic consultations for children referred by nonpsychiatric clinicians, administrative and advocacy activities, research, and training and education. After briefly reviewing the history of community child psychiatry in this chapter, I explore these roles in the diverse settings where child psychiatrists are currently employed. I then explore special issues that confront today's community child psychiatrist.

History

Historically, attention to the unique mental health needs of children and adolescents was limited. In fact, it has only been during the past century or so that children have been viewed as something more than miniature adults. In the 1890s a social movement of men and, especially, women concerned about the fate of children in the U.S. courts was born. In 1899 a law was passed containing financial authorization for special juvenile courts and judges (Lathrop 1925). This original legislation included provisions for diagnostic and treatment services. About 10 years later the Juvenile Psychopathic Institute was established and funded by Elizabeth Drummer. The original staff consisted of four or five workers, including a physician, psychologist, and social worker. Treatment included coordinating the efforts of social agencies to restore each child to a normal, functioning relationship within the community. The physician performed physical examinations with an emphasis on development and nutrition, the psychologist administered the new Binet intelligence test, and the social worker obtained detailed social and family history.

These organizations became known as child guidance clinics and survived as such through the 1950s. Psychoanalysis dominated the treatment with psychotherapy of the mother and child as the primary focus. Funding came from private individual donations, philanthropic foundations, social services agencies, and states and municipalities. In 1946 the American Association of Psychiatric Clinics for Children established their standards for clinics and provided authorized training for all disciplines. The training of child psychiatrists predominated. In these settings the psychiatrist served as clinic director, and social workers outnumbered those in other disciplines.

In the 1950s and 1960s board certification and university affiliation of child guidance clinics medicalized child psychiatry. In 1952 the American Academy of Child Psychiatry was founded as a medical organization to seek specialty board recognition, which was achieved in 1960. In the United States the social welfare and law enforcement systems developed in different directions from the medically oriented mental health system. These systems have had different sources of funding and have developed divergent authority and decision-making bases. Consequently, differences among these systems and interagency conflicts developed and persist today.

In the 1960s the Kennedy Administration rediscovered community services. In 1963 Congress approved legislation to fund the construction of community mental health centers (CMHCs) (Starr 1982). As had been true in the past, a new organization and system of mental health delivery was initiated by a new funding source. There was, however, a trend to reduce the influence of medicine in this new delivery system.

For the most part, child psychiatrists did not participate in or influence this new community movement. Child psychiatry had always been an outpatient specialty, and many maintained they were already practicing community psychiatry. Some child guidance clinics were incorporated into CMHCs. This incorporation was the way CMHCs developed strong child components. Although child and adolescent mental health services were one of the five original federally mandated services, these services often were combined with consultation services unless independent funds from child guidance clinics were available. The Community Mental Health Center Act encouraged the development of consultative practices, especially in day-care centers and schools (Rafferty and Mackie 1967), and not the provision of psychotherapy.

During the Nixon administration, Congress established Project F to provide a few million dollars for all states to help childhood mental health causes. A few small, innovative demonstration projects were developed, most involving early childhood education and treatment. Unfortunately, the few states that developed substantial regional and community child psychiatry programs experienced funding shortages in the 1970s and 1980s, resulting in curtailed services.

Interestingly, most major developments in the delivery of child mental health services in the community have been driven by parental initiatives and not by mental health professionals. These initiatives in turn drive legislative mandates, which provide necessary funding. As these directives have changed, so have the roles of the child psychiatrist.

The Role of the Community Child Psychiatrist

A child psychiatrist working in the community in the mid-1990s may see children in various settings. These settings may include child guidance clinics, CMHCs, juvenile halls, schools, other out-of-home placements, and emergency departments. A child psychiatrist may also be involved in administrative and advocacy activities, training, and education.

Child Guidance Clinics

Child guidance clinics continue to be major providers of mental health services in the community. However, they currently are more likely to be funded by governmental agencies and larger philanthropic agencies. Even though developmental and parental issues are still addressed, these clinics now serve youth who are more psychiatrically disturbed. These disturbances today typically include posttraumatic stress disorder resulting from physical abuse, sexual abuse, or violence, and organic psychiatric disorders secondary to intrauterine and postnatal insults, including psychoactive substance exposure and head traumas. These clinics are especially prone to see children with these diagnoses because of their frequent location in inner cities rife with these extraordinary stressors and traumas.

Child psychiatrists in child guidance clinics often serve in a consulting capacity. This function includes teaching, as many child guidance clinics are staffed with trainees in various disciplines, including social work, counseling, nursing, psychology, and psychiatry. Consultation often takes place in regular staff meetings with nonmedical clinicians. Individual patients, recurrent diagnostic and treatment dilemmas, and staff process issues are commonly discussed in the context of an interdisciplinary approach. Child psychiatrists in these clinics may see patients directly, but generally only the most difficult patients and those requiring medication consultations. At times, they are called on to help with planning and administrative duties or serve on the board of directors of the child guidance clinic. It is usually the preference of the individual child psychiatrist that ultimately determines his or her own role in the clinic.

Community Mental Health Centers

Children and adolescents continue to be served by CMHCs, even though these centers usually serve the general adult population primarily. Therefore, psychiatrists are less apt to have specialized training in child and adolescent psychiatry. These centers are also generally less equipped and less well staffed for youth services than child guidance clinics.

Crisis evaluations and stabilization predominate the interventions at CMHCs. Frequently children and adolescents are referred and escorted by school personnel. Sometimes psychiatric mobile response teams and police are involved in the referral process. Evaluations for possible voluntary or involuntary psychiatric hospital admissions are performed. Psychiatrists are also asked in CMHCs to perform psychotropic evaluations and follow-up medication management. Often children and adolescents are referred to other community programs to help meet their other biopsychosocial needs.

Schools

In the school system, a child psychiatrist is usually a consultant but may from time to time or per his or her preference see students directly and function as an individual therapist. The consulting is usually done in group teacher and staff conferences, often referred to as *student study teams*. Individual cases may be presented on a routine basis in formal case conferences. Sometimes the conferences are more informal, addressing multiple student and teacher issues. A child psychiatrist may be instrumental in addressing developmental and diagnostic issues, in teacher education about mental illness, and in both behavioral and psychodynamic interventions. Obviously, developmental stages and chronological ages will affect the problems encountered, and thus guide the interventions offered, by the child psychiatrist. For example, the grade school teacher may have questions regarding a hyperactive 10-year-old, whereas the high school teacher may wonder about substance abuse or sexuality.

Schools and programs for emotionally and physically disabled students present special problems for school personnel. With his or her medical training, the child psychiatrist is particularly well situated to deal with these special circumstances. Infrequently, a child psychiatrist in the schools may be involved in administration and planning. With more and more school-based mental health clinics developing in communities, the special expertise of the child psychiatrist will undoubtedly play an important part in these programs.

Juvenile Halls, Courts, and Probationary Services

Juvenile halls are another setting where a child psychiatrist may be employed. The psychiatrist must have a full understanding of the system's workings, including the procedures of probation and the courts. Unfortunately this linkage is often poorly integrated, and the child psychiatrist rarely has significant input into the juvenile offender's disposition. The psychiatrist's role is primarily to assist in behavioral management while the minor is detained. Generally, the psychiatrist has no follow-up with the minor after he or she leaves the detention center, which often results in discoordinated, inefficient, and ineffective ongoing psychiatric care. It should be remembered that even though the legal system assumes guardianship responsibility for the minor, the parents still have a wealth of information regarding him or her.

Sometimes a child psychiatrist is involved in disputes regarding dependency and may be asked to assist with questions of custody. Increasingly, child and adolescent psychiatrists with additional training in forensic psychiatry are performing these evaluations. At times the child psychiatrist may be employed at facilities designed to accommodate dependents of the court.

Alternative Residential Settings

Frequently a child psychiatrist works at out-of-home placements for youth. These facilities can range from residential treatment centers where severely psychiatrically disturbed children are placed to group homes or camps where children involved in probation or dependency reside. The goal of most of these placements is to rehabilitate the child so that he or she can return to the home community. The role of the child psychiatrist at these facilities is generally to provide psychiatric evaluations and medication management. Sometimes these interventions are court mandated. On occasion the child psychiatrist may help with staff consultation at these facilities in a manner similar to that used for consultation in schools.

Crisis Resolution

The emergency department often becomes the focus of crisis intervention in the community. Out-of-control or suicidal children and adolescents are taken to the emergency department by their parents or guardians, school personnel, or the police when their behaviors overwhelm the coping strategies of the involved social systems. The child psychiatrist in the emergency department—either medical or psychiatric—is required to ensure the safety of both the patient and others in the community. The psychiatrist must make a rapid assessment and devise an intervention plan without forsaking safety. Frequently the critical decision is whether to hospitalize the child. The child psychiatrist must be aware of the resources in the community, and in that sense he or she becomes a case manager. Needless to say, the psychiatrist must be quite resourceful and very flexible. The child psychiatrist usually functions as a consultant in the pediatric emergency department and provides liaison services to pediatricians. Increasingly, however, emergency services for children and adolescents are being designed and implemented in CMHCs and other community settings. The child psychiatrist then has an opportunity to occupy a more central role in emergency care delivery.

Administration and Management

As mentioned previously, a child psychiatrist in the community may be involved in administration or advocacy. Most public mental health agencies are led by nonmedical mental health professionals. Often, though, a psychiatrist is employed administratively as a medical director to assist with the more medical, psychiatric, and physician-related issues. Chapter 18 elsewhere in this volume provides a useful guide for the design of this role.

With child and adolescent psychiatry itself still in its early development, advocacy in childhood mental health and illnesses is seen as an integral part of this profession. The child psychiatrist should play a prominent role in the education of the community about these issues. Child psychiatrists pride themselves on being advocates for the rights and care of children and adolescents. This advocacy role has long been championed by the American Academy of Child and Adolescent Psychiatry.

Special Interests for the Contemporary Community Child Psychiatrist

Child psychiatrists encounter unique problems when working with children and adolescents in the community. These include ethnic and cultural diversity, homosexuality, gangs and violence, child abuse, poverty and homelessness, foster care, substance abuse, and disasters and emergencies.

Ethnic and Cultural Diversity

Particularly in urban areas, many community-based service agencies serve a broad constituency comprising many ethnic and cultural groups. The degree of acculturation into American society of parents and child can have a profound impact on attitudes toward and utilization of mental health services. Chapter 22 provides clear and relevant insight into the approach to be taken by a community child psychiatrist. Special children's issues include the degree to which a family culture endorses the expression of feelings and thoughts by children, and the role of extended family members in child care and dispute resolution. The clinician must always be sensitive to the range of special and unique beliefs and explore them, as they can dramatically alter the outcome of care. The clinician should be culturally sensitive and build these beliefs into both evaluation and intervention.

New immigrants may need information regarding the process of health care delivery in this country, because it may be different from their country of origin. New immigrants may be unemployed or underemployed and faced with lack of finances and insurance coverage. Language barriers should be overcome, whenever possible, by the use of clinicians who are conversant in the family's native tongue or by specially trained translators. Psychotropic medications can also have different therapeutic and untoward effects in different ethnic groups. Even though these differences are currently poorly understood, the clinician should be wary of them, particularly when faced with poor treatment response and unusual or severe side effects.

Homosexuality

Homosexual issues are important and frequently encountered by the child psychiatrist working in the community. As the average age of self-identification lowers into the mid-teens, these issues become more relevant to the child psychiatrist. Often the gay adolescent cannot discuss these feelings with parents but is more comfortable dealing with them in school or community settings. Unfortunately, schools often are ill-equipped to handle this sensitive issue. The child psychiatrist can act as an advocate for the gay adolescent and help educate the child, his or her parents, the schools, and the community. The child psychiatrist should ask in a nonjudgmental, unforced manner about the adolescent's sexual feelings and behaviors. This evaluation is particularly important in today's society because of the risk of sexually transmitted diseases, especially acquired immunodeficiency syndrome. The community child psychiatrist must be wary of the reported higher incidence of suicidal ideation in homosexual youth and their often limited support systems.

Gangs and Violence

Violence confronts all parts of society. Considering that homicide and accidents are leading causes of mortality and morbidity in adolescents, the child psychiatrist must be equipped to handle these problems, stretching far beyond the simple act of diagnosing conduct disorder or antisocial traits. Criminal behavior in youth is often associated with gang involvement. Various cults may require criminal or violent behavior as an initiation rite of passage. These behaviors pose emotional and physical dangers to the adolescent, his or her own family, and the community at large. The clinician should ask in a nonjudgmental manner about gang and cult affiliation.

The clinician should be sensitive to the role played by gangs and the impact it has on the developing child and his or her view of life. The child often has limited exposure to other coping skills and alternative prosocial activities. The child often accepts his or her own death, as well as peers' deaths, as inevitable. Unfortunately no intervention has yet been developed to successfully reduce or eliminate these violent behaviors. However, the clinician should be cautious not to see these children as hopeless and unreachable. The child psychiatrist can promote and encourage prosocial activities by taking an inventory of the child's interests and linking them with appropriate community programs. Mentoring programs may be helpful referral sources.

Child Abuse

In addition to participation in violence, the child is also often the witness of violent behavior at home or in the community. Some children are exposed to repetitive violent behaviors, whereas others experience a life-threatening behavior only once. These differences in exposure can lead to differing symptom development. A diagnosis of particular note in this population is posttraumatic stress disorder with hyperarousal, hyperstartle reflexes, and recurrent flashbacks along with possible symptoms ranging from depression and anxiety to psychosis and/or disruptive behaviors. Community-based interventions, usually provided with the active participation of the school, are likely to be the most successful.

Another form of violence or aggression is child abuse, a sad national tragedy. Approximately 2.9 million children were reported as abused or neglected in 1992, a number that undoubtedly is underreported (National Center on Child Abuse and Neglect 1992). Sexual abuse reports are increasing for both male and female victims. These emotional, physical, and sexual abuses and neglect predispose the developing child to multiple medical and mental illnesses. Victims of child abuse can present with varied symptomatology, including anxiety, depression, psychosis, and dissociation. Posttraumatic stress disorder is a common response. The clinician must constantly be aware of and search for possible signs of abuse. In fact, clinicians are mandated by law to report even suspicions of such abuses to local child protective agencies. The most important principle is to maintain the child's safety. If the clinician suspects child abuse, caregivers should be interviewed with and without the child, and the child should undergo a thorough physical examination as part of a comprehensive evaluation. Of particular importance in the organic workup is to consider head trauma, especially when there is an altered level of consciousness or change in behavior. If in doubt, the clinician should proceed with an abuse evaluation.

Runaway and missing children frequently are victims of abuse. Often with limited coping and survival skills, runaways and missing children remain abused as they live on the streets, in makeshift tenements, or with strangers. Community child psychiatrists usually come into contact with these children when they are brought in by staff from youth shelters and agencies or by a law enforcement agency as a result of being engaged in bizarre or potentially life-threatening behaviors. In addition to performing a mental status evaluation with a consequent diagnosis, the child psychiatrist must function as an advocate, ensuring that the child's daily needs of safety, food, clothing, and shelter are being met. Developmental issues are also critical for runaway youth and should be addressed by the psychiatrist and other care-providing groups.

Poverty and Homelessness

Homeless and poverty-stricken families and their children are only now beginning to receive attention from decision makers, clinicians, and researchers. In addition to lacking structure, consistency, and safety in their physical living conditions, such children's caretaker and support systems are likewise disrupted. Parents and caretakers, who are more concerned with providing the basics of food, clothing, and shelter, have less time to devote to parenting and developmental concerns. Socialization with peers and education are also disrupted, as children either are not enrolled in school or move from one school to another on a frequent basis. The rate of emotional disorders is higher in this population. Because these families are usually uninsured, they receive medical and psychiatric care at public health and mental health agencies. Once again, the child psychiatrist must act as an advocate for the child and his or her family to ensure the safety and emotional and physical well-being of the child.

Foster Care

Many children who present to child psychiatrists are in out-of-home placements, especially foster care. It is estimated that about 500,000 American children are in foster homes (Geiser 1973). Foster home placements may be transient or longer term in nature. A younger child may retain no memories of placement or incidents leading to placement. Even when parents are abusive, older children suffer from separations. All children are traumatized by impersonal treatment, lack of continuity of foster homes and social workers, and lack of connection with families of origin. Early deprivation and subsequent disruption lead to disturbances in foster children. Many children show signs of regression and transient adjustment reactions including sphincter dyscontrol, withdrawal, aggression, and sleep and appetite problems. Grief, guilt, anxiety, confusion, anger, and lowered self-esteem and depression are common psychological responses. A child psychiatrist working with foster children should provide routine monitoring of the specific placement and process, evaluations of the child's overall treatment plan, and psychotherapy for reactive or long-standing problems. Children in group homes have much in common with foster children and represent the most deprived and volatile segment of the child population. Unfortunately, many group homes have limited mental health care at their facilities, resulting in reliance on community-based agencies for such services.

Substance Abuse

Adolescent substance abuse is a major concern in the community and receives much media attention. Even though there has been a general downward trend in the prevalence of drug use since the 1980s, many adolescents continue to use illicit drugs. Drug use among American high school seniors increased in 1993 for the first time in more than a decade (Johnston et al.

1993). Eighth and 10th grade students also showed increases in their drug use. This survey found that 42.9% of high school seniors had used an illicit drug at least once in their lives. Risk factors for drug abuse include a family history of drug abuse, dysfunctional family of origin, cultural background, psychiatric diagnosis, poor school performance, and impulsive behavior.

When working with adolescents, especially those in early and middle adolescence, the clinician must recognize that many adolescents have not yet achieved Piaget's formal operational thinking stage and therefore have difficulties in understanding abstract concepts (e.g., denial and "higher power"), a common fact in the addiction field (Piaget 1962). Often the adolescent is not resisting treatment but in fact cannot understand it. Many adolescent substance abusers have concomitant high-risk behaviors, psychiatric problems, learning disabilities, impulse control and attention problems, and serious family and school problems, all of which further complicate evaluation and treatment by the child psychiatrist and other clinicians. Tolerance, craving, withdrawal, and withdrawal avoidance are less common and less severe in adolescence, making the need for detoxification relatively rare. More than any other age group, adolescents use role modeling and imitation and yield to peer pressure as part of the process of achieving independence and identity. All of these factors are important considerations in treating the adolescent substance abuser.

Of particular interest to the community child psychiatrist is the effect of ethnic and racial variables on adolescent substance abuse behavior. Native American high school seniors have the highest rates for use of marijuana, cocaine, alcohol, cigarettes, inhalants, hallucinogens, heroin, other opiates, stimulants, and sedatives and tranquilizers. White and Hispanic seniors have the second and third highest rates, respectively, of drug use, whereas African American and Asian American students have the lowest rate (Bachman et al. 1991). These differences are important considerations for the child psychiatrist developing community-based substance abuse interventions.

Comprehensive psychiatric evaluations in the substance-abusing adolescent are essential. Concomitant psychiatric disorders, known as *dual diagnoses*, learning disabilities, and school and family problems must be identified and receive appropriate attention. In addition to direct thorough questioning of the adolescent and family regarding his or her illicit drug-taking patterns, several screening instruments for adolescent substance use currently exist. These instruments include the Adolescent Alcohol Involvement Scale (Mayer et al. 1979), the Chemical Dependency Assessment Scale (Oetting et al. 1984), and the Drug Use Screening Inventory (Tarter 1990), among others (Kaminer 1994).

Once assessment is complete, the community child psychiatrist should determine the level of intervention necessary for that particular adolescent. Usual options include inpatient, outpatient, and partial hospitalization services, but other novel approaches are often indicated, such as alternative residential programs, special school or work programs, and other community services. As noted previously, dual diagnoses require appropriate psychiatric interventions, including the possible use of psychotropic medications. Substance abuse treatment should include both individual and multiple family therapy. Very commonly the adolescent is referred to group therapy, which can be relapse-prevention, psychodynamic, or self-help (e.g., Alcoholics Anonymous) in nature. Increasingly, behavioral and cognitive therapies are being used with greater success.

Preventive approaches to substance abuse are of great interest for the community child psychiatrist. The most common approaches to primary or early prevention are media campaigns and education programs. A number of empirical studies have shown that these approaches to prevention among youth are ineffective (Schinke et al. 1991). A more advanced strategy for prevention is based in social learning theory and problem behavior theory. These prevention programs are aimed at enhancing self-esteem and social skills, utilizing standardized interventions in group settings.

Disasters and Emergencies

Disasters may be physical, natural, or emotional and by their very nature are unpredictable. They can affect an entire country and be witnessed via the media, as occurred with the *Challenger* tragedy. They can strike an entire community, as in the case of earthquakes, hurricanes, or riots. They can strike individuals or families in the form of, for example, house fires. Whatever the context, the developing child is especially vulnerable to such unexpected assaults to the psyche. A common response is regressive behavior to an earlier developmental stage. A 4-year-old child may become more oppositional. A 13-year-old adolescent may resume nocturnal enuresis.

Of greater concern are long-term emotional sequelae such as depressive or anxiety disorders. It is commonly held by mental health professionals that if the parents can convey a sense of security and stability despite a chaotic environment, the child generally will fare well. The parent, however, should speak in simple, straightforward, and honest terms when discussing the circumstances with the youngster.

In states of disaster, the community child psychiatrist is called on to work at disaster relief sites themselves or at schools or other community-based agencies. The child psychiatrist must advocate strongly for the special needs of youth so that they will not be overlooked during the stressful crisis period. The child psychiatrist will see individual children or adolescents and act as a consultant to the other counseling staff, which will likely be largely composed of inexperienced volunteers. The model for this consultation is similar in nature to that provided in schools.

Emergencies, too, are unpredictable. Emergencies may or may not be life threatening, but they are extremely stressful both to the child in crisis and to those around him or her. In an emergency situation, the child's physical safety assumes first priority for the child psychiatrist and other clinicians. The psychiatrist should perform a rapid yet thorough assessment and determine the immediate course of action. He or she must assess whether medical intervention is necessary; whether the child requires constant observation for suicidal ideation or actions; and whether the child is at risk for leaving the evaluation prematurely, either on his or her own or through the actions of his or her caretaker.

The child psychiatrist should formulate a working diagnosis and a longer range treatment plan for the period after the crisis has resolved. A physical examination is required, particularly in cases involving abuse, alcohol or drug intoxication or overdose, suicide attempts, or abrupt behavioral changes. Additional sources, such as the child's therapist, social services worker, or pediatrician, should be contacted for more information. It is essential to assess the safety of the family and home situation, especially if considering returning the child to that environment. Assessing the parents' capacity to support an at-risk child in the home is critical.

If a child or adolescent poses an immediate threat to his or her own safety or to the safety of others, he or she requires inpatient psychiatric hospitalization. Hospitalization may be accomplished on a voluntary or involuntary basis. An important responsibility of the child psychiatrist is to advocate for the safety of the child. At times, third-party payers will not approve hospitalization despite the child psychiatrist's objection to sending the child home to an unsafe environment. The child psychiatrist then should know and be able to access community resources to ensure the child's safety. These resources include child protective agencies, state and local departments of social services and mental health, and legal agencies.

Suicidal ideation and behavior are common psychiatric childhood and adolescent psychiatric emergencies. Even though children under 12 years of age threaten and attempt suicide, completion of suicide in such children is rare. However, in adolescence the suicide rate is significant and increasing. In fact, in the 15- to 19-year-old age group, the suicide rate has tripled since the mid-1960s (Brent et al. 1987). Although more girls than boys exhibit suicidal behavior, five times more teenage boys commit suicide than teenage girls (Shaffer et al. 1988). Those who complete suicide are more likely to use firearms, and males are more likely than females to use violent weapons (Brent et al. 1987). A suicide attempt, regardless of the lethality, should be treated as an emergency. Any child or adolescent who attempts suicide usually does so as a last resort.

In evaluating a suicide attempt in a child or adolescent, the psychiatrist first should provide lifesaving medical measures. The patient should be in a safe environment, under observation by mental health staff. The psychiatrist must stress the seriousness of the situation in a nonjudgmental and nonpunitive manner, conveying genuine concern. A thorough psychiatric evaluation should be performed, assessing the precipitating stressor, the lethality of the attempt, the motivation, the concept of death, and the patient's current attitude. The family should be interviewed separately. A mental status evaluation is critical to assess reality testing results, mood state, judgment, and impulse control.

In assessing the child, the clinician should be aware of circumstances that carry a continued suicide risk. A negative attitude or lack of concern toward the parent is associated with increased suicide risk, as is the parent's minimization of the seriousness and belief that the suicide attempt is merely attention-getting behavior (Hoberman and Garfinkel 1988). Increased risk is associated with a family's instability and inability to cope with the child and provide a safe, supportive environment. Finally, the incidence of familial suicide attempts and serious depression must be ascertained, because suicide attempts in children correspond significantly with parental suicidal ideation.

In determining the disposition of a suicidal child or adolescent, the child psychiatrist should hospitalize the youth if there is any doubt as to whether the patient should be sent home with the caretaker. Other factors a psychiatrist must consider include the immediate potential for self-destructive behavior, concurrent psychopathologic disorder, the child's intrapsychic needs, the family's unambivalent desire for the child to live, and practical limitations of the family's ability to ensure safety. If the child or adolescent is sent home, a follow-up appointment in the near future should be made, along with provisions for recurrent emergency situations.

Homicide is another emergency that confronts community child psychiatrists. In 1985 8% of murders in the United States were committed by juveniles. Homicide is the second leading cause of death for individuals in the 15- to 24-year-old age group and the leading cause of death for young black males in that group ("Homicide" 1990). Characteristics of juveniles who commit murder include neurological impairment, psychomotor symptoms, episodic psychotic symptoms occurring sporadically without the diagnosis of schizophrenia, a history of child abuse, and a history of severe parental psychopathologic disorder and violence (Lewis et al. 1988). Furthermore, it appeared that an abusive environment in conjunction with these characteristics predisposed to severe aggression. Further risk factors include a history of fire setting, a history of cruelty to animals, labile affect, an orientation toward action, an ability to see killing as a feasible act, membership in a culture accepting of violence, a psychiatric diagnosis, intoxication with drugs or alcohol, possession of a weapon, a formulated plan of action, and a history of previously having murdered (Allen 1981). Many youngsters who kill give premonitory signs (Malmquist 1971). These clues include an object loss in a relationship that served to provide the perpetrator with a cohesive sense of self, a threat to one's sexuality, an ensuing shift in mood to hopelessness and often to self-hate, increasing restlessness and agitation, use of drugs to alter feelings and impulses, increasing somatization or recurrent medical problems, a "cry for help," and an emotional enhancement with loosening of thought processes.

The community child psychiatrist is charged in many ways with protecting the safety of the community. When an adolescent presents with homicidal ideation, the psychiatrist must consider all of the above characteristics. If there is any concern about a serious risk of violence, the psychiatrist must consider hospitalization or possibly incarceration to protect society. Most communities require that the threatened individual be notified, along with the law enforcement agency in the locale in which he or she resides.

The Future: Coordinated, Comprehensive Community-Based Services

A growing trend in community services is to provide more integrated and comprehensive services. These issues have been addressed by examining systems of care and developing what have been referred to as *wraparound* services. Traditionally, child welfare has been split among child protective, probation, and mental health delivery systems. Newer programs attempt to integrate these systems to provide increased cohesiveness. The ultimate goal is to prevent incarceration and psychiatric hospitalization and allow children to lead productive, normalized lives in their own communities. Another model, referred to as *family preservation,* attempts to maintain the child at home by providing more intensive services in the home, school, and community. Legislative action and parental mandates through advocacy have fueled these changes.

The role of the child psychiatrist historically has been underutilized in the community, and this role holds great promise in the future. Heretofore, the child psychiatrist has been marginalized by other mental health professionals. However, with the growing complexities of psychiatric illnesses and society at large, the expertise and broad training of the child psychiatrist is becoming more evident and utilized. Truly, the potential for a child psychiatrist working in the community is limited only by his or her creativity and energy.

Community child psychiatrists are facing varied challenges and opportunities in the mid-1990s. As managed care continues to affect the delivery of mental health care, the role of the child psychiatrist will evolve. The community-based child psychiatrist will continue to practice individual therapy, but his or her role in a consultative and administrative capacity undoubtedly will expand as new mental health complexities demand the broader perspective of the psychiatrist's background.

References

Allen NH: Homicide prevention and intervention. Suicide Life Threat Behav 11:167–179, 1981

Bachman JG, Wallace JM, O'Malley PM, et al: Racial/ethnic differences in smoking, drinking and illicit drug use among American high school seniors 1976–1989. Am J Public Health 81:372–377, 1991

Brent DA, Perper JA, Allman CJ: Alcohol, firearms, and suicide among youth. JAMA 257:3369–3372, 1987

Geiser RL: The Illusion of Caring: Children in Foster Care. Boston, MA, Beacon Press, 1973

Hoberman HM, Garfinkel BD: Completed suicide in children and adolescents. J Am Acad Child Adolesc Psychiatry 27:689–695, 1988

Homicide among young black males, United States, 1978–1987. MMWR Morbid Mortal Wkly Rep 39:869–873, 1990

Johnston LD, O'Malley PM, Bachman JG: Details of Annual Drug Survey. Ann Arbor, MI, University of Michigan News and Information Services, 1993

Kaminer Y: Adolescent Substance Abuse: A Comprehensive Guide to Theory and Practice. New York, Plenum, 1994

Lathrop JC: The Background of the Juvenile Court in Illinois: The Child, the Clinic and the Court. New York, New Republic, 1925

Lewis DO, Lovely R, Yeager C, et al: Intrinsic and environmental characteristics of juvenile murderers. J Am Acad Child Psychiatry 27:582–587, 1988

Malmquist C: Premonitory signs of homicidal aggression in juveniles. Am J Psychiatry 121:461–465, 1971

Mayer J, Filstead WJ: The adolescent alcohol involvement scale: an instrument for measuring adolescent use and misuse of alcohol. J Stud Alcohol 40:291–300, 1979

National Center on Child Abuse and Neglect: Study Findings: Study of National Incidence and Prevalence of Child Abuse and Neglect. Washington, DC, U.S. Department of Health and Human Services, 1992

Oetting, E, Beauvais F, Edwards R, et al: The Drug and Alcohol Assessment System. Fort Collins, CO, Mountain Behavioral Sciences Institute, 1984

Piaget J: The Moral Judgment of the Child. New York, Collier, 1962

Rafferty FT, Mackie J: The Diagnostic Check Point for Community Child Psychiatry. Washington, DC, American Psychiatric Association, 1967

Schinke SP, Botvin GJ, Orlani MA: Substance Abuse in Children and Adolescents: Evaluation and Intervention. Newbury Park, CA, Sage, 1991

Shaffer D, Gould M, Fisher P, et al: Preventing teenage suicide: a critical review. J Am Acad Child Psychiatry 27:675–687, 1988

Starr P: The Social Transformation of American Medicine. New York, Basic Books, 1982

Tarter RE: Evaluation and treatment of adolescent substance abuse: a decision free method. Am J Drug Alcohol Abuse 16:1–46, 1990

Chapter 9

Community Care of Adults With Developmental Disabilities and Mental Illness

William C. Torrey, M.D.

T he telephone rang, and a frightened, horrified voice on the other side of the line said, "David Jones keeps biting deeply into his arm here in front of me. Doctor, you've got to do something, now!" This was my introduction to the psychiatric care of people with developmental disabilities and mental illness. My first response to this charged situation was the thought, "This must be someone else's problem."

Community psychiatrists typically feel overwhelmed when they first encounter the clinical problems of people with developmental disabilities and mental illness. They face intense staff and family needs yet lack adequate training and experience to effectively address these seemingly foreign problems (Jacobson and Ackerman 1988). Without a clear approach to the psychiatric assessment and treatment of this group of patients, psychiatrists encounter many obstacles in their efforts to apply their skills. These obstacles include the following:

- Unfamiliar presenting problems (frequent behavioral disturbances) (Sovner and Hurley 1989)
- Difficulty in taking a history from the patient (Sovner 1986)

- Difficulty in obtaining relevant information from family, staff, and old records (Sovner and Hurley 1990a)
- Lack of usefulness of the standard American Psychiatric Association criteria in diagnosing this population (Sovner 1986)
- Difficulty in differentiating the effects of mental retardation (Reiss et al. 1982) and institutionalization (Menolascino et al. 1986) from the effects of mental illness
- Uncertainty about the appropriate use of medicine, given the bias against medication found in some of the literature (Findholt and Emmett 1990)

The thought that "this must be someone else's problem" has occurred to many clinicians. As with people with both mental illness and chemical dependence, persons with both developmental disabilities and mental illness fall between service systems (Fletcher 1989; Reiss 1982). They are referred away from the community mental health centers for many reasons, including the assumption that they would be better served elsewhere. This is a false assumption. Community mental health agencies are the natural place to care for the mental health needs of this deinstitutionalized population (Fletcher and Menolascino 1989; Sovner and Hurley 1989; Szymanski and Grossman 1984).

Community psychiatrists are uniquely suited to contribute to the care of people with developmental disabilities and mental illness, because the experience of working with people with severe mental illness provides the basic required skills. Community psychiatrists are familiar with community integration, the team approach to care, the clinical assessment of poor informants, the psychoeducation of patients and families, and the use of a broad range of clinical interventions (e.g., psychotherapy, social skills training, behavioral treatment, medication) with the aim of minimizing disability rather than merely eliminating symptoms. When an orientation to the specific challenges involved in the assessment and treatment of people with developmental disabilities and mental illness is added to this foundation of knowledge, community psychiatrists can overcome the obstacles to care.

In this chapter I provide an introduction to the community psychiatric care of people with developmental disabilities and mental illness. After outlining the scope of the problem, the philosophy grounding community care, and the need for a team, I present a practical approach to information collection, assessment, diagnosis, treatment planning, and treatment options for people with developmental disabilities and mental illness. In this chapter I use the terms *developmental disability* and *mental retardation* interchangeably.

The Extent of the Problem

To meet DSM-IV criteria for mental retardation, a person must have an IQ of 70 or below, concurrent impairments in adaptive functioning, and onset before the age of 18. There are four levels of severity of impairment: mild, moderate, severe, and profound (American Psychiatric Association 1994).

The population of persons with developmental disabilities and mental illness currently living in the community is both large and underserved (Landsberg et al. 1987; Menolascino 1989; Sovner and Hurley 1989). Social, political, legal, and clinical changes over the past decades have shifted care of persons with developmental disabilities away from institutions and toward the community (Braddock 1981; Stark et al. 1984). This move began later and has been more gradual for persons with developmental disabilities than for those with severe mental illness. It is, however, a strong and ongoing trend (Braddock 1981).

Community studies indicate that persons with developmental disabilities suffer from mental illness at a higher rate than the rest of the population (Borthwick-Duffy and Eyman 1990; Parsons et al. 1984). Research studies consistently demonstrate that mental illness is found in 20%–35% of developmentally disabled persons not living in institutions (Landsberg et al. 1987; Ruedrich and Menolascino 1984). The full range of mental illnesses found in the general population has been described in persons with developmental disabilities (Sovner and Hurley 1989).

Many factors leave persons with developmental disabilities at high risk to develop mental illness. These factors include constitutional vulnerabilities from central nervous system impairment (Menolascino et al. 1986) (e.g., frontal lobe damage or seizure disorders), psychological vulnerabilities such as low self-esteem (Menolascino et al. 1986), and social support vulnerabilities such as poverty of interpersonal relationships (Eaton and Menolascino 1982). Persons with developmental disabilities take these vulnerabilities into a world that has unique stresses beyond those experienced by individuals without developmental disabilities. They must deal with the stigma associated with mental retardation (Benson et al. 1985; Reiss and Benson 1985), rejection by peers (Menolascino et al. 1986), and lack of control over basic needs such as housing or employment (Deutsch 1989).

Not only are the rates of psychiatric illness high, but the disability caused by mental illness is significant (Parsons et al. 1984). Only mobility limitations rank higher than psychiatric impairments in causing secondary disability among adults with developmental disabilities (Jacobson 1982; Jacobson and Ackerman 1988). Psychiatric and behavioral disturbances are frequently the factors blocking community integration (Lindenbaum 1989), housing placement (Reid 1989), social acceptance (Reid and Ballinger 1987; Schloss 1982), and vocational success (Schalock et al. 1978).

Despite a recent increase in interest in this population among mental health professionals (Menolascino 1989), the mental health needs of persons with developmental disabilities are seriously underserved (Fletcher et al. 1989). In particular, this population is not adequately served by community mental health services (Sovner and Hurley 1989). Emotional problems in persons with developmental disabilities are often missed because diagnostically important abnormal behavior is attributed to mental retardation alone (Reiss et al. 1982). When mental illness is identified, skilled treatment is difficult to find (Menolascino et al. 1986). A national survey of services for the mentally ill mentally retarded rated availability, accessibility, and adequacy of services as poor (Jacobson and Ackerman 1988).

There is a great need for professionals trained in meeting the mental health needs of persons with developmental disabilities (Jacobson and Ackerman 1988; Landsberg et al. 1987; Parsons et al. 1984; Szymanski and Grossman 1984). Community psychiatrists can help to close the gap between need and services by applying their skills and experience to the care of this population.

Community Integration as a Guiding Principle

Community psychiatrists who work with persistently mentally ill adults are familiar with the importance of community integration in improving the lives of adults with disabilities. True community integration involves using treatment resources to support people in normal living situations rather than building separate community enclaves for persons with disabilities. For example, instead of creating work in sheltered environments, vocational efforts can focus on obtaining and supporting real jobs for real money in the general community. Police and courts must be educated to help them appropriately provide their community limit-setting functions since people learn community standards of behavior better when they are not protected from the negative consequences of their actions.

Community integration for persons with developmental disabilities includes integration into community mental health care. Persons with developmental disabilities should have the same right to the proven benefits of psychosocial and psychopharmacological interventions as others in need (Findholt and Emmett 1990; Szymanski and Grossman 1984). Protecting persons with disabilities from the dangers of the world through segregation also creates barriers to community opportunity.

The Team Approach

As is true for persons with severe mental illness, all aspects of assessment, treatment planning, and ongoing care of persons with developmental disabilities and mental illness require a team approach (Findholt and Emmett 1990; Sovner and Hurley 1983a). A team is needed because the work involved is often more than one person can accomplish. The psychiatrist, behavioral expert, and frontline staff must communicate so that all team members have the best information available and care can be coordinated.

A team approach also provides an opportunity to share perspective, expertise, and uncertainty. A community psychiatrist does not have to be a mental retardation behavioral expert to be helpful to persons with developmentally disabilities, but he or she must be able to understand and collaborate with someone on the team who is knowledgeable in this area. The clinical situations contain so much uncertainty that the perspectives of different minds and disciplines are extremely valuable. As one author reflecting on this field put it, "the reality is that no individual professional group has a monopoly of answers or wisdom" (Reid 1989, p. 366). Working as a team is more enjoyable than working alone and enables caregivers to sustain their efforts over time.

Building a working team takes time and commitment, especially when the team consists of members from several agencies. The clinical rewards are worth the effort. An ideal community team contains, at a minimum, a behavioral expert, a psychiatrist, and persons with close firsthand knowledge of the client.

Case 1

The behavioral expert on our team and I were discussing a moderately mentally retarded woman whose behavioral records show that she had recently restarted a pattern of pica, urinary incontinence, and dangerous behavior, such as lying down in a busy road. We wondered if the behavioral plan should be changed or if this might be a good time for a medication adjustment. During the discussion her case manager entered the meeting and told us that the behavior had begun on the day she learned she would be moving to a new residence. No medication or behavioral intervention change was made, and after the move, the behaviors abated.

Obtaining Reliable Information

Because psychiatric assessments and treatments are only as good as the information on which they are based, psychiatrists must insist on adequate information. Obtaining this information is often the most difficult obstacle to good care (Sovner and Hurley 1990a). Many patients have deficits in verbal skills (Sovner and Hurley 1983b) and lack facility with abstract concepts (Sovner 1986), which limits their ability to provide detailed histories. Their history must be supplemented by family members and the staff who see the patient on a daily basis.

Because family members and staff are not usually mental health experts, they do not know what information is relevant to psychiatric assessment and treatment. Typically, for example, they do not bring information about sleep pattern, appetite, weight loss, energy level, and family history of depression when requesting an evaluation for a suddenly withdrawn, weepy, noncommunicative individual (Sovner and Hurley 1983b, 1990a). Directing informants to bring specific information improves speed and accuracy of care (Sovner and Hurley 1983b), as the following vignette illustrates.

Case 2

A 42-year-old barely verbal woman was brought for follow-up 2 weeks after starting a new medication for depression. The patient looked the same, but the residential staff worker who brought her answered all questions nonspecifically by saying she was "doing great." No objective incident reports or sleep records were provided. As no reasonable determination could be made about her condition, arrangements were made for her to come back the next week with the relevant information.

Assessment

The initial assessment involves studying the information provided; reviewing old psychiatric records (which are sometimes indispensable but often useless); interviewing the patient's family or other caretakers; and, of course, examining the patient. For patients who can give a good history, the process of collecting a personal and developmental history can add diagnostically important information and help the psychiatrist build an alliance with the patient (Levitas and Gilson 1989). When the patient cannot describe his or her symptoms and functional status, the mental status examination is still important for the observable signs of mental illness (Ruedrich and Menolascino 1984).

Stereotyped maladaptive behavior such as aggression, self-injury, or hyperactivity is very often the presenting problem in persons with developmental disability (Sovner and Hurley 1989). The maladaptive behavior is a signal of distress. The lower a person's IQ, the more constricted that person's repertoire is for expressing distress (Reid 1989). The behavioral message is nonspecific, so new onset or worsening of these behaviors can be precipitated by sensory deprivation, psychological stress, stress of general medical illness, adverse drug reaction, and psychiatric illness.

Behavioral change is an important barometer of stress. Psychiatrists should not consider the behavior itself to be the problem without first making a thorough search for an underlying cause. This search requires a broad investigation of the patient's medical and psychological life history.

Psychiatrists must have a high index of suspicion for general medical problems when evaluating new-onset or worsening behavioral problems in a person with a developmental disability (Kastner et al. 1990). Even in the general psychiatric population, psychiatric symptoms have been found to be caused by undetected medical conditions at rates as high as 9% (Hall et al. 1978). This rate is probably much higher in the developmentally disabled population. Persons with developmental disability cannot express themselves as precisely as nondisabled persons and yet are at high risk for seizure disorders (Kaufman and Katz-Garris 1979) and other serious and painful medical conditions (Kastner et al. 1990).

Case 3

A 34-year-old severely mentally retarded woman with a seizure disorder was brought in because of lack of energy, sadness, irritability, and increased low-level self-injury. Staff wondered if an antidepressant would help this "depression." Workup revealed a toxic blood level of phenytoin (Dilantin). Depressive symptoms resolved after her phenytoin dose was adjusted.

Diagnosis

Establishing a valid psychiatric diagnosis in a person with a developmental disability is often difficult. Psychiatric syndromes frequently present atypically (Sovner and Hurley 1989), and the conventional diagnostic scheme is of limited usefulness in this population. The diagnostic criteria of DSM-IV often require complex self-report (i.e., suicidal ideation, auditory hallucinations), making it hard for less verbal patients to meet full criteria (Sovner and Hurley 1990b).

Persons with mild or moderate mental retardation are more likely than persons with severe or profound mental retardation to present with clear and classic psychiatric syndromes (Russell 1989). For example, it is relatively easy to diagnose the syndrome of schizophrenia in mildly mentally retarded individuals, because it presents just as it does in individuals without a developmental disability (Meadows et al. 1991). However, in nonverbal patients with severe or profound mental retardation, it is controversial whether the diagnosis can even be made (Reid 1972, 1989). New-onset withdrawal, blunted affect, bizarre behavior, and nonverbal signs of paranoia occurring in a severely mentally retarded individual at a high-risk age may well signal schizophrenia (Menolascino et al. 1985), but the level of diagnostic certainty is lower than it would be if the patient were verbal.

Making the best possible psychiatric diagnosis demonstrates a search for the underlying cause of behavioral disturbance and guides treatment. There are times, however, when some individuals with severe or profound mental retardation present with disabling maladaptive behaviors that do not fit clearly into the current diagnostic system. Stretching the concept of "atypical" too far makes the taxonomy meaningless. When a general medical or psychiatric cause cannot be found, psychiatrists should acknowledge the limits of the diagnostic system and document that they are treating disabling behaviors and not specific disorders (Gualtieri and Keppel 1985).

Behavioral problems can be so disabling or dangerous that, despite the lack of a specific DSM-IV diagnosis, psychosocial or psychopharmacological treatment is indicated. This point is illustrated in the vignette that follows.

Case 4

A 36-year-old nonverbal, severely retarded man with a history of unprovoked aggressive and self-injurious behavior had been on low-dose chlorpromazine for years. A well-designed behavioral plan was in place. His very disabling symptoms did not resemble any DSM-IV diagnosis. Concern about early signs of tardive dyskinesia found on Abnormal Inventory Movement Scale screening led to discussions with his guardian and with treatment staff. Propranolol was added to his medications before chlorpromazine was tapered over several months. One morning, with little warning, he struck a staff member and bit the face of an elderly resident, sending both to the emergency department for stitches. Chlorpromazine was restarted and propranolol tapered several months later without difficulty.

Treatment Planning

Once the psychiatric diagnosis or definition of the maladaptive behavior has been established, treatment options can be considered. Standard psychiatric treatments tend to work for standard psychiatric problems, so for classic syndromes the treatment plan is relatively straightforward (Hurley 1989; Matson 1985). For example, if a patient has a clear-cut phobia the treatment of choice is behavioral therapy using counterconditioning techniques, just as for a nonretarded patient (Hurley 1989). Diagnosable psychiatric conditions should be treated with conventional treatments before nonstandard experimental treatments are tried (Gualtieri 1989).

When maladaptive behavior such as aggression, self-injurious behavior, or overactivity does not appear to be the result of a definable psychiatric syndrome, empirical trials of reasonable interventions should be employed. Trials should be planned and systematically delivered, beginning with the most benign interventions (Eichelman 1988). Each intervention must be given sufficient time to demonstrate its degree of effectiveness (Ruedrich and Menolascino 1984).

Whether the treatment is standard or experimental, a quantifiable means for assessing its efficiency is indispensable (Eichelman 1988; Gualtieri 1989). Objective behavioral data should record psychiatrically relevant information such as sleep pattern or frequency and intensity of the maladaptive target behavior (Sovner and Hurley 1990a). Preintervention data sometimes show patterns that help determine the diagnosis and provide a baseline from which to measure the effectiveness of interventions.

Case 5

A 21-year-old woman with Down's syndrome had month-long periods of high activity several times a year. Behavioral incident reports documented an increase of irritable aggressive outbursts at these times. Sleep records showed a drop in sleep from 10 hours nightly to 5. The diagnosis of bipolar affective disorder was made, and treatment with lithium was instituted. The sleep record returned to normal, and the number and intensity of the incidents dropped off.

Treatment Options

As in the care of persons with severe mental illness, treatment options for individuals with developmental disabilities and mental illness include a broad range of possible psychosocial and psychopharmacological interventions. Because all interventions can have negative as well as positive effects on a person's life, the potential benefits and risks of intervention must always be weighed against those of not intervening.

Psychotherapy

Psychodynamic psychotherapy can be helpful to many mildly and moderately retarded individuals. It has been underused because of beliefs that verbal deficits make communication difficult and that abstract thought deficits preclude insight (Russell 1989). Several practitioners, however, report success in their work (Levitas and Gilson 1989; Szymanski 1980) and argue that the special characteristics of this population call for an adjustment in technique rather than an abandonment of the treatment modality (Levitas and Gilson 1989).

Technique must be tailored to the individual patient. Clear, simple language can be used when the patient has a limited vocabulary (Monfils and Menolascino 1984). Treatment should be active and directive, and unacceptable behavior must be clearly and consistently limited (Monfils and Menolascino 1984). For some patients the clinician's office may feel like a safe place, but for others treatment is best done at a location comfortable to the patient. Psychotherapy can be done at a location familiar to the patient, such as his or her home, or while out walking, where interpersonal anxiety is lessened by the immediate presence of the outside world. The therapist should interact with the patient as a real person so that the therapy has the feeling of a conversation about the emotional dilemmas we all confront (Levitas and Gilson 1989).

As is true of children and persons with severe mental illness, the quality of life of persons with developmental disabilities is strongly influenced by those on whom they must depend for care. This web of relationships is an important focus for treatment. Understandings gleaned from psychotherapy can be used not only to directly influence the patient, but also to modify the emotional environment in which the patient lives (Levitas and Gilson 1989).

Certain themes consistently recur in the psychotherapy of adults with developmental disabilities. Patients are commonly concerned with feelings about being retarded and what it means to be different (Bates 1984). Frequently they feel unloved and inadequate (Monfils and Menolascino 1984). Frustration in competitive endeavors is a common theme that is brought out by stressors ranging from getting little time in a softball game to being surpassed in marriage by a younger sibling (Levitas and Gilson 1989). Conflicting desires for dependence and independence can cause significant distress in the lives of retarded individuals. The issue is often quite obvious in the transference and can be resolved in therapy (Levitas and Gilson 1989). Therapy provides a private setting for the discussion of sexual concerns that may be difficult to address appropriately elsewhere (Monfils 1989).

Themes can be effectively addressed in a group format. Groups work best if they have a clear purpose, defined structure, and a compatible composition. The group format has the advantage of the potential for peer support and cohesion (Fletcher 1984; Monfils 1989). The format also makes efficient use of therapist time when this valuable resource is scarce. Group work requires an active leader who is willing to model behaviors and set appropriate limits (Monfils and Menolascino 1984).

Behavioral Interventions

Behavioral interventions have been used in the care of persons with developmental disabilities for more than 40 years (Russell 1989). As is true in the general population, these techniques can be used successfully in the treatment of phobia, depression, and anorexia in persons with developmental disabilities (Hurley 1989; Hurley and Sovner 1991). They can also be used to modify maladaptive behaviors such as pica and self-injurious behavior that cannot always be identified as a symptom of a classic mental illness syndrome (Gardner and Cole 1984).

Behavioral interventions require a client-specific assessment to understand the current factors contributing to the ongoing expression of maladaptive behavior (Gardner and Cole 1984). Once an intervention plan is developed, it can be taught to nonprofessionals such as parents and residential staff, who then implement it in the natural settings of the client's life (Russell 1989).

Modern approaches aim not only to reduce or eliminate disabling behaviors through techniques based on operant conditioning, but also to replace these behaviors through the teaching and rewarding of appropriate responses (Gardner and Cole 1984). For example, an individual who regularly throws his plate on the floor when frustrated while waiting for dessert can be conditioned not to throw his plate and can also be taught to ask assertively for what he wants.

Social skills training can be taught in the areas of assertiveness (Bregman 1985), differentiating among types of relationships (Hingsburger 1989), and dating (Valenti-Hein 1990). This can be done in groups or individually using techniques of instruction, modeling, role playing, performance feedback, and social reinforcement (Matson 1984). Emphasis is placed on teaching valued behaviors in a natural social context to promote generalized use of adaptive skills (Griffiths 1990). Some clients require direct training in recognizing and naming feelings before they can make use of skills teaching aimed at appropriate expression of emotions (Ludwig and Hingsburger 1989).

Medications

Psychiatrists should use psychotropic medication only when the potential benefits have been fully analyzed. The assessment must show that the symptomatic person has either a well-defined and drug-responsive mental illness or a behavioral disorder for which medications are likely to work (Sovner and Hurley 1983a).

Psychopharmacology studies indicate that for defined psychiatric presentations, the medications that work for individuals in the general population are likely to work for persons with developmental disability (Matson 1985). There is less psychopharmacological guidance for behavioral disorders that do not appear to be the result of recognizable DSM-IV syndromes. The literature on the drug treatment of nonspecific maladaptive behaviors consists mostly of case reports and small studies but is growing steadily. Currently there is evidence supporting the selective use of many agents, including lithium, tricyclic antidepressants, fluoxetine, benzodiazepines, buspirone, beta blockers, anticonvulsants, clonidine, and antipsychotics. Several excellent reviews have summed up what is known (Aman and Singh 1988; Farber 1987; Lapierre and Reesal 1986; Sovner 1989).

Because prediction of drug efficacy is difficult, pharmacological treatment of nonspecific maladaptive behavioral disorders usually involves empirical trials of medication (Gualtieri and Keppel 1985). The list of possible drugs should be prioritized on the basis of probability of response, side effect profile, safety, and experience with the medication (Russell 1989). Interventions should be aimed at specific target symptoms that can be monitored (Sovner and Hurley 1990a). Careful documentation of effectiveness, dose level, blood level (when appropriate), duration of trial, side effects, and reason for discontinuing the trial can save an individual with a chronic problem from multiple trials of the same ineffective medication by different psychiatrists (Sovner and Hurley 1990a).

Unless a patient has demonstrated a rapid return of symptoms when medications are discontinued, a trial period off medication should be considered after time has passed. The medication may not have been the active agent in remission, may no longer be needed, or may be causing an unrecognized side effect such as akathisia (Sovner and Hurley 1984).

Controversy surrounds the use of psychotropic drug use in persons with developmental disabilities. Concern centers mainly around the use of antipsychotic medications (Gualtieri and Keppel 1985) and evidence that they are sometimes used without adequate consideration of diagnosis, side effects, and pharmacological and nonpharmacological alternatives (Linaker 1990). Studies demonstrate that psychotropic medications are used at a high rate in this population (e.g., 25%–35% in community residential facilities) (Intagliata and Rinch 1985) and that antipsychotic medications are the most widely used psychotropic medications, with the exception of anticonvulsants (Gualtieri and Keppel 1985). Few psychopharmacologists specializing in developmentally disabled individuals recommend using antipsychotics as the treatment of first choice (Sovner 1991), but there is good evidence they are effective in some situations (Schroeder 1988). The fact that antipsychotics have been overused in this population does not mean that they are contraindicated (Gualtieri and Keppel 1985). Strong bias against the use of all psychotropic medication, which is still easy to find in the literature, ignores the fact that persons with developmental disabilities can suffer from the full range of mental illness seen in the other persons, that these illnesses can be very disabling, and that carefully used medication can enhance efforts aimed at normalization and habilitation (Schalock et al. 1985).

Medication use is no substitute for habilitative services. Drug use should not be used for staff convenience, for punishment, or at levels that interfere with habilitation (Intagliata and Rinch 1985). It can most easily be integrated into the habilitation process through a team approach aimed at finding the least restrictive form of behavioral management (Findholt and Emmett 1990).

The thoughtful application of several different kinds of intervention is the best treatment for some individuals. The final vignette describes a woman whose community psychiatric treatment has involved psychotherapy, behavioral interventions, and psychopharmacology. A multidisciplinary treatment team coordinates her care.

Case 6

A 52-year-old moderately mentally retarded woman was on high-dose antipsychotics for years at the state institution before moving to the community. She had a long history of aggression toward others and toward property, but evidence for psychosis was weak. Target symptoms were identified, and after data collection began, a behavioral plan was instituted. After she had spent a year in the community, the antipsychotic was tapered. She did not become psychotic. At first she was very anxious and broke property in the community, for which legal charges were brought. She then became sad and begged to return to the state institution (which had closed), saying she could not handle living in the community. She was diagnosed as suffering from a major depression and was treated with both an antidepressant and weekly psychotherapy by a psychiatric resident in the mental health center. In therapy, she talked about how unhappy and angry she was that she had to leave the institution where she was cared for and where little was expected of her. The therapy focused on mourning the loss of this safe and familiar environment. She gradually became more comfortable in the community, with a decrease in the intensity and frequency of her aggressive behavior.

Future Directions

I have outlined an approach to the psychiatric assessment, diagnosis, and treatment of developmentally disabled adults in the community and suggest the following key directions for the future:

1. Community psychiatrists are uniquely suited to contribute to the care of persons with developmental disabilities. Their experience caring for persons with severe mental illness prepares them for the challenges of the community care of persons with developmental disabilities. They can help developmentally disabled individuals gain access to important community resources through their established connections to psychiatric inpatient units, other mental health professionals, and other physicians. Community psychiatrists can overcome the obstacles to good care by having a practical approach in mind when the telephone rings with a referral.

2. Research into the development of a two-tiered diagnostic system would be extremely helpful (Gualtieri and Keppel 1985). Such a system would diagnose known psychiatric syndromes on the first tier and nonclassifiable behavior disturbance on the second tier. This would help researchers explore behavioral and psychopharmacological interventions for specific presentations and help clinicians identify and record exactly what is being treated.

3. Most psychiatrists need more training in the community care of persons with developmental disabilities. Formal education should begin early in residency and contain both didactic and clinical teaching. Many programs have no training at all in this area, perpetuating the notion that community care of persons with developmental disabilities does not fall within the province of psychiatry. More opportunities for fellowship training are needed to prepare clinicians and researchers to advance the knowledge base of this field.

4. Finally, political efforts are needed to forge better research and clinical alliances between mental health and mental retardation professionals. At many organizational levels, time and energy that could be applied to advancing this field are wasted in struggles over authority and responsibility. Finding ways to bypass these struggles and work together will significantly benefit persons with developmental disabilities and mental illness living in the community.

References

Aman MG, Singh NN (eds): Psychopharmacology of the Developmental Disabilities. New York, Springer-Verlag, 1988

American Psychiatric Association: Diagnostic and Statistical Manual of Mental Disorders, 4th Edition. Washington, DC, American Psychiatric Association, 1994

Bates WJ: Multimodal treatment of mental illness in institutionalized mentally retarded persons, in Handbook of Mental Illness in the Mentally Retarded. Edited by Menolascino FJ, Stark JA. New York, Plenum, 1984, pp 219–230

Benson BA, Reiss S, Layman DS: Psychosocial correlates of depression in mentally retarded adults, II: poor social skills and difficult life goals. Am J Ment Defic 89: 657–659, 1985

Borthwick-Duffy S, Eyman R: Who are the dually diagnosed? Am J Ment Retard 94:586–595, 1990

Braddock D: Deinstitutionalization of the retarded: trends in public policy. Hosp Community Psychiatry 32:607–615, 1981

Bregman S: Assertiveness training for mentally retarded adults. Psychiatric Aspects of Mental Retardation Reviews 4:43–48, 1985

Deutsch H: Stress, psychological defense mechanisms, and the private world of the mentally retarded: applying psychotherapeutic concepts to habilitation. Psychiatric Aspects of Mental Retardation Reviews 8:25–30, 1989

Eaton LF, Menolascino FJ: Psychiatric disorders in the mentally retarded: types, problems, and challenges. Am J Psychiatry 139:1297–1303, 1982

Eichelman B: Toward a rational pharmacotherapy for aggressive and violent behavior. Hosp Community Psychiatry 39:31–39, 1988

Farber JM: Psychopharmacology of self-injurious behavior in the mentally retarded. J Am Acad Child Adolesc Psychiatry 26:296–302, 1987

Findholt NE, Emmett CG: Impact of interdisciplinary team review on psychotropic drug use with persons who have mental retardation. Ment Retard 28:41–46, 1990

Fletcher RJ: Group therapy with mentally retarded persons with emotional disorders. Psychiatric Aspects of Mental Retardation Reviews 3:21–24, 1984

Fletcher RJ: The role of a day program in increasing support for dually diagnosed persons, in Mental Retardation and Mental Illness: Assessment, Treatment and Service for the Dually Diagnosed. Edited by Fletcher RJ, Menolascino FJ. Lexington, MA, DC Heath, 1989, pp 203–215

Fletcher RJ, Menolascino FJ: Introduction, in Mental Retardation and Mental Illness: Assessment, Treatment and Service for the Dually Diagnosed. Edited by Fletcher RJ, Menolascino FJ. Lexington, MA, DC Heath, 1989, pp ix–x

Fletcher RJ, Holmes PA, Keyes CB, et al: Linking research and practice: an integrated approach to the treatment of the dually diagnosed, in Mental Retardation and Mental Illness: Assessment, Treatment and Service for the Dually Diagnosed. Edited by Fletcher RJ, Menolascino FJ. Lexington, MA, DC Heath, 1989, pp 59–68

Gardner WI, Cole CL: Use of behavior therapy with the mentally retarded in community settings, in Handbook of Mental Illness in the Mentally Retarded. Edited by Menolascino FJ, Stark JA. New York, Plenum, 1984, pp 97–154

Griffiths D: Teaching social competency part 1: practical guidelines. The Habilitative Mental Healthcare Newsletter 9:1–5, 1990

Gualtieri CT: The differential diagnosis of self-injurious behavior in mentally retarded people. Psychopharmacol Bull 25:358–363, 1989

Gualtieri CT, Keppel JM: Psychopharmacology in the mentally retarded and a few related issues. Psychopharmacol Bull 21:304–309, 1985

Hall RC, Popkin MK, DeVaul RA, et al: Physical illness presenting as psychiatric disease. Arch Gen Psychiatry 35:1315–1320, 1978

Hingsburger D: Relationship training, sexual behavior, and persons with developmental handicaps. Psychiatric Aspects of Mental Retardation Reviews 8:33–37 1989

Hurley AD: Behavioral therapy for psychiatric disorders in mentally retarded individuals, in Mental Retardation and Mental Illness: Assessment, Treatment and Service for the Dually Diagnosed. Edited by Fletcher RJ, Menolascino FJ. Lexington, MA, DC Heath, 1989, pp 127–140

Hurley AD, Sovner R: Cognitive behavioral therapy for depression in individuals with developmental disabilities. The Habilitative Mental Healthcare Newsletter 10:41–47, 1991

Intagliata J, Rinch C: Psychoactive drug use in public and community residential facilities for mentally ill persons. Psychopharmacol Bull 21:268–278, 1985

Jacobson J: Problem behavior and psychiatric impairment in a developmentally disabled population, I: behavior frequency. Appl Res Ment Retard 3:121–139, 1982

Jacobson J, Ackerman L: An appraisal of services for persons with mental retardation and psychiatric impairments. Ment Retard 6:377–380, 1988

Kastner T, Friedman DL, O'Brien DR, et al: Health care and mental illness in persons with mental retardation. The Habilitative Mental Healthcare Newsletter 9:17–24, 1990

Kaufman R, Katz-Garris L: Epilepsy, mental retardation and anticonvulsant therapy. Am J Ment Defic 84:256–259, 1979

Landsberg G, Fletcher R, Maxwell T: Developing a comprehensive community care system for the mentally ill/mentally retarded. Community Ment Health J 23:131–134, 1987

Lapierre YD, Reesal R: Pharmacologic management of aggressivity and self-mutilation in the mentally retarded. Psychiatric Clin North Am 4:745–766, 1986

Levitas A, Gilson S: Psychodynamic psychotherapy with mildly and moderately retarded patients, in Mental Retardation and Mental Illness: Assessment, Treatment and Service for the Dually Diagnosed. Edited by Fletcher RJ, Menolascino FJ. Lexington, MA, DC Heath, 1989, pp 71–110

Linaker OM: Frequency of and determinants for psychotropic drug use in an institution for the mentally retarded. Br J Psychiatry 156:525–530, 1990

Lindenbaum L: A model for clinical training and supervision for mental health professionals treating dually diagnosed clients, in Mental Retardation and Mental Illness: Assessment, Treatment and Service for the Dually Diagnosed. Edited by Fletcher RJ, Menolascino FJ. Lexington, MA, DC Heath, 1989, pp 229–242

Ludwig S, Hingsburger D: Preparation for counselling and psychotherapy: teaching about feelings. Psychiatric Aspects of Mental Retardation Reviews 8:1–7, 1989

Matson JL: Social skills training. Psychiatric Aspects of Mental Retardation Reviews 3:1–5, 1984

Matson JL: Emotional problems in the mentally retarded: the need for assessment and treatment. Psychopharmacol Bull 21:258–261, 1985

Meadows G, Turner L, Campbell SW, et al: Assessing schizophrenia in adults with mental retardation: a comparative study. Br J Psychiatry 158:103–105, 1991

Menolascino FJ: Overview: promising practices in caring for the mentally retarded–mentally ill, in Mental Retardation and Mental Illness: Assessment, Treatment and Service for the Dually Diagnosed. Edited by Fletcher RJ, Menolascino FJ. Lexington, MA, DC Heath, 1989, pp 3–14

Menolascino FJ, Ruedrich SL, Golden CJ, et al: Diagnosis and pharmacotherapy of schizophrenia in the retarded. Psychopharmacol Bull 21:316–322, 1985

Menolascino FJ, Levitas A, Greiner C: The nature and types of mental illness in the mentally retarded. Psychopharmacol Bull 22:1060–1071, 1986

Monfils M: Group psychotherapy, in Mental Retardation and Mental Illness: Assessment, Treatment and Service for the Dually Diagnosed. Edited by Fletcher RJ, Menolascino FJ. Lexington, MA, DC Heath, 1989, pp 111–126

Monfils MJ, Menolascino FJ: Modified individual and group treatment approaches for the mentally retarded–mentally ill, in Handbook of Mental Illness in the Mentally Retarded. Edited by Menolascino FJ, Stark JA. New York, Plenum, 1984, pp 155–170

Parsons JA, May JG, Menolascino FJ: The nature and incidence of mental illness in mentally retarded individuals, in Handbook of Mental Illness in the Mentally Retarded. Edited by Menolascino FJ, Stark JA. New York, Plenum, 1984, pp 3–44

Reid AH: Psychosis in adult mental defectives, II: schizophrenia and paranoid psychosis. Br J Psychiatry 120:213–218, 1972

Reid AH: Psychiatry and mental handicap: a historical perspective. J Ment Defic Res 33:363–368, 1989

Reid AH, Ballinger BR: Personality disorder in mental handicap. Psychol Med 17:983–987, 1987

Reiss S: Psychopathology and mental retardation: survey of a developmental disabilities mental health program. Ment Retard 20:128–132, 1982

Reiss S, Benson BA: Psychosocial correlates of depression in mentally retarded adults, I: minimal social support and stigmatization. Am J Ment Defic 89:331–337, 1985

Reiss S, Levitan GW, Szyszko J: Emotional disturbance and mental retardation: diagnostic overshadowing. Am J Ment Defic 86:567–574, 1982

Ruedrich S, Menolascino FJ: Dual diagnosis of mental retardation and mental illness: an overview, in Handbook of Mental Illness in the Mentally Retarded. Edited by Menolascino FJ, Stark JA. New York, Plenum, 1984, pp 45–82

Russell A: Psychiatric treatment in mental retardation. Psychiatric Annals 19:184–189, 1989

Schalock RL, Foley JW, Toulouse A, et al: Medication and programming in controlling the behavior of mentally retarded individuals in community settings. Am J Ment Defic 89:503–509, 1985

Schalock RL, Harper RS, Carver G: Independent living placement: five years later. Am J Ment Defic 83:240–247, 1978

Schloss PJ: Verbal interaction patterns of depressed and nondepressed institutionalized mentally retarded adults. Appl Res Ment Retard 3:112, 1982

Schroeder SR: Neuroleptic medications for persons with developmental disabilities, in Psychopharmacology of the Developmental Disabilities. Edited by Aman MG, Singh NN. New York, Springer-Verlag, 1988, pp 82–100

Sovner R: Limiting factors in the use of DSM III criteria with mentally ill/mentally retarded persons. Psychopharmacol Bull 22:1055–1059, 1986

Sovner R: Treating mentally retarded adults with psychotropic drugs: a clinical perspective, in Mental Retardation and Mental Illness: Assessment, Treatment and Service for the Dually Diagnosed. Edited by Fletcher RJ, Menolascino FJ. Lexington, MA, DC Heath, 1989, pp 157–184

Sovner R: Prevalence of psychotropic drug therapy in institutional settings. The Habilitative Healthcare Newsletter 10:11–12, 1991

Sovner R, Hurley AD: Psychotropic drug therapy: an overview. Psychiatric Aspects of Mental Retardation Newsletter 2:17–19, 1983a

Sovner R, Hurley AD: Preparing for a mental health consultation. Psychiatric Aspects of Mental Retardation Newsletter 2:37–40, 1983b

Sovner R, Hurley AD: Discontinuing psychotropic drug therapy: rationale, guidelines, and side-effects. Psychiatric Aspects of Mental Retardation Reviews 3:41–44, 1984

Sovner R, Hurley AD: Ten diagnostic principles for recognizing psychiatric disorders in mentally retarded persons. Psychiatric Aspects of Mental Retardation Reviews 8:9–14, 1989

Sovner R, Hurley AD: Assessment tools which facilitate psychiatric evaluations and treatment. The Habilitative Mental Healthcare Newsletter 9:91–98, 1990a

Sovner R, Hurley AD: Affective disorder update. The Habilitative Mental Healthcare Newsletter 9:103–108, 1990b

Stark JA, McGee JJ, Menolascino FJ, et al: Treatment strategies in the habilitation of severely mentally retarded–mentally ill adolescents and adults, in Handbook of Mental Illness in the Mentally Retarded. Edited by Menolascino FJ, Stark JA. New York, Plenum, 1984, pp 189–218

Szymanski LS: Individual psychotherapy with retarded persons, in Emotional Disorders of Mentally Retarded Persons: Assessment, Treatment, and Consultation. Edited by Szymanski LS, Tanguay PE. Baltimore, MD, University Park Press, 1980, pp 131–147

Szymanski LS, Grossman H: Dual implication of "dual diagnosis." Ment Retard 22:155–156, 1984

Valenti-Hein DC: A dating skills program for adults with mental retardation. The Habilitative Mental Healthcare Newsletter 9:47–50, 1990

Chapter 10

Contemporary Treatment of Individuals With Chronic Mental Illness

Jerome V. Vaccaro, M.D.
Alexander S. Young, M.D.

I n another publication (Vaccaro et al. 1992c) we suggested that clinicians may be at the threshold of a major change in the care of individuals with chronic mental illnesses such as schizophrenia. The community mental health movement ushered in the belief that these individuals could be treated outside large institutions such as state hospitals. At first clinicians believed that these patients would respond to traditional office-based psychotherapeutic interventions. This view was later influenced by the community support movement, so that greater emphasis was placed on using techniques that were likely to be successful in helping these patients adapt to community living. We believe that the next paradigm shift in the community treatment of these patients will involve fuller incorporation of rehabilitative technologies, leading to greater reliance on methods and techniques such as structured functional assessment, social skills training, supported employment strategies, and other modalities.

Psychologists' understanding of psychopharmacological and psychosocial techniques continues to improve through innovation and research. More effective and less toxic medications have been discovered or are coming into widespread use, whereas rehabilitation technologies have been shown to improve social and vocational functioning. The role of the family has been strengthened, as has the alliance between professionals and consumers. Clinicians have also begun to appreciate that the design of their treatment systems has powerful effects on outcome. Finally, researchers have begun to acknowledge the importance of investigating global outcomes of treatment, including improved quality of life, reduced recidivism, skill acquisition, and vocational or occupational success.

This progress has been the result of a renewed interest in the treatment of persons with chronic mental illness. This interest has stemmed, in part, from a heightened appreciation of the enormous suffering and economic burden that accompany chronic mental illness. As attention has shifted from the "worried well" to the more severely ill, mental health organizations have struggled with ways to define this population. Labels used include *chronically mentally ill, seriously mentally ill, persistently mentally ill,* and others. People with these illnesses have been referred to as *patients, clients, consumers,* and *individuals.*

It is important to define chronic mental illness not only by diagnosis, but also by level of functioning. Indeed, the defining characteristic of these individuals is that they function poorly in interpersonal, social, and vocational spheres. They have severe deficits in functioning that often do not respect diagnostic boundaries. For the purposes of this chapter we will limit ourselves to one widely accepted definition of chronic mental illness: individuals with schizophrenia-spectrum illness and major mood disorders that result in significant functional impairment.

In this chapter we review components that should be part of any treatment program for persons with chronic mental illness (Vaccaro et al. 1993) and suggest ways that these components can be implemented, along with roles for the community psychiatrist. This begins with a discussion of treatment systems and their effect on treatment. There is evidence, for instance, that comprehensiveness and continuity of care are both clinically and economically effective. Next we examine the use of functional assessment in the development of a rehabilitation plan. We then discuss psychosocial technologies such as social skills training, vocational rehabilitation, and clinical case management. Finally, we assert the value of combining psychosocial treatments with psychopharmacological techniques. There is evidence, for instance, that combined approaches that employ psychopharmacological treatment and social skills training are effective in enhancing compliance and reducing relapse (Wirshing et al. 1991).

The Treatment System

Initially, efforts to treat chronically mentally ill individuals in community settings were limited by treatment models and techniques that did not address the specific challenges faced when chronically mentally ill individuals cope with life in the community. For example, early interventions were based on the individual psychotherapeutic paradigm, which stressed acquisition of insight, and were usually office-based, appointment-driven interventions. Psychiatrists now accept that these interventions, when used as the primary or sole modality, are ineffective in improving the course of serious mental illness (Gunderson et al. 1984). During this era, the locus of care shifted, but complementary shifts in treatment focus had not occurred, nor were appropriate models of care articulated or implemented (Stein 1988). The community support era ushered in a new focus, emphasizing the need to assist chronically mentally ill individuals as they struggle to live in the community. This change in focus implied that new models of treatment and rehabilitation were needed.

Currently accepted models of chronic mental illness hold that these conditions relapse and remit. Furthermore, the needs of individuals with these illnesses are varied and extensive. For example, when individuals with schizophrenia are reliably compliant with medication regimens, their annual relapse rates are still more than 40%. Combined approaches that link pharmacotherapy with other psychosocial interventions such as social skills training can further reduce this rate to about 20% (Hogarty et al. 1986). Studies suggest that this rate can be further reduced and quality of life enhanced when case management is added to this matrix of services (Vaccaro et al. 1992a).

Many mental health systems of care are better equipped to treat acute episodes of illness than they are to provide lifelong care for chronic illnesses. This is particularly true in those systems where there are ineffective links among the various treatment system components. This has resulted in public mental health systems that are widely regarded as both inefficient and ineffective. Reactions to these perceptions have included management of mental health financing and the development of practice guidelines (Chapters 2 and 18). Public Law 99-660, which mandated that state mental health systems implement coordinated systems of community mental health care, also addressed these concerns. This has been implemented through the development of local mental health authorities, integrated entitlement programs, and capitated payment systems (Lehman 1989). Most of these result, on the clinical level, in some form of continuous treatment team (Torrey 1986). These multidisciplinary teams continuously follow cohorts of patients across treatment settings, creating "functional bridges" among treatment and rehabilitation services.

Diagnostic and Symptomatic Assessment

Through the use of structured instruments and specific probes, diagnosis of chronic mental illness has become progressively more refined. Schizophrenia has been overdiagnosed in some populations and underdiagnosed in others. This resulted from unclear or conflicting diagnostic schemes; disagreement regarding boundaries among these illnesses; neglect; and, in some cases, bias. Clinicians now have available a reasonably clear diagnostic system, DSM-IV (American Psychiatric Association 1994), which is widely used in clinical settings, and structured diagnostic instruments that accompany this manual (Structured Clinical Interview for Diagnosis). These structured instruments have heretofore been used primarily in research settings but are simple and clear enough to use in clinical settings. In addition, we have instruments that can be used for the routine monitoring of psychiatric symptoms. For instance, the Brief Psychiatric Rating Scale (BPRS) (Overall and Gorham 1988) is appropriate for clinical use, and various self-report instruments have been developed.

It is our view that these instruments are underutilized in clinical settings. We advocate the use of standardized instruments in clinical settings for diagnostic and symptom assessment, as they can guide treatment efforts. For example, a psychiatrist can use a modified version of the BPRS to monitor psychotic symptoms and tailor the dose of an antipsychotic medication. This facilitates the treatment of focal and well-defined symptoms and overcomes the problems inherent in treating a globally characterized illness. This is depicted in the following case vignette.

> Joe is a 34-year-old man with a schizophrenic illness. He has been unhappy with past medication regimens, complaining that he has experienced troublesome side effects with several classes of neuroleptics. He is seen by a psychiatrist, who performs a careful assessment of his symptoms using questions from the BPRS that gauge the frequency and intrusiveness of auditory hallucinations. On the first visit the psychiatrist learns that Joe hears voices commenting on his

behavior throughout the day and that they trouble him greatly and cause him to act in a bizarre manner. The psychiatrist begins by prescribing a low dose of medication and gradually titrates this dose upward until the voices are heard rarely (less than once per week), are "not very loud," and do not cause any behavioral problems. This careful approach is greatly appreciated by Joe and leads to full compliance with the prescribed regimen.

Functional Assessment and Rehabilitation Planning

It has become clear that the patient must play an active role in his or her recovery (Strauss et al. 1987). Efforts to rehabilitate individuals with chronic mental illnesses will fail unless they are linked to 1) the life goals and roles that patients identify for themselves, 2) the skills patients possess that help them achieve these goals, and 3) the behavioral deficits or disturbances that may impede personal growth and progress. These data make up the functional assessment. Functional assessment steers psychiatric treatment and rehabilitation through its many phases, allowing the practitioner to target interventions to the patient's state of impairment and disability. Once impairments such as psychiatric symptoms or cognitive deficits are identified, specific interventions, such as pharmacotherapy, skills training, or social prostheses, can be linked to targeted problems.

Depending on the nature of the service setting and the roles of psychiatrists and other caregivers, the psychiatrist's contribution to and participation in the process of functional assessment will vary. In any case, it is important that the psychiatrist at least be familiar with the concept and some of the instruments used in functional assessment. In most settings the psychiatrist will contribute information to the functional assessment but will neither be the sole assessor nor the individual responsible for its coordination. Typically, the psychiatrist is asked to assess the level of disability and handicap created by the patient's symptoms and medication side effects; the interference with functioning caused by specific behavioral disturbances; and cognitive impairments that impede rehabilitation. We recommend that psychiatrists read basic information about functional assessment (Vaccaro et al. 1992b), obtain and review functional assessment instruments (preferably those used in the psychiatrist's own setting), and negotiate roles for themselves with other key individuals.

Social Skills Training

Social skills training is a form of psychotherapy that is informed by behavioral and learning theories. It is the most highly structured form of psychosocial treatment for individuals with chronic mental illness. Goals are explicitly stated (e.g., to teach medication management or conversational skills), sessions are planned in advance, procedures such as role playing and structured problem solving are employed, and in vivo and homework exercises are used to enhance generalization of skill usage to other life areas. Group formats are most effective, as they provide opportunities for vicarious learning and a built-in "buddy system" for completing homework (Liberman et al. 1986).

Controlled studies have yielded convergent findings regarding the efficacy of social skills training (Benton and Schroeder 1990). It has been found that individuals learn the skills taught and retain this knowledge and skill over extended periods of time and that their relapse rates are reduced, particularly when combined with sound pharmacotherapy. To spur widespread use of this technology, user-friendly, modularized social skills training packets have been developed. These include training manuals, video-assisted programs, and use of other novel approaches.

In addition to such highly prescriptive approaches, less structured approaches to social skills training have been characterized in the literature. Hierholzer and Liberman (1986) articulated an approach in which the principles and practice of social skills training are employed to teach participants the problem-solving skills they need to negotiate daily living. This "successful living group" format can be used to set treatment and rehabilitation goals.

It is our view that the psychiatrist should be proficient in the provision of social skills training, even though he or she may not provide this service with great frequency in most settings. If psychiatrists are to lead clinical efforts for these patients, then their clinical competencies must be broad and include familiarity, through direct experience, with the multiple treatment modalities used with this population. This competency may be obtained by attending professional training seminars in this area coupled with co-leading social skills training groups with more experienced skills trainers.

Vocational Rehabilitation

For the most part, vocational rehabilitation involving persons with serious mental illness has been ignored or relegated to obscurity in mental health systems. Early approaches stressed hospital-based work programs as the main-stays of intervention. This sheltered approach was hindered by virtue of its "dead-end" jobs that offered no future and taught few marketable work skills. Later, the community mental health movement of the 1960s created an op-portunity to move hospital-based vocational programs toward more main-stream activities. However, this potential was never realized. Thus, transitional employment programs, such as those in Fountain House–type psychosocial re-habilitation centers, evolved independently and often without much input from mental health or rehabilitation professionals. This isolation still exists, with most psychiatric treatment systems neglecting the area of vocational rehabilitation.

Vocational rehabilitation has entered a renaissance marked by the emer-gence of the supported employment movement. The federally sponsored supported employment initiative springs from the understanding that indi-viduals with psychiatric disabilities require ongoing services, such as train-ing in the skills necessary to maintain employment, once they secure competitive employment. It deemphasizes the importance of what has been labeled "prevocational" training, advocating instead a "place-train" ap-proach. Patients are placed in employment settings and then offered train-ing necessary to maintain their positions. In its fully applied form, individuals are offered services indefinitely, with "job coaches" visiting them at their workplaces to help them learn and retain the technical, interpersonal, and problem-solving skills they need to sustain employment. Job coaching con-sists of three types of interventions: skill development, service coordination, and employer consultation. During the continuing phases of employment, participants are visited by a job coach, who guides the worker in the use of the work and social and independent living skills he or she has learned.

Although still in its early stages, empirical work in the vocational rehabilita-tion arena has evolved to a point where important directions for future develop-ment can be summarized. Transitional employment programs have increased the length of continuous time that seriously mentally ill individuals are able to sustain employment. Programs that employ job coaching have demonstrated some efficacy in helping seriously mentally ill individuals maintain employ-ment and improve their instrumental role functioning. In summary, clearer models of supported employment and job coaching have to be articulated and tested among diagnostically and functionally distinct groups of patients.

Clinical Case Management

It is generally accepted that persons with chronic mental illness require cer-tain supports to live in the community. These supports must prospectively anticipate their needs, advocate for and provide linkage to services to meet these needs, coordinate care, and teach community living skills. Assertive forms of clinical case management have been shown to be effective in coordinating care, minimizing relapse and recidivism, and maintaining community tenure (Test 1992). Case managers provide services in the community, often outside their offices, and stress the prospective anticipation of patient needs coupled with active and assertive intervention.

Although case management is widely regarded to be a desired service for individuals with chronic mental illness, models of delivery vary widely. Different case management definitions place varying emphasis on advocacy, service linkage, counseling, and skills development. In addition, integration of innovative rehabilitation technologies (e.g., social skills training) with case management has not been fully realized or tested. Research in the field of case management has been carried out, but the limited number of published empirical studies have serious methodological problems, and most do not adequately define the form and process of the case management they report.

Family Interventions

As a result of the deinstitutionalization movement, most individuals with serious mental illness currently rely heavily on their families for emotional sustenance, financial support, and guidance in daily living. Not surprisingly, the burden of caring for an adult relative who requires supervision and whose behavior may be chaotic, incomprehensible, or hostile often results in extreme family distress. The recognition that families serve a vital role in supporting the rehabilitation of persons with serious mental illnesses has spurred enthusiasm for providing both the patient and his or her relatives with treatment to maximize community reintegration.

This interest has been strengthened by studies that have established that family attitudes can influence the prognosis of relatives with chronic mental illness. These attitudes have been termed *expressed emotion* (EE). Relatives and other care providers (for example, investigators have examined this construct among residential care facility and hospital staff) can be classified as either high or low EE based on the presence, during a structured interview (Vaughn and Leff 1976), of critical or hostile comments and descriptions of overinvolved, self-sacrificing behavior. Many cross-cultural prospective studies have established that patients from high-EE families tend to relapse

50%–100% more frequently in the 9 months following an acute exacerbation than those from low-EE families (Parker and Hadzi-Pavlovic 1990). Some have hypothesized that negative affect or intrusiveness triggers relapses and that contact with families with high levels of ambient stress precipitates more relapses. Others have argued that EE signifies the extreme burden of caring for the chronically mentally ill, and that it is not at all surprising that high levels of EE are normative in many Western societies. Although most EE research has focused on individuals with schizophrenia, studies indicate that there is probably a similar effect on the course of bipolar illness. In one study, Koenigsburg et al. (1993) documented the validity of this construct among families of diabetic patients.

Some early reports suggested that families bore responsibility for their relatives' relapses, and that families might somehow be inherently high in expressed emotion. More contemporary views, however, hold that this over-simplified position regarding etiology is unwarranted. Thus, the emergence of "high expressed emotion" may be seen as a response of a taxed care system to a debilitating and demoralizing illness. This uncertainty regarding etiology has not dampened enthusiasm for developing interventions to reduce high EE levels and improve family coping with the pernicious effects of chronic mental illness. Family-based interventions can have a significant, positive impact on persons with serious mental illness and frequently on their relatives as well (Hogarty et al. 1986). Indeed, relapse rates in patients assigned to family treatment are typically only one-third to one-half of those in patients participating in alternative treatment groups. Although the validated family intervention programs are diverse, they share several important characteristics (Vaccaro et al. 1993):

- Embedding the family intervention in a comprehensive psychiatric rehabilitation program
- Providing basic information on the symptoms, treatments, etiology, and prognosis in serious mental illness
- Advocating psychotropic medication compliance
- Minimizing insight or family systemic change as a therapeutic goal
- Strongly emphasizing the development of patients' and relatives' realistic expectations for recovery and stress management skills

The findings from investigations of these skills-oriented, family-based interventions have been very impressive. They highlight the mutually beneficial effects of effective psychopharmacological interventions and structured psychosocial programs with clearly defined, realistic goals.

Combining Psychosocial and Pharmacological Therapies

The optimal use of pharmacotherapy for individuals with chronic mental illness requires that it be tightly linked with other services in a comprehensive psychosocial treatment system. It is also clear, however, that effective treatment requires that the psychiatrist use the latest medications and techniques. Psychopharmacological interventions have become more refined, and studies indicate that low-dose and targeted strategies offer clear advantages over more standard approaches. Collaboration among informed patients, their families, and the psychiatrist decreases relapse and enhances outcome. In addition, there is evidence that combined therapies offer synergistic benefits, reducing relapse rates to as low as half the rate for either therapy alone. In recent years, we and other collaborators have developed and tested techniques to teach patients the skills they need to act as effective collaborators in such strategies as those involving reduced dosages or targeted dosing of neuroleptics (Liberman et al. 1993). The following case vignette illustrates this point.

> Bill is a 23-year-old man with a 5-year history of schizophrenia. He resisted taking medication because of the side effects he had experienced, including severe akathisia, tremors, and muscle stiffness. He acknowledged that these medications had diminished his psychotic symptoms and improved his attention and concentration, but resisted efforts to increase his compliance with prescribed regimens. He also related that some of his psychotic symptoms, particularly auditory hallucinations, persisted at a low level despite altered doses and types of medications. Bill had been hospitalized an average of three times per year for psychotic exacerbations since the onset of his illness. He communicated his perception that all efforts to treat him "missed the boat" and that staff had not attended to his goals and ambitions.
>
> At this point, staff engaged Bill in a goal-setting process in which he identified goals of living independently without being hospitalized, taking little or no medication, and eventually getting a job. His psychiatrist and social worker supported these goals and set out to establish clear and measurable landmarks to gauge his success in the pursuit of these aims. With this accomplished, they worked with Bill to identify his strengths and the obstacles he faced in attaining his goals. Bill said that the most frustrating problem was his lack of understanding about his illness and its treatment, as this led to frequent relapses and concomitant life disruption.

Bill's psychiatrist and social worker next enrolled him in a class designed to increase his understanding of his illness and the medications used to treat it. He gained a working knowledge of the way in which these medications caused the side effects he found so intolerable, and he learned skills that would help him effectively negotiate the type and dosage of his medication with his physician. Following this, he worked with his psychiatrist and chose a low-dose alternative treatment that involved taking injections of long-acting neuroleptics every 4 weeks. Finally, he was taught ways in which he could manage the persisting auditory hallucinations he experienced. This led Bill to feel a sense of mastery over his illness, and he remained compliant with medications for the next year. He experienced two minor relapses, sought help from treatment personnel early in the course of these relapses, and did not require rehospitalization.

The key features of the preceding example were that Bill's goals and personal desires were solicited, respected, and incorporated into the treatment plan; his resistance to medication was confronted in a straightforward, nonjudgmental, problem-solving manner; and he was taught skills he needed to become an effective collaborator in his own treatment and rehabilitation. This occurred in a multidisciplinary treatment team context, and Bill was seen continuously by the same group of treatment providers. This process may be separated into overlapping stages.

First, *the patient must be fully educated about the indications for the medication he or she is being prescribed and the benefits to be expected.* This should be accomplished using clear, simple language and repeating information over a number of sessions to ensure adequate learning. For example, a patient should be specifically told the symptomatic relief to be expected, such as diminished auditory hallucinations, improvement of mood (e.g., lessened dysphoria), and the time it will take to see these effects. Overly vague or global statements such as "you'll feel better," "your depression will go away soon," or "your illness will improve" should be avoided without clarifying remarks that provide greater detail and accuracy.

Next, *the patient should be taught about the side effects of his or her medication, using the same level of detail used for beneficial effects.* For example, the clinician should explain the full array of side effects in a supportive, reassuring manner, giving details about their relative frequencies and likelihood of occurrence. Finally, the patient should be taught the necessary skills so that he or she is able to negotiate successfully with the psychiatrist about choice of medication, dosing, and other related matters. With this approach, patients are more likely to comply with recommendations and approach the psychiatrist with their concerns.

Table 10–1.   Common symptoms and signs that precede relapse in schizophrenia

Sleep disturbance	Greater sensitivity to criticism
Difficulty concentrating	Distractibility
Irritability	Increased use of alcohol or other drugs
Confusion	

Once the patient is fully educated about the prescribed medications, the psychiatrist can use the same approaches to *develop an effective relapse prevention strategy.* We have had considerable success in this regard when dividing this segment of treatment into several phases. In the first phase the patient identifies prodromal symptoms that precede relapses. A list such as that in Table 10–1 is used to prompt dialogue and stimulate the patient's memory of events. Once a set of "warning signs" is articulated, the patient is taught to monitor these regularly and record this monitoring on a daily basis. During visits with the psychiatrist, these forms are reviewed, and patterns indicative of relapse are detected in advance of full relapse, allowing for early intervention. Also during this process, the patient identifies any persisting symptoms so that the psychiatrist-patient team can test psychopharmacological and psychosocial strategies to reduce the symptoms. If the symptoms are resistant to treatment, the team develops alternative coping strategies to counteract the disabilities caused by the symptoms.

Psychopharmacology and Rehabilitation

Significant advances have been made in the pharmacotherapy of previously refractory depression, bipolar illness, and schizophrenia. The treatment of depression has been advanced by the development of new medications, such as the selective serotonin reuptake blockers, that cause markedly fewer side effects. Efficacy has also been improved by the judicious use of combinations of antidepressant medications (Bernstein 1988). The treatment of bipolar illness has benefited from significant advances in the understanding of the use of lithium (Gitlin 1992) and from the widespread use of new agents, such as carbamazepine and valproate.

Although the treatment of mood disorders has improved, advances in the pharmacotherapy of schizophrenia are of even more importance to the community practitioner. Traditional neuroleptics have been available for more than 30 years, but only recently have their side effects begun to be fully appreciated (Marder et al. 1991). Elucidating these side effects has been difficult because neuroleptics are known to improve some positive and negative symptoms while causing others. Traditional neuroleptics can cause parkinsonism, apathy, anhedonia, dysphoria, akathisia, and sexual dysfunction. Although parkinsonism and akathisia can sometimes be controlled with medication, other side effects are generally more resistant to treatment. Fortunately, these side effects are generally dose-dependent and occur most often at doses above 10–15 mg of haloperidol per day. Higher doses than this are rarely indicated for more than a few days. High doses, including those used in "rapid neuroleptization," are counterproductive and can lead to treatment noncompliance and worsening of psychosis (Van Putten et al. 1992). In addition, social and vocational functioning may worsen on higher doses of neuroleptics (Hogarty et al. 1988).

Because neuroleptics may have adverse effects at moderate doses, clinicians should carefully assess treatment effect and titrate dosages accordingly. Optimal doses for patients can be found by weighing beneficial and adverse effects. It is not uncommon for the optimal dose to be below that needed to remove all positive symptoms. Maximal functioning may be achieved even when the patient continues to have some psychotic symptoms. Therefore, it is crucial that patients be taught to recognize symptoms and side effects and to communicate these to their physicians. Although such education can be time consuming, it is feasible (Liberman et al. 1986).

Depot neuroleptics may also be used to increase compliance. These should be considered in all individuals with schizophrenia and not simply reserved as the treatment of last resort for the noncompliant patient. Patients should be told that depot agents make medication compliance easier and often reduce the exposure to neuroleptics by facilitating precise dose reduction. Clinicians need to be aware that patients must continue oral medications for several months after starting a depot agent, as three to five doses of a decanoate preparation may be needed before a steady state is reached.

Novel Neuroleptics and Rehabilitation

Although neuroleptic nonresponse can be difficult to accurately define, it is apparent that 10%–40% of persons with schizophrenia get little or no benefit from traditional neuroleptics. These "nonresponders" are often given extremely high doses of neuroleptics in an effort to control symptoms or sedate the patient. A small group of patients may actually need these doses to achieve adequate concentrations of neuroleptic at receptor sites, but most experience disabling side effects.

When confronted with a patient who is nonresponsive at typical doses, several strategies should be considered. First, behavioral control can often be achieved with a combination of low-dose neuroleptic and a potent benzodiazepine (such as clonazepam). In addition, Kuehnel et al. (1992) have had success with the use of behavioral therapies to compensate for persistent psychosis. These behavioral therapies make use of a token economy, brief time-outs, social skills training, and relaxation techniques. It is often necessary to lower neuroleptic doses before rehabilitation is possible, as troublesome side effects such as decreased cognitive abilities impair learning.

An emerging approach to neuroleptic refractoriness is the use of novel agents such as clozapine. Clozapine has been shown to be effective in about one-third of patients refractory to traditional neuroleptics. Until relatively recently it has been used in only a fraction of eligible patients. Several factors prevent its more widespread use. First, it is relatively expensive, leading public agencies at the federal, state, and local levels to resist shifting scarce resources to funding clozapine use. Discrimination has contributed to this: although clinical technologies of equal or lower effectiveness for physical illnesses are readily funded (e.g., coronary bypass surgery), public agencies are used to treating the seriously mentally ill with small budgets. Clozapine is also difficult to use and more dangerous than traditional neuroleptics. Therefore, psychiatrists have shied away from it because of the training, time, and risk that accompanies its use.

Many patients on clozapine experience symptom reduction, including fewer psychotic symptoms and less of the dysphoria, apathy, and anhedonia that accompany the use of traditional neuroleptics. These symptom reductions make rehabilitation essential, as individuals who have had positive and negative symptoms for many years suddenly find themselves symptomatically improved, but without the necessary skills for successful community living. We have even seen some patients who discontinue clozapine when they find themselves unprepared for life. These individuals are ideally suited for social skills training, vocational rehabilitation, and other psychosocial technologies.

Summary and Conclusions

The treatment and rehabilitation of individuals with chronic mental illness have undergone rapid change since the mid-1980s. We currently accept that these individuals are able to regain at least a modest degree of social and occupational functioning if optimal care is provided. To design and implement such care, we believe that the treatment setting and system, as well as the content of the treatment, are key to success. Treatment systems should ensure that care is provided continuously and without interruption across service settings, and should employ a comprehensive array of interventions.

The comprehensive array of interventions should be arranged in a user-friendly format, so that patients and their families are able to access care that is appropriate to their contemporary needs. This set of available services includes pharmacotherapy linked with psychosocial interventions including clinical case management, social skills training, vocational rehabilitation, and family support and treatment.

The psychiatrist's role in the community-based care of individuals with chronic mental illnesses will vary somewhat based on the availability of other services and the value placed on the psychiatrist's contributions. We advocate that the psychiatrist lead through clinical competence, which suggests that the psychiatrist must have knowledge of and skill in delivering the many treatment modalities we have described. He or she may not actually deliver these treatments but might supervise other clinicians in their work, assist in the design of effective clinical programs, and offer medical interventions that enhance and do not impair psychosocial interventions. Finally, the psychiatrist should advocate both for an effective services mix and a more productive role for the psychiatrist in community settings.

References

American Psychiatric Association: Diagnostic and Statistical Manual of Mental Disorders, 4th Edition. Washington, DC, American Psychiatric Association, 1994

Benton MK, Schroeder HE: Social skills training with schizophrenics: a meta-analytic evaluation. J Consult Clin Psychol 58:741–747, 1990

Bernstein JG: Drug Therapy in Psychiatry, 2nd Edition. Chicago, IL, Year Book Medical, 1988

Gitlin MJ: Lithium: serum levels, renal effects, and dosing strategies. Community Ment Health J 28:355–362, 1992

Gunderson JG, Frank AF, Katz HM, et al: Effects of psychotherapy in schizophrenia, II: comparative outcome of two forms of treatment. Schizophr Bull 10:564–598, 1984

Hierholzer R, Liberman R: Successful living: a social skills and problem-solving group for the chronic mentally ill. Hosp Community Psychiatry 37:913–918, 1986

Hogarty GE, Anderson CM, Reiss DJ, et al: Family psychoeducation, social skills training, and maintenance chemotherapy in the aftercare treatment of schizophrenia, I: one-year effects of a controlled study on relapse and expressed emotion. Arch Gen Psychiatry 43:633–642, 1986

Hogarty GE, McEvoy JP, Munetz M, et al: Dose of fluphenazine, familial expressed emotion, and outcome in schizophrenia: results of a two-year controlled study. Arch Gen Psychiatry 45:797–805, 1988

Koenigsburg HW, Klausner E, Pelino D, et al: Expressed emotion and glucose control in insulin-dependent diabetes mellitus. Am J Psychiatry 150:1114–1115, 1993

Kuehnel T, Liberman R, Marshall B, et al: Optimal drug and behavior therapy for treatment-refractory institutionalized schizophrenics. New Dir Ment Health Serv 53:67–78, 1992

Lehman AF: Strategies for improving services for the chronic mentally ill. Hosp Community Psychiatry 40:916–920, 1989

Liberman RP, Mueser K, Wallace CJ, et al: Training skills in the severely psychiatrically disabled: learning coping and competence. Schizophr Bull 12:631–647, 1986

Liberman RP, Wallace CJ, Blackwell G, et al: Innovations in social skills training for the seriously mentally ill: the UCLA Social & Independent Living Skills Modules. Innovations & Research 2:43–59, 1993

Marder SR, Wirshing WC, Van Putten T: Drug treatment of schizophrenia: overview of recent research. Schizophr Res 4:81–90, 1991

Overall J, Gorham D: The Brief Psychiatric Rating Scale (BPRS): recent developments in ascertainment and scaling. Psychopharmacol Bull 24:97–99, 1988

Parker G, Hadzi-Pavlovic D: Expressed emotion as a predictor of schizophrenic relapse: an analysis of aggregated data. Psychol Med 20:961–965, 1990

Stein LI: It's the focus, not the locus. Hocus pocus (letter)! Hosp Community Psychiatry 39:1029, 1988

Strauss JS, Harding CM, Hafez H, et al: The role of the patient in recovery from psychosis, in Psychosocial Treatment of Schizophrenia: Multidimensional Concepts, Psychological, Family, and Self-Help Perspectives, Edited by Strauss JS, Boker W, Brenner HD. Lewiston, NY, Hans Huber Publishers, 1987, pp 160–166

Test MA: Training in community living, in Handbook of Psychiatric Rehabilitation, Edited by Liberman RP. New York, Macmillan, 1992, pp 153–170

Torrey EF: Continuous treatment teams in the care of the chronic mentally ill. Hosp Community Psychiatry 37:1243–1247, 1986

Vaccaro JV, Liberman RP, Wallace CJ, et al: Combining social skills training and assertive case management: the Social and Independent Living Skills program of the Brentwood Veterans Affairs Medical Center. New Dir Ment Health Serv 26:33–42, 1992a

Vaccaro JV, Pitts DB, Wallace CJ: Functional assessment, in Handbook of Psychiatric Rehabilitation. Edited by Liberman R. New York, Macmillan, 1992b, pp 78–94

Vaccaro JV, Liberman RP, Roberts LJ: Schizophrenia: from institutionalization to community reintegration, in The Mosaic of Contemporary Psychiatry in Perspective. Edited by Kales A, Pierce CM, Greenblatt M. New York, Springer-Verlag, 1992c, pp 269–280

Vaccaro JV, Young AS, Glynn S: Community-based care of individuals with schizophrenia: combining psychosocial and pharmacologic therapies. Psychiatr Clin North Am June:387–399, 1993

Van Putten T, Marder SR, Mintz J, et al: Haloperidol plasma levels and clinical response: a therapeutic window relationship. Am J Psychiatry 149:500–505, 1992

Vaughn CE, Leff JP: The measurement of expressed emotion in the families of psychiatric patients. Br J Soc Clin Psychol 15:157–165, 1976

Wirshing WC, Eckman T, Liberman RP, et al: Management of risk of relapse through skills training of chronic schizophrenics, in Advances in Neuropsychiatry and Psychopharmacology, Vol 1: Schizophrenia Research. Edited by Tamminga C, Schultz S. New York, Raven, 1991, pp 255–267

Chapter 11

Substance Abuse: Assessment and Treatment in Community Psychiatry

Michael J. Bohn, M.D.
Michael T. Witkovsky, M.D.

I n this chapter we present a practical approach to the assessment and treatment of patients with alcohol and drug use disorders in the community mental health center (CMHC) setting. This approach emphasizes a multidimensional assessment to facilitate appropriate patient-treatment matching and stresses a flexible pharmacological and psychosocial treatment plan. It can be adapted to different stages of treatment of the patient with an alcohol or drug use disorder.

Background

Community surveys in the United States and other developed countries have reported that alcoholism and drug abuse are among the most highly prevalent psychiatric disorders. In the Epidemiologic Catchment Area (ECA) study of more than 20,000 U.S. residents, the lifetime prevalence of abuse and dependence was 13% for alcohol and 8% for drugs (Robins et al. 1984). The corresponding 1-month prevalence figures were 2.8% and 1.3% for alcoholism and drug abuse, respectively (Regier et al. 1988). Among those

ECA respondents treated in ambulatory settings, 44.8% received treatment in an outpatient mental health clinic or crisis center for a mental health or addiction-related reason, accounting for a projected 56.3 million visits annually (Narrow et al. 1993). Similar findings have been reported in other surveys regarding service utilization (Manderscheid et al. 1993).

Mental illnesses and substance use disorders frequently occur in the same individual. In the ECA study, almost one-third of those with a substance use disorder also met criteria for a concurrent psychiatric disorder (Regier et al. 1990). Among clinical populations of alcoholics (Hesselbrock et al. 1985) and drug addicts (Rounsaville et al. 1982; Weiss et al. 1986), the prevalence of coexisting psychiatric disorders, particularly anxiety, and affective, and antisocial personality disorders, is even higher. Approximately half of visits to mental health centers were devoted to care of individuals who had both a mental illness and a substance use disorder.

Thus, a primary goal of community psychiatrists and other mental health practitioners is the comprehensive assessment of all patients seeking mental health services to detect and treat concurrent substance use disorders. This in turn should facilitate the coordinated treatment of both types of disorders.

Assessment

Assessment of the alcoholic or drug-abusing patient is an ongoing process and must build on a trusting and nonjudgmental relationship with the patient. Careful studies have demonstrated that a calm, empathic, and detailed inquiry significantly increases the accuracy of information reported by the patient and enhances treatment outcome (Miller and Sovereign 1989). In contrast, harsh confrontation can powerfully increase the use of both denial and minimization and often contributes to treatment dropout.

The first purpose of assessment is to reliably establish the diagnosis and thereby facilitate initial treatment planning. DSM-IV criteria (American Psychiatric Association 1994) for substance use disorders can be reliably applied in the interview of patients, including the majority of those with coexisting psychiatric conditions (Bryant et al. 1992). The interviewer should include questions regarding the quantity, frequency, and routes of administration of a variety of types of beverage alcohol; agents in each major drug class; and prescription sedatives, opioids, and stimulants. The frequency of heavy drinking (e.g., consumption of six or more drinks/day) should also be obtained, as heavy drinking increases the risk of trauma (Kranzler et al. 1990). Both the motivations for alcohol and/or drug use and the negative

ment. Persistence of a major depressive disorder, however, is associated with

consequences of substance use should be evaluated. A history of significant tolerance, substance-specific withdrawal syndromes, and use of the substance to prevent or alleviate withdrawal symptoms should be assessed. Dependent patients frequently report a history of uncontrolled and continued use of the substance in the face of repeated adverse physical, psychological, or social consequences of its use. Even in the absence of physical dependence, the patient's drinking or drug use may lead him or her to neglect hobbies, work, or other rewarding activities. In addition to information provided by the patient, reports from reliable collateral informants should be elicited.

Physical examination remains a mainstay in evaluation of the patient with a substance use disorder. Intoxication may be revealed by ataxia due to sedatives, whereas miosis may indicate opiate intoxication. Withdrawal from sedatives or alcohol is suggested by hypertension, diaphoresis, and tremor, whereas opiate withdrawal is marked by mydriasis, rhinorrhea, and piloerection. Physical examination should include a search for conditions resulting from substance use (e.g., infectious or alcoholic hepatitis). Urine or blood testing (e.g., drug screening or serum gamma-glutamyltransferase [GGT] level determination) should be routinely considered to corroborate the history and physical examination findings.

Specific psychiatric disorders are common among alcoholics, opiate addicts, and cocaine abusers. These include depressive and anxiety disorders and antisocial personality disorder (ASP). Thus, patients with a substance use disorder should be routinely assessed for symptoms of these concurrent disorders. In addition to their high prevalence, symptoms of these disorders confer a poor prognosis following inpatient or outpatient substance abuse treatment (McLellan et al. 1983). Knowledge about comorbid psychopathology can improve patient-treatment matching. For example, alcoholics with these psychiatric symptoms respond more favorably to cognitive-behavior treatment for alcoholism and less favorably to interpersonal psychotherapy for alcoholism. Conversely, patients with few of these symptoms respond more favorably to interpersonal psychotherapy than to cognitive-behavior alcoholism treatment (Kadden et al. 1989).

Beyond the global importance of symptoms of psychiatric distress, assessment of particular psychiatric disorders is important to improved substance abuse treatment planning. Depressive and anxiety symptoms are common among substance abusers, but most of the depression and anxiety seen in alcoholics and drug abusers is secondary to substance use itself. Depressive and anxiety symptoms typically resolve spontaneously during the first 3-4 weeks of abstinence, even without specific psychiatric treatment. Persistence of a major depressive disorder, however, is associated with a poor prognosis among alcoholic and opiate-dependent men (Rounsaville et al. 1986, 1987). However, major depression appears to confer a relative protection from relapse in alcoholic women (Rounsaville et al. 1987).

In contrast to mood and anxiety disorder symptoms, ASP typically begins prior to the onset of a substance use disorder and does not remit with abstinence. Sociopathic patients have great difficulty establishing trust, tolerating strong affect, and accepting feedback from peers. This makes them prone to drop out of treatment programs that rely heavily on psychosocial treatments emphasizing these factors. Indeed, ASP has repeatedly been associated with high relapse rates among alcoholics and drug abusers (Alterman and Cacciola 1991; Rounsaville et al. 1986, 1987). Development of trust early in psychotherapy with a sociopathic drug abuser can enhance treatment outcome (Woody et al. 1985). Among alcoholics, a high degree of sociopathy predicts superior outcomes following skills training, whereas interactive treatment is more effective for those with lower degrees of sociopathy (Kadden et al. 1989; Litt et al. 1992).

A variety of physical conditions occur at high rates among alcoholics and drug addicts. Thorough assessment of these conditions is important to improve the patient's health, reduce motivation for relapse owing to physical distress, and increase the capacity for social functioning. Evidence suggests that even among chronic public alcoholics with severe alcohol-associated medical conditions, coordinated treatment involving medical care, case management, and alcohol relapse prevention techniques can substantially improve morbidity and lessen homelessness and mortality (Sisson and Azrin 1989; Willenbring et al. 1991).

The patient's current motivations for seeking treatment should be assessed, including external motivations such as legal mandates, threatened job dismissal, and family discord. Current evidence indicates that patients who are persuaded, encouraged, or even coerced into treatment by meaningful persons, such as spouses, children, or supportive employers are more likely to remain in treatment and have a better prognosis than those not so pressured. Thus, an external motivation may provide opportunities for support and deterrence against a pattern of relapse. Minimally, the therapist can initiate a process to enhance the patient's own motivation to change by exploring both internal and external motivating factors.

The patient's own goals in seeking treatment should be given significant weight in treatment planning. For example, some patients are unwilling to endorse abstinence as an initial treatment goal and may experience considerable satisfaction after substantially reducing their drinking. With continued encouragement and development of alternative leisure activities, they may experiment with increasingly prolonged periods of abstinence and ultimately find little reason to continue drinking.

Prior substance use and relapses should be assessed. Relapses are often associated with interpersonal conflict, social pressure, physical discomfort, negative or positive affect, and craving for alcohol or drugs (Marlatt and Gordon 1980).

Family, social, employment, and legal problems should also be assessed. Stressful events such as unemployment or family discord increase the risk of relapse (Kosten et al. 1986; Vaillant 1983), particularly when social support is poor. Self-help groups such as Alcoholics Anonymous (AA) provide social support, which is often invaluable in maintaining abstinence.

Treatment

Many patients who have substance use disorders appear poorly motivated to change their addictive behavior. Short-term outcome following treatment for addictive disorders often involves brief (and occasionally prolonged or problematic) relapses to alcohol or drug use. Relapse can be viewed as less defeating for both practitioner and patient when appreciated from within the following model describing changes in addictive behavior (Prochaska and DiClemente 1986): The substance abuser begins in a state of *precontemplation,* in which they do not perceive a problem is present. They progress through an ambivalent stage of *contemplation,* in which they acknowledge that a problem is present but have low motivation for change. The next is a stage of *determination,* in which they decide to change their behavior or seek treatment. They may then enter a stage of *action,* beginning treatment and altering their substance use, typically by attempting at least brief periods of abstinence. In the *maintenance* stage, the challenge is to avoid a return to use or a problematic relapse. *Relapse,* which is common and often demoralizing, poses a challenge to recover quickly and return to the process of action and maintenance. Viewed broadly, the goal of substance abuse treatment is to increase the motivation to change and to have the patient progress toward the maintenance stage of change.

There are a variety of effective treatment approaches for alcoholism and drug abuse (Hester and Miller 1989; Hubbard et al. 1989). In discussing treatment options, we begin by describing effective pharmacological and psychosocial treatment approaches applicable at various stages of treatment. We then discuss principles that are important in planning integrated treatment based on the patient's current motivation and needs. Third, we discuss the importance of a multidimensional assessment of patient outcome during treatment. Finally, we discuss broadly the role of the community mental health center and particularly the role of the community psychiatrist in care of the patient with a substance use disorder.

Pharmacological Treatment

Current data indicate that psychotropic medications are useful in 1) treatment of intoxication resulting from opiates, stimulants, or hallucinogens; 2) detoxification from alcohol, sedatives, and opiates; 3) reduction of the risk of relapse among patients dependent on alcohol and opiates; and 4) treatment of selected comorbid psychiatric conditions among patients with substance use disorders.

Any potentially intoxicated patient should have a thorough medical examination, including a toxicological examination if clinically indicated, together with supportive measures and gavage. Patients with opiate intoxication as a result of intentional or accidental overdose should be monitored for potentially fatal respiratory depression and should be treated aggressively with repeated 0.4-mg intravenous (iv) doses of naloxone if respiratory depression occurs. For amphetamine or phencyclidine intoxication, which typically are manifested by marked agitation and psychosis, lorazepam 1 mg iv and haloperidol 1 mg iv are often effective (Chang and Kosten 1992).

Treatment of alcohol withdrawal, which is characterized by signs of anxiety and autonomic hyperactivity, is primarily directed toward relief of distress and prevention of withdrawal seizures and delirium. Frequent monitoring, supportive measures such as fluid and thiamine replacement, and avoidance of stimulation are often helpful. In most cases of mild or moderate withdrawal, these measures alone are effective. More severe cases benefit from treatment with benzodiazepines (e.g., diazepam 10 mg orally every 1–4 hours), with subsequent judicious tapering of the dose over 3–5 days. Carefully monitored outpatient detoxification of uncomplicated alcohol withdrawal can be accomplished safely and at substantial cost savings compared with inpatient detoxification. Effective medications useful in outpatient detoxification include diazepam 10 mg orally every 1–4 hours or oxazepam 15 mg every 6 hours.

Similar pharmacotherapeutic treatment is often sufficient for sedative withdrawal, which can be life threatening. Barbiturate withdrawal should be more aggressively treated with pentobarbital and phenobarbital following establishment of initial barbiturate dose requirements (Wesson et al. 1992).

Opiate withdrawal, characterized by autonomic hyperactivity and a flu-like syndrome, is rarely life threatening. Inpatients can be treated with a brief course of methadone 10–40 mg daily initially, with the dose tapered over 3–13 days. Outpatients can be treated with clonidine 0.1–0.2 mg every

4 hours for up to 1 mg on day 1, followed by tapering over 2–7 days. Care must be exercised to avoid hypotension following the initial clonidine dose (Kleber 1994). Successful opiate detoxification will lessen patient distress and reduce the short-term relapse risk of opiate addicts.

Medications may also assist appropriately selected alcoholics and drug abusers to avoid a relapse. Although medications appear to enhance outcomes for patients receiving psychosocial substance abuse rehabilitation, current evidence indicates that, when used alone, medications are minimally effective in reducing substance abuse relapses.

Disulfiram is effective in reducing alcoholic relapses among abstinent alcoholics. Disulfiram's efficacy is largely due to the potential for a disulfiram-alcohol reaction (DER) following drinking. A typical dose is 250 mg daily. This medication appears to be best suited for patients without medical contraindications (including rubber allergy, severe liver disease, or angina pectoris) who are both well motivated and not taking other medications. Supervised administration of this medication or use of other means to enhance compliance is critical to its efficacy. Because it is an irreversible inhibitor of aldehyde dehydrogenase, disulfiram-treated patients should be cautioned that they may have a DER if they drink during the 1- to 2-week period following their last dose. Patients taking disulfiram should undergo periodic monitoring of serum transaminase levels and should be monitored for emergence of peripheral neuropathy and psychosis, which have been reported.

When combined with psychosocial rehabilitation for alcoholism, the oral opiate antagonist naltrexone in a dosage of 50 mg/day appears to reduce drinking relapses and may reduce the desire for a drink in some subjects (O'Malley et al. 1992; Volpicelli et al. 1992). To avoid induction of opiate withdrawal, patients receiving naltrexone treatment should have abstained from opiates for 2 weeks. Patients with severe hepatic dysfunction and those requiring opiate treatment for relief of pain (e.g., following elective surgery) should not be treated with naltrexone.

Pharmacotherapy can also substantially enhance the long-term stability of detoxified opiate addicts. The opiate agonists methadone and *l*-alpha-acetyl-methadol (LAAM), the mixed agonist/antagonist buprenorphine, and the antagonist naltrexone are effective in preventing relapse to intravenous opiate use (O'Brien 1994; Senay 1994). At adequate doses (e.g., 60 mg daily), methadone maintenance reduces use of (and craving for) intravenous opiates such as heroin. This in turn reduces human immunodeficiency virus (HIV) infection risk and is associated with increased employment, reduced illegal activity, and improved social functioning. Naltrexone, in dosages of 50 mg daily to 150 mg every 3 days, blocks the effects of exogenous opiates such as heroin and is effective in reducing opiate use following opiate detoxification. However, methods to ensure compliance, similar to those described for disulfiram, are often needed for this medication to be effective among opiate addicts.

Antidepressants may also improve outcomes for appropriately selected abstinent substance abusers. Some alcoholic patients have a primary major depression (i.e., one that antedates their alcoholism or that has been present during periods of prolonged abstinence). For such patients, treatment with adequate doses of a tricyclic antidepressant such as desipramine 150–250 mg/day has been shown to reduce both symptoms of depression and the risk of alcoholic relapse (Mason and Kocsis 1991). Persistently depressed opiate addicts benefit from imipramine treatment at similar doses, demonstrating both reduced heroin use and reduced depressive symptoms (Kleber et al. 1983). Despite favorable reports from early and uncontrolled studies, evidence indicates that antidepressants are not more effective than placebos in treatment of cocaine-dependent patients (Meyer 1992). In treatment of substance abusers with antidepressants, it is important to closely monitor serum antidepressant levels, particularly because alcoholics and drug abusers often smoke and have hepatic dysfunction, which may speed their metabolism of antidepressants.

Psychosocial Treatment

As with pharmacological treatments, a full description of the variety of effective psychosocial treatments for alcoholism and drug abuse is beyond the scope of this chapter. We will limit our discussion to four approaches that are commonly employed in outpatient treatment of alcoholism and drug abuse. We will discuss 1) brief prescriptive counseling, 2) motivational enhancement therapies, 3) 12-step treatments, and 4) cognitive-behavior therapies (including relapse prevention skills training). Clearly, many effective treatments consist of combinations of these types, and flexibility in treatment of substance abusers is often invaluable.

Brief prescriptive counseling.   Brief counseling is primarily useful in treatment of heavy drinkers who are not physically dependent on alcohol (Heather 1989). Most commonly, the physician/therapist and patient review the objective evidence of the harmful effects that drinking has produced. This may involve review of abnormal laboratory results such as an elevated serum GGT level or mean corpuscular volume, job difficulties, family arguments, and other objective data. The patient is then advised to attempt a reduction in drinking or a period of experimental abstinence from alcohol. If the patient agrees to a goal of reduced drinking, the specific circumstances surrounding episodes of drinking are identified, alternative activities that may be substituted for drinking are suggested, and methods for counting drinks and planning days of abstinence are negotiated. Typically, brief counseling involves one to six sessions during a 6- to 24-month period. These brief intervention methods yield a substantial treatment effect, evidenced by reduced GGT level and other laboratory abnormalities, as well as reductions in drinking, work abstinence, hospital use, and death.

Motivational enhancement therapies. Motivational interviewing is a substantially different, nonprescriptive approach. It is intended to enhance the patient's awareness of the consequences of his or her substance use and to create cognitive dissonance, which may enhance his or her motivation to reduce or stop substance use (Miller and Rollnick 1991). Objective data from the assessment are presented without conclusion. Labels such as *alcoholic* are deemphasized. Resistance is met with reflection designed to highlight the risks and benefits of continued or reduced substance use. The responsibility for the patient's behavior is seen as a matter of personal choice, autonomy is not challenged, and recommendations are not made. Goals, including moderation of use, are negotiated, and the patient is nondirectively encouraged to monitor him- or herself and to return for future planning sessions. Although many of the principles employed in this approach are broadly applicable in treatment of the substance abuser, this approach may have particular usefulness for socially stable patients who are ambivalent regarding abstinence and for those who have relatively mild problems due to their substance use.

Twelve-step treatments. Interpersonal approaches commonly rely on group formats to facilitate mutual self-examination of patients, often emphasizing principles of AA and related 12-step groups. This approach is particularly suited to patients for whom abstinence is the goal and those who are relatively articulate, self-reflective, spiritually oriented, and possess at least moderate social skills. Twelve-step groups view substance abuse as a disease over which the individual is powerless, urge patients to accept the label of being alcoholic or an addict, and then help the patient seek renewal through self-reflection and spiritual awakening. Self-disclosure, confrontation of apparent denial, and involvement with other abstinent substance abusers (as peers or sponsors) are commonly encouraged. Therapists facilitate members' exploration of their reactions to behavior of other group members. Typically, members are urged or required to attend 12-step group meetings frequently, in addition to attendance at therapist-facilitated groups.

Patients with coexisting mental illnesses may find it difficult to participate in 12-step groups such as AA. Despite the publication of AA literature indicating that medically monitored treatment with psychotropic medications is necessary for sober recovery of many alcoholics, many AA members have discouraged their mentally ill peers to discontinue psychotropic medications, often with adverse results. Thus, it is particularly important that psychiatrists and other mental health providers attend local AA groups and educate AA members. The indications for psychotropic treatment, risks of unmonitored medication discontinuation, and need for open dialogue regarding the benefits and risks of ongoing psychotropic medication treatment of substance abusers with coexisting psychiatric disorders should be addressed. In some cases, it is useful for CMHCs to assist in the establishment of new self-help groups specifically oriented to the needs of mentally ill substance abusers.

Cognitive-behavior therapies.   A broad variety of cognitive-behavior strategies have proven useful in treatment of patients dependent on alcohol, cocaine, opiates, and a variety of other drugs. In relapse prevention treatment (Monti et al. 1989), high-risk situations are identified and antecedents to drinking or drug use are reviewed. Emergency coping strategies, including avoidance of high-risk situations (e.g., conditioned cues for craving or use) and limiting access to alcohol and drugs, are emphasized. Therapists provide training in cognitive methods for reducing craving, anxiety, depression, and anger and teach behavioral methods to improve time management and pursuit of sober, pleasant leisure activities. In addition, assertiveness, communication, and other social skills, including drink and drug refusal, are practiced. Homework is prescribed following rehearsal of these skills, and self-efficacy is monitored. Specific problems encountered, including brief relapses, are viewed as opportunities to learn from one's mistakes, rather than as indications of powerlessness or failure. This treatment is probably most effective for socially stable patients who do not have marked cognitive impairment and for those with coexisting sociopathy or other psychiatric conditions.

For more chronically ill or unemployed patients, these methods have been successfully enhanced by a community reinforcement approach (Sisson and Azrin 1989). In this approach, members join a job club, are involved in a recreational center, take disulfiram or other medication to reduce substance abuse, and are involved in couples communication skills counseling with their spouse. All these treatments are contingent on continued abstinence. Considerable success has been achieved using this method with recidivist alcoholics. Evidence suggests that a comprehensive treatment approach involving the addition of psychiatric and psychosocial treatment markedly enhances the effectiveness of methadone maintenance treatment (McLellan et al. 1993).

Planning Integrated Treatment

To be effective, treatment planning must address the objective treatment needs of the patient, the patient's own internal motivation, and the readiness of the patient to make a change in his or her life. The first step in treatment planning must be the assessment of the self-acknowledged substance abuser. In addition, other patients presenting in the CMHC should be evaluated for substance use disorders, as approximately 20%–30% have undetected alcohol or drug use disorders. Several brief yet sensitive screening questionnaires have been developed and used in this population, including the Michigan Alcoholism Screening Test (Selzer 1971) and the Drug Abuse Screening Test (Skinner 1982).

Treatment results may be improved by considering the patient's stage of readiness to change his or her substance abuse patterns. Patients in the precontemplation stage have little internal motivation to reduce their alcohol or drug use, and treatment should focus on the development of a trusting relationship during a period of systematic, regular examination of the effects of alcohol or drug use on the patient's life. Motivational enhancement strategies may be useful for treatment of patients at the contemplation stage, particularly if there is no evidence of severe physical or cognitive dysfunction. In addition, the psychiatrist must be prepared to prevent or treat intoxication, withdrawal states, and behavioral crises such as suicide attempts in such patients. Maintenance of abstinence can be facilitated by any of the psychosocial or pharmacological approaches described above. None of the pharmacotherapies is incompatible with a particular psychosocial approach, although 12-step approaches must often be modified if methadone-maintained patients are to be accepted by the group. Patient preference, staff training and beliefs, and pretreatment assessment of comorbid psychopathology should guide treatment modality selection. For those patients who have substantial acute physical or psychiatric illness or those who have failed aggressive outpatient treatment, residential or hospital treatment may be indicated. There is no substantial benefit from routine inpatient treatment of alcoholics or drug addicts, although the cost of treatment is much higher than for outpatient treatment.

Monitoring Outcome

It is particularly important to monitor not only alcohol and drug use but also other areas of patient functioning during and following substance abuse treatment. Improvement in alcohol or drug use and associated problems is often related to improvement in psychiatric symptoms but is only weakly related to improvement in social functioning, employment, and legal difficulties for many patients. Thus, self-reported consumption of alcohol and drugs, supplemented by objective evidence (e.g., urine toxicological testing, serum GGT) or collateral informant reports should be monitored, as should health status; psychological symptoms; and legal, employment, and family relationship problems. Follow-up interviews are time consuming and difficult but provide information about the effectiveness of treatment and are essential to improving treatment approaches.

Role of the CMHC and Community Psychiatrist

Despite the high prevalence of alcoholism and drug abuse in the CMHC setting, some CMHC staff view the treatment of substance abuse problems as lying outside their domain. This schism has several origins. Psychiatrists and other community mental health practitioners have typically received little training in diagnosis and treatment of substance use disorders. Historically, funding and advocacy for mental health and substance abuse treatment have been separated. Philosophical differences have widened the gap. Ironically, many mental health professionals who find little difficulty accepting relapses as part of chronic mental illnesses have viewed relapses to alcohol and drug use as evidence of the lack of efficacy of substance abuse treatment per se. Conversely, substance abuse treatment providers have too often viewed even prescribed use of psychotropic medications as indicative of ongoing drug abuse and have rigidly insisted on an initial commitment to abstinence as a condition of provision of any outpatient substance abuse treatment. Finally, many professionals continue to view alcoholism and drug abuse as "willful misconduct," resulting in therapeutic nihilism.

The primary role of the psychiatrist in the CMHC setting is to facilitate the identification and assessment of the needs of the substance abuser and to act as a member of the treatment team. Psychiatrists and other community mental health providers can play a significant role in staff development, enhancing both the psychiatric assessment and treatment skills of substance abuse counselors and the substance abuse assessment and treatment skills of mental health treatment providers. Psychiatrists are particularly well suited to assist in the development of conjoint or integrated treatment plans for mentally ill substance abusers. As such, appropriate medical and psychotropic treatment and monitoring are common roles for the psychiatrist.

Among the most significant of medical treatment needs of substance abusers is the risk of HIV infection and acquired immunodeficiency syndrome (AIDS). Intravenous drug abuse, alcoholism, and chronic mental illness are commonly associated with needle sharing and high-risk sexual behaviors. Psychiatrists should train patients and staff in risk reduction techniques; assist in identification of infected individuals; and provide assessment and treatment for HIV-associated psychiatric conditions, including major depression, substance abuse, anxiety disorders, and dementia (Fernandez and Ruiz 1992).

It is essential that the psychiatrist be familiar with and collaborate with vocational rehabilitation, occupational therapy, and other professionals to achieve a comprehensive treatment program for substance abusers. The CMHC may assist the patient by facilitating ongoing liaison with other community agencies and organizations, such as AA and other self-help groups, halfway houses, and detoxification centers. Clearly, a major role of the CMHC is to provide uninterrupted and longitudinal care for those with substance use disorders. This may necessitate assertive case management and outreach for isolated, homeless, or highly recidivist substance abuse patients.

Summary

In this chapter we have discussed the high prevalence of substance use disorders, which are often complicated by significant psychiatric comorbidity. Individuals with these disorders utilize substantial mental health and addiction treatment resources, often in the community mental health setting. Effective treatment planning first hinges on accurate identification of individuals at risk and assessment of their frequently multiple areas of poor functioning. Appropriate selection of both psychosocial and pharmacological strategies depends on assessment of both substance use and other psychiatric disorders. Treatment matching can then contribute to improved patient outcomes and cost savings. The community psychiatrist can thus play an integral role as a member of a coordinated treatment team caring for the patient with a substance use disorder.

References

Alterman AI, Cacciola JS: The antisocial personality disorder diagnosis in substance abusers: problems and issues. J Nerv Ment Dis 179:401–409, 1991

American Psychiatric Association: Diagnostic and Statistical Manual of Mental Disorders, 4th Edition. Washington, DC, American Psychiatric Association, 1994

Bryant KJ, Rounsaville B, Spitzer RL, et al: Reliability of dual diagnosis: substance dependence and psychiatric disorders. J Nerv Ment Dis 180:251–257, 1992

Chang G, Kosten TR: Emergency management of acute drug intoxication, in Substance Abuse: A Comprehensive Textbook, 2nd Edition. Edited by Lowinson JH, Ruiz P, Millman RB, et al. Baltimore, MD, Williams & Wilkins, 1992, pp 437–444

Fernandez F, Ruiz P: Neuropsychiatric complications of HIV infection, in Substance Abuse: A Comprehensive Textbook, 2nd Edition. Edited by Lowinson JH, Ruiz P, Millman RB, et al. Baltimore, MD, Williams & Wilkins, 1992, pp 775–787

Heather N: Brief intervention strategies, in Handbook of Alcoholism Treatment Approaches: Effective Alternatives. Edited by Hester RK, Miller WR. New York, Pergamon, 1989, pp 93–116

Hesselbrock MN, Meyer RE, Keener JJ: Psychopathology in hospitalized alcoholics. Arch Gen Psychiatry 42:1050–1055, 1985

Hester RK, Miller WR: Handbook of Alcoholism Treatment Approaches: Effective Alternatives. New York, Pergamon, 1989

Hubbard RL, Marsden ME, Rachal JV, et al: Drug Abuse Treatment: A National Study of Effectiveness. Chapel Hill, NC, University of North Carolina Press, 1989

Kadden RM, Cooney NL, Getter H, et al: Matching alcoholics to coping skills or interactional therapies: posttreatment results. J Consult Clin Psychol 57:698–704, 1989

Kleber HD: Opioids: detoxification, in The American Psychiatric Press Textbook of Substance Abuse Treatment. Edited by Galanter M, Kleber H. Washington, DC, American Psychiatric Press, 1994, pp 191–208

Kleber HD, Weissman MM, Rounsaville BJ, et al: Imipramine as treatment for depression in addicts. Arch Gen Psychiatry 40:649–653, 1983

Kosten TR, Rounsaville BJ, Kleber HD: A 2.5-year follow-up of depression, life crises, and effects on abstinence among opioid addicts. Arch Gen Psychiatry 43:733–738, 1986

Kranzler HR, Babor TF, Lauerman R: Problems associated with average alcohol consumption and frequency of intoxication in a medical population. Alcohol Clin Exp Res 14:119–126, 1990

Litt MD, Babor TF, DelBoca FK, et al: Types of alcoholics: application of an empirically derived typology to treatment matching. Arch Gen Psychiatry 49:609–614, 1992

Manderscheid RW, Rae DS, Narrow WE, et al: Congruence of service utilization estimates from the Epidemiologic Catchment Area Project and other sources. Arch Gen Psychiatry 50:108–114, 1993

Marlatt GA, Gordon JR: Determinants of relapse: implications for the maintenance of behavior change, in Behavioral Medicine: Changing Health Lifestyles. Edited by Davidson P, Davidson S. New York, Brunner/Mazel, 1980, pp 410–452

Mason BJ, Kocsis JH: Desipramine treatment of alcoholism. Psychopharmacol Bull 27:155–161, 1991

McLellan AT, Luborsky L, Woody GE, et al: Predicting response to alcohol and drug abuse treatments: role of psychiatric severity. Arch Gen Psychiatry 40:620–625, 1983

McLellan AT, Arndt IO, Metzger DS, et al: Are psychosocial services necessary in substance abuse treatment? JAMA 269:1953–1959, 1993

Meyer RE: Pharmacotherapy for cocaine dependence revisited. Arch Gen Psychiatry 49:904–907, 1992

Miller WR, Rollnick S: Motivational Interviewing: Preparing People to Change Addictive Behavior. New York, Guilford, 1991

Miller WR, Sovereign RG: The check-up: a model for early intervention in addictive behaviors, in Addictive Behaviors: Prevention and Early Intervention, Edited by Løberg T, Miller WR, Nathan PE, et al. Amsterdam, The Netherlands, Swets & Zeitlinger, 1989, pp 219–231

Monti PM, Abrams DB, Kadden RM, et al: Treating Alcohol Dependence. New York, Guilford, 1989

Narrow WE, Regier DA, Rae DS, et al: Use of services by persons with mental and addictive disorders: findings from the National Institute of Mental Health Epidemiologic Catchment Area Program. Arch Gen Psychiatry 50:95–107, 1993

O'Brien CP: Opioids: antagonists and partial agonists, in The American Psychiatric Press Textbook of Substance Abuse Treatment. Edited by Galanter M, Kleber H. Washington, DC, American Psychiatric Press, 1994, pp 223–236

O'Malley S, Jaffe AJ, Chang G, et al: Naltrexone and coping skills therapy in the treatment of alcohol dependence: a controlled study. Arch Gen Psychiatry 49:881–887, 1992

Prochaska JO, DiClemente CC: Toward a comprehensive model of change, in Treating Addictive Behaviors: Processes of Change. Edited by Miller WR, Heather N. New York, Plenum, 1986, pp 3–27

Regier DA, Boyd JH, Burke JD, et al: One-month prevalence of mental disorders in the United States. Arch Gen Psychiatry 45:977–986, 1988

Regier DA, Farmer ME, Rae DS, et al: Comorbidity of mental disorders and other drug abuse: results from the Epidemiologic Catchment Area study. JAMA 264:2511–2518, 1990

Robins LN, Helzer JE, Weissman MM, et al: Lifetime prevalence of specific psychiatric disorders in three sites. Arch Gen Psychiatry 41:949–958, 1984

Rounsaville BJ, Weissman MM, Kleber HD, et al: Heterogeneity of psychiatric diagnosis in treated opiate addicts. Arch Gen Psychiatry 39:161–166, 1982

Rounsaville BJ, Kosten TR, Weissman MM, et al: Prognostic significance of psychopathology in treated opiate addicts: a 2.5-year follow-up study. Arch Gen Psychiatry 43:739–745, 1986

Rounsaville BJ, Dolinsky ZS, Babor TF, et al: Psychopathology as a predictor of treatment outcome in alcoholics. Arch Gen Psychiatry 44:505–513, 1987

Selzer ML: The Michigan Alcoholism Screening Test: the quest for a new diagnostic instrument. Am J Psychiatry 127:1653–1658, 1971

Senay EC: Opioids: methadone maintenance, in The American Psychiatric Press Textbook of Substance Abuse Treatment. Edited by Galanter M, Kleber H. Washington, DC, American Psychiatric Press, 1994, pp 209–221

Sisson RW, Azrin NH: The community reinforcement approach, in Handbook of Alcoholism Treatment Approaches: Effective Alternatives. Edited by Hester RK, Miller WR. New York, Pergamon, 1989, pp 242–258

Skinner HA: The Drug Abuse Screening Test: Guidelines for Administration and Scoring. Toronto, Ontario, Canada, Addiction Research Foundation, 1982

Vaillant G: The Natural History of Alcoholism. Cambridge, MA, Harvard University Press, 1983

Volpicelli JR, Alterman AI, Hayashida M, et al: Naltrexone and the treatment of alcohol dependence. Arch Gen Psychiatry 49:876–880, 1992

Weiss RD, Mirin SM, Michael JL, et al: Psychopathology in chronic cocaine abusers. Am J Drug Alcohol Abuse 12:17–29, 1986

Wesson DR, Smith DE, Seymour RB: Sedative-hypnotics and tricyclics, in Substance Abuse: A Comprehensive Textbook. Edited by Lowinson JH, Ruiz P, Millman RB, et al. Baltimore, MD, Williams & Wilkins, 1992, pp 271–279

Willenbring ML, Ridgely MS, Stinchfield R, et al: Application of Case Management in Alcohol and Drug Dependence: Matching Techniques and Populations. Rockville, MD, ADAMHA, 1991

Woody GE, McLellan AT, Luborsky L, et al: Sociopathy and psychotherapy outcome. Arch Gen Psychiatry 42:1081–1086, 1985

Chapter 12

Dual Diagnosis in Seriously and Persistently Mentally Ill Individuals: An Integrated Approach

Kenneth Minkoff, M.D.

T he goal of this chapter is to provide a clear and pragmatic approach to the assessment, diagnosis, and treatment of dual-diagnosis patients in community mental health care systems. The emphasis will be on utilizing a unified conceptual framework (Minkoff 1989) in which substance disorders and major mental illnesses can each be viewed as examples of primary biological chronic mental illnesses that both fit into a disease and recovery (or illness and rehabilitation) model of treatment. Clinical examples will illustrate the application of this model to assessment, diagnosis, and treatment.

Prevalence

Patients with the dual diagnosis of serious mental illness and substance disorder (abuse or dependence) have become increasingly prevalent in community mental health service systems since the mid-1980s. Measures of the prevalence of substance disorders in chronically mentally ill populations have ranged from 32% to 65% for abuse and from 15% to 40% for dependence (Alterman 1985; Caton et al. 1989; Drake et al. 1989; Pepper et al. 1981; Safer 1987; Schwartz and Goldfinger 1981). The Epidemiologic Catchment

Area (ECA) study found that 47% of individuals with a lifetime diagnosis of schizophrenia had met criteria for a substance disorder. These figures rose to 55% for schizophrenic patients in treatment and 62% for patients with affective disorder (Regier et al. 1990). Clearly, these figures suggest that the presence of dual diagnosis in treatment populations is so common that it must be expected, rather than considered an exception. If caffeine and nicotine are included as substances of abuse, this statement can be made even more strongly.

Terminology

Numerous terms have been used (with great variability in different locations) to describe this population, including *dual diagnosis, dual disorder, comorbidity, mentally ill chemical abuser and addict (MICAA), chemical-abusing mentally ill, mentally ill substance abuser,* and *psychiatrically ill substance abuser.* There is no consensus on a single label, and in fact, the terms are often used with great inconsistency. It is not uncommon, for example, for the term *dual diagnosis* to be applied to substance-dependent individuals with coexisting psychiatric symptoms (e.g., depression, anxiety, hallucinations), even when such symptoms do not warrant a separate diagnosis of psychiatric illness. Consequently, it is advisable that all terms be carefully defined and patient populations clearly specified.

Reasons for the High Prevalence of Dual Diagnosis

Although increased awareness has certainly heightened recognition of this problem, the real increase in this population has been due to the combined effects of deinstitutionalization and the expanded acceptance and availability of drugs—particularly cocaine and potent hallucinogens—in American culture during the 1970s and 1980s. For mentally ill patients in the community, drug and alcohol use may represent an effort to alleviate or self-medicate symptoms of mental illness or medication side effects (Schneier and Siris 1987), to facilitate socialization (Bergman and Harris 1985), and to develop an identity more acceptable than that of mental patient (Drake et al.

1991a, 199b; Lamb 1982). People with schizophrenia report that substance use relieves dysphoria, boredom, anxiety, isolation, and emptiness more consistently than psychotic symptoms—not unlike non–mentally ill substance abusers. (Dixon et al. 1990; Noordsy et al. 1991). In addition, many patients were heavy drug and alcohol users prior to the onset of mental illness (Caton et al. 1989) and in many cases continue to abuse substances even though such abuse may have contributed to the onset of their psychotic illness. Consequently, as Drake et al. (1991a) pointed out, the reasons for initial use and the immediate benefits of use "should be differentiated from the factors that sustain . . . use" after problems arise. In fact, much of the literature reflects the view that substance abuse and dependence are autonomous and self-sustaining primary disorders, rather than secondary to the underlying illness or dysphoria that may contribute to the initial reasons for use (Lehmann et al. 1989; Minkoff 1989; Osher and Kofoed 1989).

Course and Outcome

Longitudinal data regarding outcome for dual-diagnosis patients is sparse (Turner and Tsuang 1990). Nonetheless, most cross-sectional studies indicate that, in general, substance abusing mentally ill patients do worse, with more severe psychiatric symptoms (F. C. Osher, R. E. Drake, D. L. Noordsy, et al., unpublished manuscript, 1991); more disruptive, self-destructive, and violent behavior (Drake et al. 1989; McCarrick et al. 1985), including criminality (Safer 1987); more problems with housing instability and homelessness (Drake and Wallach 1989; Minkoff and Drake 1994); and more noncompliance with medication and treatment (Drake and Wallach 1989). They have been described as "system misfits" (Bachrach 1987) who are nonresponsive to traditional interventions and are more at risk for relapse, rehospitalizations, treatment rejection, and treatment failure.

Barriers to Care

After initial recognition of the contribution of dual diagnosis to the problems of the young adult chronic patient (Pepper et al. 1981), Alcohol, Drug Abuse and Mental Health Administration (ADAMHA) commissioned a nationwide review of the research, treatment, and training needs of this population. The resulting reports (Ridgely et al. 1986, 1987) made it clear that a major contributor to poor outcome was the failure of the treatment system to address dual diagnosis appropriately. The alcohol and drug abuse treatment systems and the mental health system are organized separately at the federal, state, and local levels (Ridgely et al. 1990) and often have competing philosophies concerning the role of self-help, the use of medication, and the roles of various mental health professionals. Each system has tended to identify the disease it treats as "primary" and symptoms of the other as "secondary" and thus to focus treatment on only the primary illness. Dual-diagnosis patients are often given "ping pong therapy"; they are extruded from each system because of the presence of comorbidity (Ridgely et al. 1990). At best, care is rarely integrated; instead, patients may receive sequential treatment (that is, stabilized in one system and then referred to the other) or parallel treatment in both systems with little coordination. Caregivers have typically been trained in only one field (mental health or chemical dependency), and frequently the case management approach of mental health clinicians (with aggressive outreach to be responsible for providing help for the patient and his or her needs) clashes with the detachment approach of addiction counselors, who let the patient "hit bottom" in order to assume responsibility for him- or herself and for asking for help for his or her own needs. Most community mental health centers (CMHCs), in particular, have had few available resources for integrated treatment of dual-diagnosis patients, although this is slowly but steadily beginning to change (see later discussion).

Unified Conceptual Framework: Disease and Recovery Model

According to Minkoff (1989), major mental illnesses and substance dependence can both be viewed as examples of chronic biological mental illnesses which, despite differences in specific symptoms and treatments, share significant common characteristics that define the process of treatment and recovery. Specific parallels are listed in Table 12–1. These include both characteristics of the illness itself (i.e., chronicity, incurability, progression, treatability, lack of control of thought, behavior, and emotion) and characteristics of the individual's (and family's) reaction to the illness (i.e., denial, minimization, shame, guilt, stigma, sense of failure, denial of chronicity,

Table 12–1.   Common features of psychosis and addiction

A biological illness
Hereditary (in part)
Chronic
Incurable
Leads to lack of control of behavior and emotions
Affects the entire family
Symptoms can be controlled with proper treatment
Disease of denial
Disease progresses without treatment
Facing the disease can lead to depression and despair
Disease is often seen as a "moral issue" resulting from personal weakness
    rather than biological causes
Feelings of guilt and failure
Feelings of shame and stigma
Physical, mental, and spiritual disease

control by "will power"). The basic tasks of treatment for either type of
illness are to stabilize acute symptoms, engage the patient in a program of
treatment (e.g., medication for psychosis, Alcoholics Anonymous [AA] for
alcoholism) to prevent relapse, and then to foster rehabilitation and growth
over time, thus, for each illness there are parallel phases of recovery, as listed
in Table 12–2. Individual patients do not proceed through these phases in
parallel, however. Instead, patients tend to stabilize one illness at a time;
engagement in treatment for the other illness may not take place until years
later. Thus, there is no one type of treatment program for dual-diagnosis
patients. Specific treatment interventions depend on careful assessment of
specific diagnoses and the phase of recovery, degree of severity, extent of
disability, and motivation for treatment for each (Minkoff 1991).

Assessment

Assessment of dual-diagnosis patients is often a complex, open-ended process (Lehmann et al. 1989) "with diagnoses considered tentative in the face
of changing data" (Kofoed, 1991, p. 44). Nonetheless, five basic principles
can be pragmatically applied to assessment of dual-diagnosis patients in community settings:

Table 12–2. Parallels in the recovery process for addiction and mental illness

Addiction	Mental illness
Phase 1: Acute stabilization	

1. Detoxification
   a. Usually inpatient, may be involuntary.
   b. Usually requires medication.
   c. 3–5 days (alcohol).
   d. Includes assessment for other diagnoses.
	1. Stabilization of acute psychosis
	   a. Usually inpatient, may be involuntary.
	   b. Medication.
	   c. 2 weeks to 6 months.
	   d. Includes assessment for effects of substance and for addiction.

Phase 2: Engagement	
1. Engagement of the patient in ongoing treatment is crucial for recovery to proceed.	1. Engagement of the patient in ongoing treatment is crucial for recovery to proceed.
2. Engagement begins with empathy, then proceeds through the phases of education and empathic confrontation before the patient commits to ongoing active treatment (Osher and Kofoed 1989).	2. Engagement begins with empathy, then proceeds through the phases of education and empathic confrontation before the patient commits to ongoing active treatment (Osher and Kofoed 1989).
3. Education about substance use and abuse and dependence, and empathic confrontation of adverse consequences are tools to overcome denial. Patient must admit powerlessness to control drug use without help (e.g., Alcoholics Anonymous [AA] and other collaterals).	3. Education about mental illness and the adverse consequences of treatment noncompliance are tools to overcome denial. Patient must admit powerlessness to control symptoms without help (e.g., medication).
4. Educating the family and involving them in confrontation of the patient's denial facilitates engagement.	4. Educating the family and involving them in setting limits on noncompliance facilitates engagement.
5. Engagement may take place in a variety of treatment settings, including outpatient, day treatment, inpatient, and residential.	5. Engagement may take place in a variety of treatment settings, including outpatient, day treatment, inpatient, and residential.

Table 12–2. Parallels in the recovery process for addiction and mental illness *(continued)*

Addiction	Mental illness
Extended inpatient or day treatment rehabilitation (2–12 weeks) may be needed.	Extended inpatient or day treatment rehabilitation (1–6 months) may be needed.
6. Engagement may initially be coerced through a legal mandate (probation, etc.).	6. Engagement may initially be coerced through a legal mandate (guardianship, etc.).
7. Multiple cycles of relapse usually occur before engagement in ongoing treatment is successful ("revolving door" syndrome).	7. Multiple cycles of relapse usually occur before engagement in ongoing treatment is successful ("revolving door" syndrome).

Phase 3: Prolonged stabilization

Addiction	Mental illness
1. Continued abstinence (1 year).	1. Continued medical compliance (1 year).
a. Patient consistently attends abstinence support programs (e.g., AA), usually 3–5 times per week (initially, 90 meetings in 90 days).	a. Patient consistently takes prescribed medication and attends treatment sessions regularly.
b. Patient usually participates voluntarily, but ongoing compliance may be coerced or legally mandated (e.g., probation).	b. Patient usually participates voluntarily, but ongoing compliance may be legally mandated (e.g., medication guardianship).
c. Ongoing education about addiction, recovery, and skills to maintain abstinence.	c. Ongoing education about mental illness, recovery, and skills to prevent relapse.
d. Need to focus on asking for help to cope with urges to use substances and drop out of treatment.	d. Need to focus on asking for help to cope with continuing symptoms and urges to discontinue treatment.
e. Must learn to accept the illness and deal with shame, stigma, guilt, and despair.	e. Must learn to accept the illness and deal with shame, stigma, guilt, and despair.
f. Must learn to cope with negative symptoms: social,	f. Must learn to cope with negative symptoms: impaired

(continued)

Table 12–2.   Parallels in the recovery process for addiction and
mental illness *(continued)*

Addiction	Mental illness
affective, cognitive, and personality development.	cognition, affect and social skills, and lack of motivation/energy.
g. Family needs ongoing involvement in its own program of recovery (Alanon) to learn empathic detachment and how to set caring limits.	g. Family needs to be involved and learn to detach and set limits (Alliance for the Mentally Ill).
h. May need intensive outpatient treatment and/or 6–12 months residential placement.	h. May need extended hospital, day treatment, or residential placement.
i. Continuing assessment.	i. Continuing assessment.
j. Risk of relapse continues.	j. Risk of relapse continues.

Phase 4: Recovery (1–30 years)

Addiction	Mental illness
1. Continued sobriety	1. Continued stability
a. Voluntary, active involvement in treatment.	a. Voluntary, active involvement in treatment.
b. Stability precedes growth: no growth is possible unless sobriety is fairly secure. Growth occurs slowly, 1 day at a time.	b. Stability precedes growth: no growth is possible unless stabilization of psychosis is solid (may be symptomatic, but stable). Growth occurs slowly, 1 day at a time.
c. Continued work in the AA program on growing, changing, dealing with feelings (12 steps, step meetings).	c. Continued medication, but reduction to lowest level needed for maintenance. Continued work in treatment program, with increasing work on feelings in therapy, processing the impact of illness.
d. Thinking continues to clear.	d. Thinking continues to clear.
e. New skills for dealing with feelings, situations.	e. New skills for dealing with feelings, situations.

Table 12–2. Parallels in the recovery process for addiction and mental illness *(continued)*

Addiction	Mental illness
f. Increasing responsibility for illness; recovery program brings increasing control of one's life.	f. Increasing responsibility for illness; recovery program brings increasing control of one's life.
g. Increasing capacity to work and to have relationships.	g. Increasing capacity to work and relate (vocational rehabilitation, clubhouse programs).
h. Recovery is never "complete" but is always ongoing.	h. Recovery is never "complete" but is always ongoing.
i. Eventual goal is peace of mind and serenity (e.g., "Serenity Prayer").	i. Eventual goal is peace of mind and serenity (e.g., "Serenity Prayer").

1. Developing a positive relationship is usually the first step in the assessment process.
2. Denial and minimization significantly impede assessment of both disorders; patients' statements about having "no problem" should not be accepted at face value.
3. Considering that psychiatric illness and substance disorders are both primary diagnoses, each disorder should receive equally thorough and intensive assessment.
4. Assessment involves not only diagnosis, but also level of severity, extent of disability, and motivation for treatment for each disorder (Kofoed 1991; Minkoff 1991).
5. Each disorder, when active, exacerbates symptoms of the other. Active substance intoxication and withdrawal syndromes tend to worsen psychiatric symptoms; similarly, substance use tends to become more out of control in patients who are actively psychotic or manic. Therefore, assessment of comorbidity is best done when the patient is at baseline.

With regard to implementation of these principles in community mental health settings, it is advisable to develop protocols that define the process and content of evaluation for all patients and are based on the presumption that dual diagnosis is an expectation. Two types of protocols are required: one for assessment of substance disorders in chronic psychiatric patients, and one for assessment of psychiatric disorders in substance-dependent patients.

Assessment of Substance Disorders in Chronic Psychiatric Patients

The first step in this protocol is to develop a positive rapport with the patient—at baseline—to diminish denial and minimization through explicitly conveying a nonjudgmental attitude about the patient's substance use. A sample format for the interview, based on a revision of the Michigan Alcohol Screening Test (Seizer 1971) that includes some questions specific for dual-diagnosis patients, is shown in Table 12–3. Note the emphasis on asking neutral questions about the patient's positive as well as negative drug and alcohol experiences and about the positive as well as negative effects of substances on symptoms, medication compliance, and treatment efforts. Some elements of this approach are illustrated in the following vignette.

> A.B., a 21-year-old young man with paranoid schizophrenia, was referred by his community residence program to his medicating psychiatrist (who saw him monthly) for assessment of his substance abuse. The residence staff had caught him smoking marijuana on two occasions and suspected he was using it more often. A.B. angrily denied this.
>
> *Physician:* (neutrally) The halfway house has spoken to me about their concerns about your using drugs.
>
> *A.B.:* (sullen and angry) So what?
>
> *Physician:* (empathic) So I bet you think they're being a real pain.
>
> *A.B.:* (surprised) Yeah—I don't know why they have such a problem with drugs. You know, they want to restrict me! (Indignantly)
>
> *Physician:* I know what you mean. It's awful to be 21 years old and have people trying to run your life. I really support your right to make choices about your own life—including drug use. That's the best way for you to feel in control of your recovery.
>
> *A.B.:* Yeah! (smiling)
>
> *Physician:* So tell me . . . What do you enjoy about using drugs?

The assessment proceeds relatively smoothly from this point. Eventually, the discussion can focus on the negative effects of substance use and the relative merits of choosing to use drugs (and get in trouble at the halfway house) versus gaining the potential rewards of maintaining abstinence.

Assessment of Psychiatric Symptomatology in Patients With Active Substance Dependence

This process is particularly challenging, because many substance intoxication and withdrawal syndromes (e.g., alcoholic paranoia, hallucinosis, or affective status; alcohol or benzodiazepine withdrawal hallucinations; cocaine-induced paranoid psychosis or withdrawal depression; marijuana-induced chronic schizophrenic-like apathy, motivation, and loosening of thought; and hallucinogen-induced psychosis) can mimic psychiatric disorders. A protocol for assessing new patients might require a brief period of abstinence (1–4 weeks; usually 2 weeks) before applying standard DSM-IV mental status criteria (American Psychiatric Association 1994) for psychiatric diagnosis of psychotic symptoms, and a longer period of abstinence (4–12 weeks) for diagnosis of nonpsychotic depression or anxiety. For many patients, hospitalization may be indicated for the purpose of controlling substance dependence in order to obtain a valid diagnosis. However, other patients may have to be assessed in the outpatient setting.

A 34-year-old man with known cocaine dependence and no prior psychiatric history was brought in to the clinic by his brother because of a 2-week history of paranoid psychosis (feelings of being followed by drug dealers and police bugging his apartment). The patient had no insurance, refused hospitalization, and was not committable. He requested medication for relief of paranoia. The physician informed the patient and his brother that accurate diagnosis and safe pharmacotherapy could ensue only if the patient abstained from cocaine use. If the patient could remain abstinent for 24 hours with his brother's supervision, medication could begin the next day.

The patient returned the next day and was begun on trifluoperazine 5–10 mg daily. Ongoing abstinence was monitored by urine drug screens every 3–4 days. The patient's psychosis cleared completely (no residual symptoms) in 2 weeks. At this point, the medication could be discontinued. If psychosis were to recur, a presumptive diagnosis of non-drug-induced paranoid psychosis would be made; if psychosis did not recur, the psychosis would be considered drug-induced. Referral for ongoing addiction treatment should be made, if the patient is willing, in either case.

Note that if this patient were known to have a history of paranoid schizophrenia treated with neuroleptics, he would be managed differently. Antipsychotics would be begun (or increased) immediately and maintained indefinitely, regardless of cocaine use. Tapering of medication should occur, if at all, only after 6–12 months of cocaine abstinence. It is unlikely in most cases that the schizophrenia diagnosis would turn out to be incorrect.

Note also, however, that diagnoses do occasionally change. Patients with drug-induced psychoses may spontaneously become psychotic after months

Table 12–3.   Alcohol and drug use assessment

1. Tell me about your drinking/drugging pattern. What do you drink? Do you drink/drug every day? How many drinks? How much alcohol do you put in each drink? Do you measure the alcohol?

2. How much alcohol do you consume in a week?

3. Was there ever a time in your life when you worried about your alcohol or drug intake? Have you ever tried to control the amount/frequency?

4. Have you ever taken any drugs? (Mention pot, cocaine, speed, acid, PCP, tranquilizers.) Has a physician ever prescribed tranquilizers for you? (Get medication name and dosage.)

5. Does anyone in your family have a problem with drinking or taking drugs?

6. Is anyone in your family concerned about your drinking?

7. What do you do to relax or unwind or calm down? What do you do if you can't get to sleep at night?

8. Have you ever taken a drink/drug in the morning?

9. Do you have any health problems that may relate to alcohol/drugs? (Suggest specific problems.)

10. Are your caregivers concerned about your drinking or drugging?

11. Have you gotten in trouble at your treatment program because of alcohol or drugs? Have you been suspended or dropped from the program?

12. Have alcohol and drugs led to emergency department visits? To hospitalizations?

13. Have you ever lost time from work because of drinking or because you were sick from drinking?

14. Have you ever been in a motor vehicle accident or other dangerous situation where alcohol or drugs were involved? Who was driving? Were alcohol or drugs involved?

15. Have you ever been arrested for driving under the influence?

16. Do you know what a blackout is? Have you ever had a blackout after drinking? How often?

17. Does it annoy you if someone tells you that you drink too much?

18. Has there been an increase in the amount of drugs or alcohol you use in the past 6–12 months?

19. Do you seem to be able to "hold your liquor" better than others you know? Does it take more alcohol or drugs to get you "feeling good" than others?

20. Have you ever tried to cut down on the amounts or kinds of alcohol and/or drugs? (See question 3.)

21. Have you ever tried to quit?

22. Have you ever felt guilty after drinking or drugging?

23. Have you ever lied about drinking or the amounts you drank?

24. Have you ever "gotten drunk" even when you planned not to?

25. If you do drink or use drugs, what do you like about it? What, if anything, do you not like?

26. Do you find that drugs and alcohol are helpful or unhelpful in dealing with your mental illness? In what ways?

27. What effect does getting drunk or high have on your symptoms? How about when you're coming down, hung over, or crashing?

After asking these questions, ask yourself (the interviewer) how you feel. Do you feel the person has been defensive or uncomfortable at the questions? Does your "gut" feeling tell you there's more to the story than he or she is letting on? If so, there probably is.

of abstinence, and patients with apparent mental illness may spontaneously "clear up" after extended abstinence. Thus, assessment in these patients is always an ongoing process.

Diagnostic Criteria

The purpose of assessment is to establish clear diagnoses that predict treatment interventions. Unfortunately, the absence of clear diagnostic criteria for patients with comorbid mental illness and substance disorder frequently results in fuzzy diagnosis (and fuzzy treatment) of both disorders. The goal of this section is to recommend diagnostic criteria that may be applied consistently and practically in community mental health settings.

Diagnosis of Substance Disorders in Patients With Chronic Mental Illness

DSM-IV criteria for substance abuse and dependence can be applied readily to chronically mentally ill individuals. Substance abuse is defined as any harmful use of a substance that persists for 12 months and has never met criteria for substance dependence. Based on the ample data supporting the negative effect of even mild substance use (including caffeine and nicotine) on the course of serious and disabling psychotic conditions (Drake et al. 1989; McCarrick et al. 1985), it can be stated that any persistent and regular use of substances can be considered to be abuse; abstinence is recommended to enhance the recovery of psychotic disabled patients.

The DSM-IV criteria for substance dependence focus not on withdrawal and tolerance, but on the presence of uncontrolled craving leading to continued use in the face of clearly harmful consequences (e.g., loss of friends, family, money, or housing; increase in symptoms or hospitalizations; or legal difficulties). Any evidence of lack of control in the face of harmful consequences should result in a diagnosis of substance dependence, even if the lack of control is not constant or continuous.

A 28-year-old man with schizophrenia continues to drink to intoxication monthly, shortly after he receives his Supplemental Security Income check. He runs out of money and frequently becomes suicidal and more paranoid when he drinks. Frequent promises that "I've learned my lesson and I'll never do it again" have not resulted in any behavior change. This patient should be given a diagnosis of alcohol dependence.

Note that if the patient exhibited the same behavior but reported that he enjoyed drinking and did not wish to stop (no lack of control), and also reported more limited negative consequences, he would then be given a diagnosis of alcohol abuse. In either case, the patient should be considered to have two primary disorders: primary mental illness and primary substance abuse or dependence.

Diagnosis of Psychiatric Disorders in Patients With Substance Dependence

Following the protocol described earlier, patients with substance dependence who remain psychotic (or who still require medicine to control psychosis) after 2 weeks of abstinence should be given the appropriate DSM-III-R diagnosis for their psychotic illness. This also applies to mania, obsessive-compulsive disorder, posttraumatic stress disorder, and dissociative disorders. Most organic mental disorders (e.g., adult attention-deficit disorder) can also be diagnosed through neuropsychological testing after 2 weeks of abstinence. Note that all such patients have two primary disorders: primary substance dependence and primary mental illness.

For nonpsychotic depression, diagnostic criteria are less clear-cut. Anhedonia, insomnia, and depressed affect are common in early sobriety. Ideally, patients should have 3 months of active recovery (abstinence plus counseling and/or AA) or demonstrate dysfunctionality before major affective disorder is diagnosed and antidepressant medication initiated. Similarly, common anxiety symptoms are almost always an expectable part of recovery from substance dependence. Panic attacks are also frequent in early recovery and may be so disabling that they require nonbenzodiazepine medication. However, 95% of panic symptoms are secondary to substance dependence and resolve after 1 year of recovery. Consequently, a diagnosis of primary panic disorder should be made with great caution. (Note: The terms *primary* and *secondary* should not be used in the dual-diagnosis population to reflect sequence of onset. "Secondary" symptoms [of substance abuse or psychosis] resolve when the "primary" illness is at baseline; if symptoms persist, there are two primary disorders.)

A 41-year-old divorced man with a 15-year history of alcohol dependence was admitted to a psychiatric unit following a suicide attempt. The patient reported that he had recently lost his job owing to absenteeism, and his wife had insisted he move out. He insisted that alcohol was not his "real problem." "I only drink because I'm depressed; I've been depressed for years." The family gave an extensive drinking history associated with intense mood swings.

After 2 weeks in the hospital, the patient reported continued anhedonia and depression, along with insomnia and poor appetite. However, there was no psychosis, no rumination, and no inability to participate in unit activities. The patient's mood was observed to be somewhat reactive to interpersonal support, and his level of depression was observed to be proportional to the extent of his losses.

Consequently, the patient was advised that his presumptive diagnosis was primary alcohol dependence with secondary depression. No medication was prescribed, and the patient was referred for intensive alcohol rehabilitation. Three months later, the patient was sober in an alcoholic halfway house and euthymic.

Note that if symptoms of depression persisted or recurred at this point, reconsideration of antidepressant medication would be indicated.

Treatment

Discussion of treatment will begin by identifying specific interventions for patients in the first three phases of treatment and recovery identified in Table 12–2: acute stabilization, engagement, and prolonged stabilization (active treatment/relapse prevention). This will be followed by a broader discussion of the dual-diagnosis "system of care" and examination of the role of different types of program models in the treatment of dual-diagnosis patients.

Phases of Treatment and Recovery

Acute stabilization/psychopharmacology.   Acute stabilization of dual-diagnosis patients often requires simultaneous detoxification from addictive substances and medication of acute psychotic illness. Psychiatrists faced with this situation are frequently concerned about the interactive effects of various medications (e.g., neuroleptics) with substances of abuse or with detoxification regimens. The following rules are a useful guide to practice:

- *Rule 1:* Acute treatment of major mental illness (schizophrenia, major affective disorder, obsessive-compulsive disorder, etc.) should proceed in standard fashion, regardless of the presence of coexisting substance dependence or withdrawal. This may include use of oral or parenteral benzodiazepines to control acute agitation.
- *Rule 2:* Even if it is not clear whether acute psychotic symptoms are due to drug intoxication (with the exception of anticholinergic medications

such as scopolamine), acute pharmacological stabilization of psychosis should proceed if necessary. Discontinuation of acute antipsychotic medication can be considered once the psychosis has cleared for 2 weeks.

- *Rule 3:* Pharmacological detoxification is not required for all substance-dependent patients. Cocaine and amphetamine addicts, marijuana addicts, and intermittent alcohol users may not experience withdrawal syndromes that require pharmacological intervention.
- *Rule 4:* Mentally ill patients who demonstrate physiological withdrawal syndromes can (and should) undergo detoxification using the same protocols used for non–mentally ill addicts. Inpatient detoxification is strongly recommended for dual-diagnosis patients.
- *Rule 5:* Maintenance medications (other than benzodiazepines) should not be discontinued during detoxification or early sobriety (up to 6–12 months) unless a careful assessment has determined that the medication was originally prescribed inappropriately (e.g., neuroleptics prescribed for "anxiety" or antidepressants prescribed for "mood swings" in an active alcoholic). Maintenance benzodiazepines should be discontinued by switching to the equivalent amount of phenobarbital and then tapering slowly.

A 31-year-old man with schizoaffective disorder and maintained on depot fluphenazine, imipramine, and clonazepam 1 mg qid is admitted to an acute inpatient unit as a result of continuous alcohol dependence and exacerbation of psychosis. The patient undergoes detoxification from alcohol using oxazepam, while continuing his other medication. Supplemental oral fluphenazine is used to control paranoia. Once detoxification is completed (5 days), the oral fluphenazine is gradually eliminated, and clonazepam is switched to 30 mg qid of phenobarbital and then tapered at 15 mg per day. Intramuscular fluphenazine and imipramine are maintained indefinitely.

Engagement.   Dual-diagnosis patients commonly become engaged in community-based treatment for their mental illness before accepting that they have a substance abuse problem or need substance abuse treatment. Continued substance abuse by these patients while in outpatient, day treatment, or community residential settings often is disruptive to both the patient and the treatment environment. Caregivers often feel very frustrated in their efforts to "break through" a patient's denial or minimization of his or her substance disorder and "get the patient sober." Efforts to provide the patient with more services so he or she will not abuse alcohol or drugs are rarely successful and often leave caregivers feeling that they are "enabling" the patient to continue using the substance. At the same time, angry threats and confrontations or attempts to coerce sobriety often lead to resentment, passive-aggressive struggles, and noncompliance. The purpose of this section is to describe a more successful approach to engagement, as follows:

- *Step 1:* Acknowledge that you are powerless to "get anyone sober." Dual-diagnosis patients must choose abstinence.
- *Step 2:* Develop a relationship based on empathic detachment, demonstrating consistent caring and concern for the patient, but also respecting the patient's need to make his or her own decisions and choices and to accept the consequences of those choices.
- *Step 3:* Develop an education process to help the patient learn more about substances in order to make better choices about substance use. The educational process can occur individually or in peer group discussions. Sciacca (1991) has described a replicable model for introducing substance abuse engagement and education groups into any mental health setting. Patients who are completely in denial of substance use may be included in these groups so that they might acquire useful knowledge or offer help to others. The group leader encourages open discussion of substance use in a nonjudgmental manner through providing reading material, videos, and outside speakers. The group as a whole is encouraged to evaluate both outside data and their own experiences with substances to make better choices about substance use. Generally, over a period of months, the group begins to evolve a culture encouraging, first, control of substance use and, later, abstinence. If such groups are not available, the same process can occur during individual sessions, although with greater difficulty.
- *Step 4:* Await opportunities in which confronting the patient with the negative consequences of his or her substance use may provide leverage to encourage the patient to accept substance treatment. Confrontation, as used here, does not mean verbal attack. Successful confrontation of a dual-diagnosis patient is always based in a caring relationship, involves genuine (not contrived) consequences of the patient's substance abuse, and requires the power to enforce those consequences comfortably.

A 23-year-old man had been a patient in a day treatment program for 2 years and was very attached to the program. He had always abused substances, but in the preceding 6 months, his substance use had begun to interfere with his treatment. He had twice disrupted activities as a result of intoxication and had been caught selling drugs to another patient. The substance abuse policy of the program defined these behaviors as clear violations, and he had been confronted with the consequences of progressively longer suspensions. Each time he had been suspended, he had been offered the choice of accepting hospitalization for addiction treatment, but had turned it down. After his third offense of being disruptively intoxicated, staff decided that his unpredictable behavior was creating an unsafe environment for other patients. He was told, gently and caringly, that he must accept addiction treatment or be dropped from the program. He defiantly declared he did not need day treatment, and staff reluctantly let him go. Two weeks later, he called and said he missed the program and had changed his mind. Inpatient addiction treatment was arranged.

Note that the success of this confrontation depended on 1) the program having a clear policy defining substance violations and consequences (see Table 12–4) and 2) staff genuinely believing that the patient had to be dropped for the safety of the program if he did not accept treatment. If the confrontation had not been based on observable disruptive behaviors or if the threat of termination had been intended only to manipulate the patient, the intervention would not have worked. In addition, it must be clearly noted that all confrontations do not "work." This patient may well have decompensated and required rehospitalization for psychosis rather than agreeing to address his substance use. This is why staff must be certain that the continued substance abuse–related behavior is genuinely intolerable before initiating such a confrontation.

Allowing patients to bear the negative consequences of their substance use is an important tool in promoting motivation for recovery. However, such detachment must not become punitive or destructive. For example, patients who are suspended or dropped from community residences should not be put out on the street. Such patients should be offered hospitalization or transitional living arrangements while awaiting return to the residence. Only if patients refuse such suggestions and are noncommittable should they be let go.

Active treatment to maintain stabilization (sobriety).   Active treatment begins once the patient 1) decides to discontinue substance use and 2) decides he or she needs help to do so. Usually substance-dependent patients will try to stop on their own before realizing that they need help; in fact, inability to stop on one's own can be regarded as pathognomic of substance dependence.

Active treatment may begin in either an inpatient or outpatient setting, depending on how much containment the patient needs to attain initial abstinence. In most respects the treatment of substance dependence in the mentally ill population is very similar to treatment of non–mentally ill addicts. The content of the treatment is the same; however, allowances must be made for the cognitive limitations imposed by psychiatric disability. There are two major ingredients to active treatment:

1. Teaching the patient about the disease of substance dependence and the skills he or she will need to maintain abstinence.

Table 12–4.   Development of substance abuse policies and contracts for dual-diagnosis patients in treatment programs

---

Principle

The Substance Abuse Policy must be designed to fit the needs of the program. It can be flexible, but must be applied consistently to all patients. Too much flexibility will undermine the power and effectiveness of the policy.

Step 1:   Identify whether the policy for your program is to have all patients be totally abstinent or merely abstinent on the premises.

Step 2:   Define a "violation," and develop a progressive hierarchy of interventions for patients who have repeated violations.

Step 3:   Include a method for verification of substance use.

Step 4:   Require the patient, *not* the staff, to be responsible for his or her own sobriety and the success of his or her substance abuse treatment.

Step 5:   At the point of suspension or termination, always define the conditions for return to the program.

Sample policy

Residents may use substances *off* premises in moderation, although abstinence is encouraged. However, any use or possession *on* premises, and/or any use that leads to being intoxicated on premises, and/or leads to any behavior that is dangerous to self or others in the program will be regarded as a violation. Confirmation of substance use by urine screen can be requested by staff *at any time;* refusal is the same as a positive result. Consequences are as follows:

- First offense in a 6-month period: 24-hour suspension and offer of referral for substance treatment.
- Second offense (if less than 6 months since first offense): 3- to 7-day suspension and offer of referral.
- Third offense (if less than 6 months since second offense): 30-day suspension, plus mandatory successful completion of a substance abuse treatment program before return to the house.
- Fourth offense: Minimum of 60-day suspension, plus mandatory treatment, plus a minimum of 60 days of complete abstinence prior to return to the house, plus an abstinence contract in the house.
- Fifth offense: Minimum of 90-day suspension, plus 3 months of abstinence before return to house.
- Sixth offense: Termination, plus 6 months of documented abstinence before being eligible for reconsideration.

Note.   This contract depends on observable behavior and requires the patient to take responsibility for participation in treatment while in the residence (e.g., going to Alcoholics Anonymous meetings). Note also that the specific lengths of punishment and numbers of steps are fairly arbitrary and can be adjusted according to the needs, comfort, and enforcement capability of each program.

Reprinted from Minkoff K: "Intervention Strategies for People With Dual-diagnosis." *Innovations and Research* 2(4):11–17, 1993. Used with permission.

2. Introducing the patient to supportive programs of recovery and teaching him or her how to develop and use these supports to maintain abstinence.

Skill building. Carroll et al. (1991) have identified the following specific skills associated with relapse prevention:

- Addressing ambivalence about abstinence
- Reducing accessibility and availability of substances
- Developing coping strategies for high-risk situations
- Addressing conditioned cues for craving
- Exploring apparently irrelevant decisions that lead to relapse
- Modifying life-style and social context
- Dealing with potential abstinence violation effects ("I slipped, so I might as well keep using")

To address these issues in psychiatrically disabled persons, more concrete skill-building approaches are required (Evans and Sullivan 1990). This may include simplified written exercises, writing out index cards listing specific responses for each situation, and role playing. Development of new social networks can be facilitated by encouraging involvement in psychiatric rehabilitation as well as in addiction recovery groups. Because mentally ill patients are particularly sensitive to feelings of failure, a nonjudgmental approach to relapses or slips is essential so the patient feels comfortable discussing his or her slip and returning to treatment quickly.

A patient reported that urges to drink were triggered by feelings of isolation. With staff assistance, the patient listed five telephone numbers he could call (e.g., AA members, crisis hotline) when he had these feelings. These numbers were listed on an index card labeled "Dealing With Loneliness" that the patient was told to carry in his wallet. A staff counselor helped the patient develop a script for each telephone call and then sat with him while he made practice calls to each of the five numbers.

Programs of recovery and support. Twelve-step programs of recovery (AA, Narcotics Anonymous [NA], etc.) are the predominant support systems available for individuals seeking to maintain abstinence and are the cornerstone of almost all inpatient and intensive outpatient addiction treatment programs. Although significant numbers of dual-diagnosis patients can attain and maintain abstinence through outpatient dual-diagnosis education and treatment groups provided in the mental health setting (Drake et al. 1991b; Kofoed et al. 1986; Sciacca 1991), many patients require more intensive (e.g., inpatient) addiction treatment and utilization of generic community self-help programs (Minkoff 1989). A major advantage of generic 12-step programs is that they are widely available and free of charge. Dual-diagnosis patients with substance dependence are likely to need nearly daily support and reinforcement to maintain abstinence; dual-diagnosis group therapy 1–2 times per week may be insufficient.

Minkoff (1989) has described areas of special preparation that dual-diagnosis patients require in order to utilize AA most effectively. These include specific training on what to talk about—and what not to talk about—in AA meetings (e.g., AA is not a place to get medication advice; also, it is not helpful to talk about hearing voices leading to the urge to drink, but one can talk about "upsetting thoughts" instead); assistance in selecting specific meetings to attend; development of contacts among non–mentally ill addicts; training in making a telephone call to ask for help or obtain a ride; and teaching that asking for help means help to "get through the day" without using, not help to "feel fine," to borrow money, or to find a place to live (Table 12–5). Although concerns have been raised about the cognitive complexity of 12-step ideas, AA can be a very simple program: don't drink, go to meetings, and ask for help to stay sober. Patients should be encouraged to "keep it simple" by just following those basic precepts. Furthermore, although individual AA members may be opposed to the use of psychotropic medications, patients should be educated that AA, in general, supports the appropriateness of adherence to a prescribed medication regimen. In some areas, "double trouble" AA meetings have begun to emerge as a specific resource for dual-diagnosis patients who attend AA but wish to have a place

Table 12–5.   Areas of special preparation for dual-diagnosis patients to utilize 12-step programs

1. Training in what to talk about (e.g., urges to drink, upsetting feelings, loneliness and isolation)
2. Training in what not to talk about (e.g., medication questions, hearing voices, bizarre ideas)
3. Assistance in selecting meetings
4. Development of contacts with new mentally ill alcoholics and addicts
5. Training in making telephone calls to ask for help
6. Training in obtaining rides to meetings
7. Training in what "asking for help" means (e.g., help to get through the day without using, not help to feel good, borrow money, or find a place to live)
8. Education about Alcoholics Anonymous' acceptance of prescribed medication

to discuss medications and illness in a 12-step context. Where such meetings do not exist, staff-led dual-diagnosis relapse prevention (Osher and Kofoed 1989) or abstinence support (Sciacca 1991) groups can be developed in CMHC settings. In a similar vein, Sciacca (1991) has developed MICAA-NON support groups for families of dual-diagnosis patients. In some communities, inpatient detoxification or rehabilitation programs are simply not available for treatment of addiction in psychiatric patients. In these settings, clinicians must develop the capacity to provide such services in psychiatric settings, either as a component of an inpatient psychiatric unit or as an intensive outpatient addiction day treatment module within existing day programs.

The following case example illustrates the utility of AA for a dual-diagnosis patient who found it easier to relate to peers than to professionals.

> A 26-year-old man with 10-year history of schizophrenia and 12-year history of substance dependence has lived in a succession of community residences since age 18 and has been sober in AA for 3 years (except for two "slips" in which he drank one or two beers). Although he takes medication regularly, he has difficulty acknowledging the severity of his psychiatric disability and his poor social and vocational skills. He also has difficulty accepting his need for a community residence and feels very humiliated at any efforts by staff to help him to improve, which in turn leads to angry outbursts.
>
> By contrast, he is very eager to participate in AA, which he feels is a more "normal" environment and where he feels more like a peer than a patient. He identifies more readily as an alcoholic and drug addict and feels less stigmatized. Although he behaves inappropriately at times in AA meetings, he has a sponsor and a number of other AA contacts from whom he can accept constructive feedback, and his clear willingness to try to "work the program" helps other AA members to tolerate his behavior. Thus, AA has become a tool not only for maintaining sobriety, but also for enhancing social rehabilitation.

Dual-Diagnosis System of Care

Treatment interventions cannot be discussed independently of the program settings in which those interventions occur, yet designing community treatment programs for dual-diagnosis patients presents considerable challenges. Addiction programs (outpatient or inpatient) are often ill equipped to deal with psychotic patients who require medication, and mental health programs are often similarly ill equipped to treat patients who require an abstinent environment and/or an addiction recovery support system to get sober. Creation of specific hybrid or integrated treatment programs has been described in the literature (McLaughlin and Pepper 1991; Minkoff 1989; Ridgely et al. 1987), but such programs cannot accommodate the diversity or the magnitude of the dual-diagnosis population (Minkoff 1991).

Minkoff (1991) has proposed a model for describing how a comprehensive care system can address the needs of the dual-diagnosis population as a whole. This model combines limited reliance on hybrid programs providing simultaneous addiction and psychiatric treatment (integrated treatment) with broader utilization of modified generic program elements (within each service system) that provide individual episodes of psychiatric or addiction treatment (parallel or sequential treatment) linked by continuous case management. The role of each individual program will vary according to the illness treated most actively, the phase of treatment, the level of severity and disability, and the motivation for treatment associated with each illness. Consequently, the care system defines a role for both "abstinence-mandated" and "abstinence-encouraged" programs, and for programs that provide various levels of care and case management and require various levels of patient responsibility. Figure 12–1 illustrates the location and function of different program elements within the comprehensive care system.

Application to Community Mental Health Practice

Using this system model, any individual community mental health program can define its own role in the treatment of dual-diagnosis patients, identify referral resources for patients who need treatment elsewhere, and develop long-range strategies to design new programs to address identified system gaps. Most community mental health programs are likely to concentrate on developing 1) engagement-oriented groups for chronically mentally ill patients with substance abuse and dependence (Sciacca 1991), 2) a limited number of active treatment and relapse prevention groups (Osher and Kofoed 1989), and 3) a case management system to facilitate continuity of care and linkage and referral to other programs (Kline et al. 1991). These referral resources may include inpatient programs for detoxification and acute stabilization of mental illness; inpatient and outpatient programs for addiction rehabilitation treatment that accept stable mentally ill individuals; and residential programs that provide 1) a sober environment and addiction recovery support for stable mentally ill individuals with capability of living independently (modified traditional addiction halfway house), 2) substance education and abstinence encouragement for disabled mentally ill abusers and addicts not yet motivated toward sobriety (modified traditional mental health community residence), or 3) a sober environment and addiction

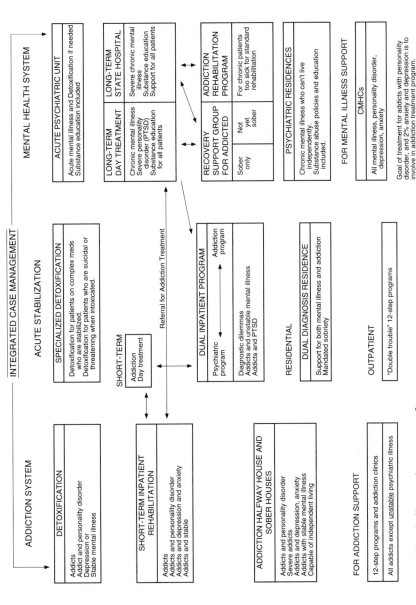

Figure 12–1. Dual-diagnosis system of care.

recovery support for disabled mentally ill addicts motivated toward abstinence (integrated dual-diagnosis sober residence). In most communities, however, many of these resources are not yet available and must be developed.

Innovative Program Models

Within the overall comprehensive care system, innovative integrated program models have been developed that enhance treatment capability with dual-diagnosis patients overall and are potentially replicable in other settings. Evaluation of these and other model programs is currently in progress.

Continuous treatment teams.   The New Hampshire continuous treatment teams (Drake et al. 1991b) provide intensive case management, direct treatment, and outreach to dual-diagnosis clients. Each team is composed of both addiction and mental health clinicians and a consulting psychiatrist. The team construct facilitates continuity even when individual team members leave.

Integrated inpatient program.   The Caulfield Center is a 21-bed voluntary psychiatric hospital in Massachusetts that treats patients with addiction alone, mental illness alone, or dual diagnosis. The unit has a full psychiatric program, a full addiction program, and psychiatric mixed and addiction mixed programs, each of which utilizes a psychoeducational approach and a disease-recovery model. Patients move through different treatment program schedules as their needs change but maintain the same treatment team throughout. This program is useful for patients who present a diagnostic dilemma, addicts with unstable mental illness, and addicts who present with suicidality or another "psychiatric" problem (Minkoff 1989).

Integrated residential program.   Harbor House is an addiction therapeutic community in New York City that has been modified by adding a psychiatric treatment team to address mental illness. The program is specifically designed for homeless dual-diagnosis patients who are willing to make a commitment to abstinence and to follow program requirements (McLaughlin and Pepper 1991).

Summary

In this chapter I have discussed the growing prevalence of dual diagnosis, noting that dual diagnosis is becoming an expectation rather than an exception. Dual-diagnosis patients clearly have poorer outcomes than patients with a single diagnosis, and treatment is hindered by numerous barriers to integration of psychiatric and addiction treatment. Both mental illness and substance dependence can be considered as examples of primary biological chronic mental illnesses, each of which fit into a disease-recovery model that can be used to define the process of assessment, diagnosis, treatment, and recovery. Phases of treatment include acute stabilization, engagement, prolonged stabilization (active treatment and relapse prevention), and recovery/rehabilitation. Each phase defines specific interventions for each illness, and within a comprehensive care system, individual program models will vary according to the illness most actively treated and the phase of treatment, level of disability, and motivation for treatment of each illness. Specific innovative integrated model programs have been developed for case management, inpatient, outpatient, and residential care.

Currently, as dual diagnosis becomes more widely recognized and successful treatment technologies continue to be developed and disseminated, the ability to treat dual-diagnosis patients in community mental health settings will slowly but steadily expand. In the near future it is likely that program evaluation research will further define current innovative program models, and additional creative strategies will emerge.

References

Alterman AI: Substance abuse in psychiatric patients, in Substance Abuse and Psychopathology. Edited by Alterman AI. New York, Plenum, 1985

American Psychiatric Association. Diagnostic and Statistical Manual of Mental Disorders, 4th Edition. Washington, DC, American Psychiatric Association, 1994

Bachrach LL: The context of care for the chronic mental patient with substance abuse. Psychiatr Q 58:3–14, 1987

Bergman HC, Harris M: Substance use among young adult chronic patients. Psychosocial Rehabilitation Journal 9:49–54, 1985

Carroll KM, Rounsaville BJ, Keller DS: Relapse prevention strategies for the treatment of cocaine abuse. American Journal of Drug and Alcohol Abuse 17:249–266, 1991

Caton CLM, Grainick A, Bender S, et al: Young chronic patients and substance abuse. Hosp Community Psychiatry 40:1037–1040, 1989

Dixon L, Haas G, Welden P, et al: Acute effects of drug abuse in schizophrenic patients: clinical observations and patients' self-reports. Schizophr Bull 16:69–79, 1990

Drake RE, Wallach MA: Substance abuse among the chronically mentally ill. Hosp Community Psychiatry 40:1041–1046, 1989

Drake RE, Osher FC, Wallach MA: Alcohol use and abuse in schizophrenia: a prospective community study. J Nerv Ment Dis 177:408–414, 1989

Drake RE, McLaughlin P, Pepper B, et al: Dual diagnosis of major mental illness and substance disorder: an overview, in Dual Diagnosis of Major Mental Illness and Substance Disorder. Edited by Minkoff K, Drake RE. San Francisco, CA, Jossey-Bass, 1991a, pp 3–12

Drake RE, Antosca LM, Noordsy DL, et al: New Hampshire's specialized services for the dually diagnosed: an overview, in Dual Diagnosis of Major Mental Illness and Substance Disorder. Edited by Minkoff K, Drake RE. San Francisco, CA, Jossey-Bass, 1991b, pp 57–68

Evans K, Sullivan JM: Dual Diagnosis: Counselling the Mentally Ill Substance Abuser. New York, Guilford, 1990

Kline J, Harris M, Bebout RR, et al: Contrasting integrated and linkage models of treatment for homeless, dually diagnosed adults: an overview, in Dual Diagnosis of Major Mental Illness and Substance Disorder. Edited by Minkoff K, Drake RE. San Francisco, CA, Jossey-Bass, 1991

Kofoed L: Assessment of comorbid psychiatric illness and substance disorders: an overview, in Dual Diagnosis of Major Mental Illness and Substance Disorder. Edited by Minkoff K, Drake RE. San Francisco, CA, Jossey-Bass, 1991

Kofoed L, Kania J, Walsh T, et al: Outpatient treatment of patients with substance abuse and coexisting psychiatric disorders. Am J Psychiatry 143:867–872, 1986

Lamb HR: Young adult chronic patients: the new drifters. Hosp Community Psychiatry 33:465–468, 1982

Lehmann AF, Myers CP, Corty E: Assessment and classification of patients with psychiatric and substance abuse syndromes. Hosp Community Psychiatry 40:1019–1025, 1989

McCarrick AK, Manderscheld RW, Bertolucci DE: Correlates of acting-out behaviors among young adult chronic patients. Hosp Community Psychiatry 44:259–261, 1985

McLaughlin P, Pepper B: Modifying the therapeutic community for the mentally ill substance abuser: an overview, in Dual Diagnosis of Major Mental Illness and Substance Disorder. Edited by Minkoff K, Drake RE. San Francisco, CA, Jossey-Bass, 1991, pp 85–94

Minkoff K: An integrated treatment model for dual diagnosis of psychosis and addiction. Hosp Community Psychiatry 40:1031–1036, 1989

Minkoff K: Program components of a comprehensive integrated care system for seriously mentally ill patients with substance disorders: an overview, in Dual Diagnosis of Major Mental Illness and Substance Disorder. Edited by Minkoff K, Drake RE. San Francisco, CA, Jossey-Bass, 1991

Minkoff K, Drake RE: Homelessness and dual diagnosis, in Treating the Homeless Mentally Ill. Edited by Lamb HR. Washington, DC, American Psychiatric Press, 1994

Noordsy DL, Drake RE, Teague GB, et al: Subjective experience related to alcohol use among schizophrenics. J Nerv Ment Dis 179:410–414, 1991

Osher FC, Kofoed L: Treatment of patients with psychiatric and psychoactive substance abuse disorders. Hosp Community Psychiatry 40:1025–1030, 1989

Pepper B, Kirshner MC, Ryglewicz H: The young adult chronic patient: overview of a population. Hosp Community Psychiatry 32:463–469, 1981

Regier DA, Farmer ME, Rae DS, et al: Comorbidity of mental disorders with alcohol and other drug abuse. JAMA 264:2511–2518, 1990

Ridgely MS: Creating integrated programs for severely mentally ill persons with substance disorders: an overview, in Dual Diagnosis of Major Mental Illness and Substance Disorder. Edited by Minkoff K, Drake RE. San Francisco, CA, Jossey-Bass, 1991, pp 29–42

Ridgely MS, Goldman HH, Talbott JA: Chronic Mentally Ill Young Adults With Substance Abuse Problems: A Review of the Literature and Creation of a Research Agenda. Baltimore, MD, Mental Health Policy Studies, University of Maryland School of Medicine, 1986

Ridgely MS, Osher FC, Talbott JA: Chronic Mentally Ill Young Adults With Substance Abuse Problems: Treatment and Training Issues. Baltimore, MD, Mental Health Policy Studies, University of Maryland School of Medicine, 1987

Ridgely MS, Goldman HH, Willenbring M: Barriers to the care of persons with dual diagnosis: organizational and financing issues. Schizophr Bull 16:123–132, 1990

Safer D: Substance abuse by young adult chronic patients. Hosp Community Psychiatry 38:511–514, 1987

Schneier FR, Siris SG: A review of psychoactive substance use and abuse in schizophrenia: patterns of drug choice. J Nerv Ment Dis 175:641–652, 1987

Schwartz SR, Goldfinger SM: The new chronic patient: clinical characteristics of an emerging subgroup. Hosp Community Psychiatry 32:470–474, 1981

Sciacca K: An integrated treatment approach for severely mentally ill individuals with substance disorders: an overview, in Dual Diagnosis of Major Mental Illness and Substance Disorder. Edited by Minkoff K, Drake RE. San Francisco, CA, Jossey-Bass, 1991, pp 69–84

Seizer ML: The Michigan Alcoholism Screening Test: the quest for a new diagnostic instrument. Am J Psychiatry 127:89–94, 1971

Turner WM, Tsuang MT: Impact of substance abuse on the course and outcome of schizophrenia. Schizophr Bull 16:87–95, 1990

Chapter 13

HIV Infection and the Community Psychiatrist

Robert M. Goisman, M.D.

F ew illnesses in history have caused as much devastation in as short a period of time as the acquired immunodeficiency syndrome (AIDS). Caused by the human immunodeficiency virus (HIV), AIDS was essentially unknown in 1980. Since its identification in 1981 (Centers for Disease Control [CDC] 1981a, 1981b), it has been responsible for 191,824 deaths in 310,680 cases known in the United States (CDC 1993). The total number of HIV-infected Americans is currently estimated to be 1–1.5 million (Chesney and Folkman 1994).

Moreover, the nature of this illness, including its routes of transmission, risk factors and demographics, and symptomatology, carries the potential for enormous psychological pain even before it kills. Issues of guilt, sexuality, prejudice, religion, allegiance to family, stigmatization, the fear of losing one's mind, death and dying, the economics of chronic illness, and access to health care are all stirred up by this disease.

The author wishes to thank Stephen M. Goldfinger, M.D., of Massachusetts Mental Health Center and Harvard Medical School, Boston, Massachusetts, for his consultation, support, and critical review of earlier drafts of this manuscript.

Given this, the need for community psychiatrists to have an understanding of the HIV epidemic in all of its manifestations is clear. In this chapter I first present a theoretical model, derived from public health, with which to understand AIDS. Reflecting the multifaceted role of the community psychiatrist, I then discuss in turn diagnosis, treatment, and prevention issues.

Primary, Secondary, and Tertiary Prevention

Caplan (1964), in his classic text on community psychiatry, adapted a public health model to psychiatry to acquaint practitioners with issues regarding the health of populations, as compared with that of individuals. In his model *primary prevention* was defined as the attempt to lower "the rate of new cases of [a] . . . disorder in a population . . . by counteracting harmful circumstances before they have had a chance to produce illness" (p. 26); this is the generally used definition of prevention and refers to attempts to decrease the incidence of an illness through specific preventive efforts. *Secondary prevention* refers to "programs which reduce the disability rate due to a disorder by lowering the prevalence of the disorder in the community" (p. 89); this occurs by lowering the rate of new cases or by shortening the duration of currently existing cases through rapid assessment and treatment. *Tertiary prevention* "aims to reduce the rate in a community of defective functioning" from a given disorder through reductions in "the rate of residual defect" (p. 113) (i.e., rehabilitation or other methods of managing sequelae).

These concepts have immediate relevance for AIDS and the community psychiatrist. The role of primary prevention, often challenged in an era of funding cutbacks, is immediately reaffirmed here; when dealing with an illness this devastating, the desirability of yearly reducing the number of new cases is obvious. Also, with the advent of specific therapeutics for some aspects of AIDS, the role of secondary prevention for timely diagnosis and intervention is much more important now than in the beginning of the epidemic. Finally, some degree of palliation and support for AIDS sufferers is clearly possible, so that even with a usually fatal outcome there is an opportunity to provide true tertiary prevention in the sense of reducing residual defect.

Thus, Caplan's model antedates the AIDS epidemic by 20 years but provides a useful way to organize the various opportunities for intervention open to the community psychiatrist. In the remainder of this chapter I describe a number of these arenas, using this model as an organizing principle.

Diagnosis

I begin by discussing secondary prevention in the form of accurate diagnosis and triage. Miller and Riccio (1990) have identified four relationships between HIV infection and psychopathology:

1. Noncognitive psychopathology in an HIV-infected individual
2. Neuropsychiatric symptomatology associated with known HIV-related central nervous system (CNS) disease
3. HIV infection or frank illness in someone with preexisting psychopathology
4. HIV-related content in the psychopathology of a noninfected individual

Of these, type 2 refers most closely to what is often called *AIDS dementia*; I discuss this illness first and then return to the other categories.

AIDS Dementia

An early case of HIV dementia was described by Nurnberg et al. (1984) in a man with Pneumocystis carinii pneumonia who developed an organic delusional syndrome with depressive and paranoid features. Nurnberg et al. described two possible pathogenetic paths for this syndrome: opportunistic CNS involvement owing to immune compromise, and immunodepression secondary to grief and stress. A third possible mechanism, primary CNS infection with HIV, was not therein discussed but began to be reported the next year (Shaw et al. 1985).

The most common cerebral pathologic abnormality affecting HIV-infected patients is a subacute encephalitis, probably caused by primary HIV infection of the CNS (Fenton 1987). This may begin as acute meningoencephalitis from HIV-containing macrophages crossing the blood-brain barrier and then releasing the virus within the CNS (S.W. Perry 1990). The term *AIDS dementia complex* (ADC) is frequently used to describe clinical dementia attributed to such primary infection. This is the most common neurological sequela of AIDS and may be the most prominent or only clinical sign of the illness (Fenton 1987; Navia and Price 1987; S.W. Perry 1990). There may also be treatable types of CNS dysfunction resulting from agents other than direct HIV infection (Ostrow et al. 1988) (i.e., an AIDS delirium as well as a dementia) (Fernandez 1988). Ostrow et al. (1988) and Fernandez (1990) have described differential diagnoses for such deliria, including CNS reactions to primary AIDS treatment such as zidovudine (AZT).

Significant central or peripheral nervous system symptoms have been reported in 23%–39% of AIDS patients (Catalan 1988). Symptoms are virtually protean and may include subtle cognitive, behavioral, and/or motor dysfunction; the differential diagnosis of such symptoms as decreased concentration and recent memory, mental slowing, social withdrawal, and apathy is complex and may point to comorbid dementia and depression or to either diagnosis alone. Fenton (1987) summarized reports of AIDS dementia cases strongly resembling schizophreniform disorder, acute paranoid psychosis, psychotic depression, and hypomania, and S. W. Perry (1990) noted that early manifestations may remain occult to mental status examination, measures of depression, neurological examination, and even patient history. Motor disturbances such as tremor, slowing of rapid alternating movements, and ataxia (Fenton 1987; Navia and Price 1987) are diagnostically helpful if present.

Electroencephalography may reveal nonfocal, diffuse slowing, and computed tomographic (CT) scanning may disclose cortical atrophy (Fenton 1987; S. W. Perry 1990), but the diagnosis is often best confirmed by a progressive course, with mutism, incontinence, coma, and death from intercurrent infection often occurring in weeks to months after the onset of symptoms. Sidtis and Price (1990) have proposed a staging system for ADC that provides a uniform manner in which to describe the neuropsychiatric progression of the disease.

The clinician should consider AIDS dementia as a possibility with the onset of acute major mental illness in a patient otherwise at high risk for AIDS, or when a patient with previously diagnosed AIDS newly develops a "functional psychosis" (Fenton 1987). A reasonable approach to such a patient has been outlined by Ostrow et al. (1988) and includes subjective and objective neuropsychiatric screening, careful premorbid psychiatric and psychosocial history taking, and neurological consultation, with lumbar puncture or other more specialized procedures considered on a case-by-case basis. The Mini-Mental State Exam (Kokmen et al. 1987) has been recommended as a 15-minute screening procedure easily adaptable to a community outpatient setting and is helpful when positive (Fernandez 1988).

The following case illustrates some of the challenges posed by patients in the following situation.

> A 35-year-old single man was referred to his catchment area clinic for evaluation of his mental status. He had a 12-year history of schizoaffective disorder well controlled on lithium and perphenazine. About 5 years prior to this referral, he had been diagnosed as HIV positive; over the preceding 2 years he had gradually shown signs of increasing dementia, with agitation, decreased recent memory, and gait impairment. He was actually doing well on his previous

psychotropic regimen plus benztropine, in addition to zidovudine and other AIDS medications, but his primary care physician had felt uncomfortable in managing his psychiatric medications without consultation.

In this case the only concrete intervention needed was to suggest a decrease in benztropine because the patient was complaining of severe dry mouth. Furthermore, the clear history of major "functional" mental illness preceding onset of AIDS made differential diagnosis relatively easy. The real issue lay in assisting the primary care physician, with whom the patient had a very supportive relationship but who feared she was in "over her head." Once the differential diagnosis was clarified and the minor medication change suggested, it became clear that a referral for ongoing psychiatric care was not necessary.

Noncognitive Psychiatric Impairment

To return to Miller and Riccio's (1990) categorization, AIDS patients are at risk for psychiatric impairment of various noncognitive ("functional") types. Of these, mood disorders would intuitively seem prevalent; adjustment disorder with depressed or anxious mood may be the most common (Fernandez 1988), with actual major depression occurring in perhaps 17%–20% of AIDS patients (Fernandez 1988; Miller and Riccio 1990). The term *adjustment reaction* (Miller and Riccio 1990) is often applied to transient psychosocial distress of a focal nature but here assumes ominous proportions and requires thoughtfulness and a serious approach to the patient. The risk of suicide is profound—perhaps as much as 66 times that of the general population (Marzuk et al. 1988)—and ongoing (Frierson and Lippmann 1988); in a study of 91 psychiatrically hospitalized HIV-positive patients, suicidal attempt or ideation was the most common reason for admission (Wiener et al. 1994). Some have wondered, however, whether the increased suicide risk correlates more with AIDS-risky behaviors than with seropositivity itself (Starace 1993).

Anxiety, probably most resembling generalized anxiety disorder (King 1989) but at times including panic attacks (Faulstich 1987) or obsessive-compulsive phenomena (Fenton 1987), would again be expected to be prevalent. The diagnostician should have a broad differential diagnosis for this symptom, including narcotic, alcohol, or sedative withdrawal; cocaine or other stimulant intoxication; ADC; advanced AIDS-related encephalopathy; and side effects of steroid or zidovudine chemotherapy (Fernandez 1990).

Regarding "functional" psychoses, mania has been described (Miller and Riccio 1990), although whether this syndrome occurs in the absence of organic pathology is a matter of debate, and true schizophrenia-like or paranoid psychoses are reported rarely (Miller and Riccio 1990). The possibility of early ADC being etiologically responsible for such symptoms, especially if of recent onset, is significant (Halstead et al. 1988).

The neuropsychiatric consequences of AIDS treatment itself have been summarized by Katz (1994). The antiretroviral medications didanosine (ddI), dideoxycytidine (ddC), and starudine (D4T) can cause significant insomnia, asthenia, vivid dreams, or increased energy to the point of anxiety, with other neuropsychiatric side effects occurring in fewer than 3% of patients. Among the medications used to treat opportunistic infections, the antitubercular drug cycloserine causes psychosis, somnolence, depression, and confusion often enough that Katz regarded it as relatively contraindicated in patients with seizures, depression, severe anxiety, psychosis, or excessive concomitant alcohol intake. (See Katz [1994] and also Myers et al. [1993] for a more extended discussion of these and other issues in medical treatment of HIV.)

HIV Infection With Preexisting Psychopathology

Among premorbid psychiatric illnesses affecting HIV-infected patients, substance abuse is of obvious importance and may have been a cause of acquisition of the virus. Alcohol abuse and nonintravenous drug use can facilitate spread of the illness by causing behavioral disinhibition and impaired judgment, as well as perhaps by causing some degree of immune suppression (Bakti 1990), whereas intravenous drug use may directly transmit the virus, especially if needles are shared. Premorbid histories of substance abuse have been found to be prevalent among HIV-positive individuals (S. Perry et al. 1990).

There is a growing literature on HIV risk in patients with chronic mental illness (Brady and Carmen 1990; Goisman et al. 1991) that attempts to delineate aspects of chronic psychiatric impairment predisposing to AIDS acquisition and/or transmission. These factors are not specific to any particular Axis I illness, although obviously DSM-IV schizophrenia (American Psychiatric Association 1994), schizoaffective disorder, and bipolar illness are included; instead, these factors apply to the class of individuals who are chronically mentally ill, especially young adults (Pepper 1985). Such factors may include an increased incidence of high-risk sexual activity, decreased ability to give or remember an accurate history, low self-esteem, increased likelihood of substance abuse, poor sexual refusal assertion skills, inability to see cause-effect patterns, and increased vulnerability to exploitative relationships (Brady and Carmen 1990; Goisman et al. 1991). Four studies reported HIV seropositivity incidences of 5.5%–7.2% in subpopulations of chronic mental illness patients (Empfield et al. 1989, 1993; Goldwurm et al.

1988; Stewart et al. 1994), whereas Torres et al. (1990) found a seropositivity incidence of 62% among high-risk homeless males in New York. These risk factors are exemplified in the following vignette:

> A community mental health center decided to undertake an AIDS education program with some of its chronically mentally ill patients living in a halfway house on the center premises. As part of the program, explicit histories of patients' current sexual and substance use activities were taken. The halfway house staff thus learned that one patient, a 45-year-old single woman with a 25-year history of paranoid schizophrenia, was regularly having sexual intercourse with a number of male halfway house residents in exchange for their buying Coca-Cola and cigarettes for her.

In this case, both the woman and her partners tested HIV negative. However, the assessment both illustrated the reality of halfway house life and uncovered a specific set of AIDS-risky behaviors to which interventions needed to be directed.

Thus, as much as HIV infection can cause neurological or psychiatric morbidity, it also may represent a complication of preexisting psychopathology. Teasing apart the causal chain may have great significance for the proper management of the patient but may be exceedingly difficult for the primary clinician to carry out in a community setting .

HIV-Related Themes in Noninfected Individuals

A more subtle consequence of the HIV epidemic is the impact of AIDS on the psychopathology of noninfected individuals. This does not refer to the tremendous burden of illness that AIDS imposes on those emotionally involved with its victims (Miller and Riccio 1990), but rather the appearance of AIDS-related concerns that are in some way disproportionate, unrealistic, or otherwise unusual in a noninfected individual. These concerns may manifest themselves as preoccupations or as frank psychiatric symptomatology.

Perhaps the most dramatic example of this type of psychopathology is the occurrence of delusional material or other manifestations of psychosis with AIDS-related content. Mahorney and Cavenar (1988) described three cases, two of major depression with mood-congruent psychosis and one of manic bipolar disorder, in which the delusion of having AIDS, accompanied in two cases by a demand to be tested for it, were clearly symptomatic of underlying Axis I disorders and disappeared when the disorders were adequately treated. Similarly, Spivak et al. (1990) described a patient with initial preoccupations about his HIV status who went on to develop frank paranoid schizophrenia with AIDS-related delusions.

Almost as dramatic are cases of AIDS-related obsessions. These are somewhat heterogeneous from a descriptive standpoint, overlapping with obsessive-compulsive disorder and somatoform disorder, but in general these patients present with a fear, usually ego-dystonic, that they are at risk for AIDS, have contracted the illness, or need an HIV antibody test. Some authors (Catalan 1988; Faulstich 1987; Miller and Riccio 1990) have described this group as the "worried well"; these patients are indeed worried but do not at all feel well (Field 1993), so Fenton's term, "AIDS panic" (1987) may be closer to clinical reality. Miller and Riccio (1990) have identified a useful constellation of features commonly found in the histories of such patients: difficulties in sexual adjustment, covert sexual activities, guilt about sex, a relative absence of AIDS-risky sexual behavior, and a previous psychiatric history.

The heterogeneity of this group is illustrated by some of the case reports in the literature (Brotman and Forstein 1988; Lippert 1986). At least one case of mixed factitious disorder presenting as AIDS has been reported (Bialer and Wallack 1990). The clinician should be aware of the prevalence of this syndrome and be prepared to respond in an individualized fashion. An example of such a case is the following.

A 50-year-old depressed married man, the father of two adolescent girls, was admitted to an inpatient unit after an overdose on amitriptyline. While in the hospital, his medication was changed to fluoxetine; he improved and was discharged to his local mental health center for outpatient care. The precipitant for the overdose was his recurrent fear of having contracted AIDS from being raped by two men 8 years previously. Since that time he had had about 50 HIV antibody tests at various facilities, received his general medical care at a clinic specializing in AIDS, frequently called AIDS hot lines around the country frantically seeking reassurance that he did not have AIDS, and was pressuring his daughters to totally abstain from all sexual activity "so that they don't end up sick like me."

Clinically, this man met criteria for major depression with comorbid obsessive-compulsive disorder. He was switched to clomipramine and became less depressed than he had been on fluoxetine, and his outpatient psychiatrist proposed behavior therapy involving him and his wife using an exposure and response-prevention paradigm. The patient half-heartedly went along with the treatment for a while but could never quite decide whether his problem was that he might have AIDS or that he could not stop thinking that he might have AIDS; in DSM-IV terms, he had obsessive-compulsive disorder with "poor insight."

Treatment

Caplan's (1964) concepts of secondary and tertiary prevention are useful in delineating both the limitations of and the opportunities for successful clinical intervention with AIDS-affected individuals. Reductions in duration of illness and in residual defect, both within an individual and within the community as a whole, are reasonable goals for psychiatric intervention in this situation, even when eradication of the infectious agent is not. To be effective in this important role, the community psychiatrist must be prepared to utilize both psychopharmacological and psychosocial methods for treatment and for rehabilitation. In this section I delineate some aspects of each that have been reported to be useful.

Psychopharmacological Treatment

For AIDS patients with medication-responsive psychiatric syndromes, the general consensus is that patients should not reflexively be excluded from proper medication trials, but that drug sensitivity may be increased and dosage ranges lower than usually advisable (Fenton 1987; Fernandez 1990; Miller and Riccio 1990). In treating depression, for example, 10 mg of a tricyclic antidepressant at bedtime is a reasonable starting dosage, and although undertreatment is as much to be avoided as overtreatment (Miller and Riccio 1990), 100 mg daily may be all that is needed as well as all that is tolerated (Fernandez 1990).

In terms of specific clinical syndromes, perhaps the most urgent indication is for agitation secondary to delirium, dementia, or psychosis. When definitive treatment of the underlying cause and conservative environmental management are insufficient, behavioral control can often be achieved with low doses of high-potency neuroleptics (e.g., haloperidol 1–5 mg. daily or an equivalent dosage of fluphenazine) (Ostrow et al. 1988). Fernandez (1990) recommended the use of intramuscular or even intravenous haloperidol, alone or with lorazepam. However, high-potency neuroleptics may be associated with frequent dystonic reactions or even with neuroleptic malignant syndrome, and therefore lower potency antipsychotics or benzodiazepines are recommended by some (Fenton 1987; S.W. Perry 1990). Fernandez (1990), in contrast, believed that oral benzodiazepines may lead to behavioral disinhibition.

Treatment of persistent psychotic ideation apart from acute management of agitation can also include the use of neuroleptics (Halstead et al.

1988).When delusional preoccupation with AIDS is due to a primary, functional psychosis rather than secondary to or comorbid with AIDS, treatment should proceed according to therapeutic standards for the underlying disorder; the cases of AIDS delusions described by Mahorney and Cavenar (1988) responded to electroconvulsive therapy (ECT) and to lithium, according to their diagnoses.

For depressive symptoms, tricyclic antidepressants are often helpful as long as side effects are carefully monitored. Some authors recommend avoiding strongly anticholinergic medications because of their greater chance of inducing atropine psychosis (Fernandez 1990; Ostrow et al. 1988); imipramine, for example, might be preferable to amitriptyline (Hintz et al. 1990). Others recommend amitriptyline if its side effect profile would be useful (e.g., in an agitated patient with diarrhea) (S. W. Perry and Markowitz 1986). Fluoxetine (Fernandez 1990; Field 1993; Hintz et al. 1990; Levine et al. 1991), sertraline (Field 1993), and bupropion (Fernandez 1990) have also been reported to be effective. Other somatic treatments recommended have included alprazolam (e.g., 0.25 mg tid with increases as tolerated) (Fernandez 1990; Ostrow et al. 1988), psychostimulants (e.g., methylphenidate 5 mg once or twice daily) (Fernandez 1990; Ostrow et al. 1988; S.W. Perry 1990), and electroconvulsive therapy (Schaerf et al. 1989). Monoamine oxidase inhibitors have generally not been recommended because of their side effect profile (Fernandez 1990).

Drug treatment of AIDS-related anxiety symptoms does not differ substantially from that recommended for anxiety in general. Benzodiazepines are generally the simplest agents to use (Fernandez 1990; Ostrow et al. 1988); some prefer shorter acting agents such as alprazolam over longer acting ones such as diazepam (Fernandez 1988) to avoid toxicity, whereas others recommend those of intermediate length of action (Ostrow et al. 1988). Buspirone is a potentially useful alternative (Fernandez 1990). Antidepressants have more side effects but may be justifiable if prescribed according to the above guidelines, especially if true panic symptoms are present. Fernandez (1990) recommended neuroleptics for panic as well.

Psychosocial Treatment

The preceding are concrete, psychopharmacological recommendations for specific problems. In contrast, discussing psychosocial interventions for AIDS patients may to some extent be more general, less data-based, and more inextricably bound with fear, guilt, shame, grief, and other emotions often experienced by those with this illness. This discussion will include specific therapy techniques, general or system-wide psychosocial interventions, and comments on the role and feelings of the therapist in doing this work.

Although to date there is not an extensive literature on psychodynamic psychotherapy with AIDS patients, a few authors have made important comments in this area. Schaffner (1990) has described some emotional themes that appear to emerge commonly in such psychotherapy, including shock at the initial diagnosis, denial, guilt, anger and frustration, isolation, grief, changes in libido or general need for intimacy, and various reactions to discussing the illness or one's possible death with one's partner or family. He regards empathic discussion of these issues as the basis of psychotherapy with AIDS patients, observing that because there are no "standard" psychiatric signs and symptoms for this illness, treatment is better described by addressing these emotional challenges, which are likely to be shared by most AIDS patients.

Similarly, Rogers (1989) has argued that the psychodynamic issues raised by this disorder are neglected because of the urgency of the biomedical and public health aspects of the epidemic. She has described a case in considerable detail in which many of the themes mentioned by Schaffner (1990) emerged in the context of a young man presenting for treatment of panic disorder with agoraphobia. Rogers, in particular, has advocated for psychodynamic understanding as a way to decrease the polarization between caregiver and patient that may have overly influenced the mental health field.

In a useful early review, S. W. Perry and Markowitz (1986) recommended helping the patient place the illness and the manner in which it was acquired into his or her life course and character style. They also delineated three general principles in dealing with AIDS patients in an outpatient setting: recognizing that the patient may have regressed into a "sick role" and actually be less characterologically dependent than may be initially apparent; allowing the patient to focus on physical symptoms rather than "forcing" the patient too quickly into a psychological discussion; and keeping in mind the power of clarification, abreaction, and suggestion.

In other reports Holland and Tross (1985) recommended exploration of feelings regarding sexual practices and guilt, and a ventilative as well as psychoeducational stance on the part of the therapist. Wolcott (1986) stressed the need to discuss any internalized homophobia that may become evident as the illness progresses. Adler and Beckett (1989) discussed the issue of HIV transmission and the role of projective identification in the outpatient therapy of AIDS patients, and Ostrow et al. (1988) described the power of the listening, empathic, nonjudgmental stance; they have found that, when asked by a physician, "What can I do for you?", the typical response of an AIDS patient is, "I want you to listen to me and not be afraid of me" (p. 20).

More specific treatment recommendations are found in the cognitive-behavior therapy literature. Some authors have recommended stress management techniques such as relaxation training, hypnosis, and guided imagery for relief of ongoing anxiety, instead of or in addition to antianxiety medication (Faulstich 1987; Perry and Markowitz 1986; Wolcott 1986). Schmaling and DiClementi (1991) have described a specific cognitive therapy approach with HIV-seropositive patients. This includes working with denial; accepting, not challenging, some distorted cognitions if accompanied by euthymia, good social support, and no compromise of medical care; "prescribing" activities in a flexible and realistic way; and challenging depressive cognitions by seeing them as examples of thinking errors (e.g., selective abstraction) or of the depressive "cognitive triad" (negative view of self, world, and future) (Beck et al. 1979). (See Chesney and Folkman [1994] for a comprehensive review of such cognitive-behavioral interventions.)

Similarly, S. Perry (1991) has adapted cognitive therapy techniques to the specific situation of AIDS patients beginning, remaining on, or deciding to stop zidovudine therapy. Levine et al. (1991) have described a group therapy program for depressed HIV-seropositive patients that draws on cognitive therapy techniques as well as on fluoxetine, psychodynamic group process, and psychoeducation as treatment modalities. Beckett and Rutan (1990) have described a more process-oriented group with some similar features.

By the nature of this illness, it is almost inconceivable to manage a patient with AIDS without adequate psychosocial as well as medical backup from a general hospital. Baer et al. (1987) discussed some issues in establishing an inpatient psychiatric unit for AIDS and ARC patients. Lauer-Listhaus and Watterson (1988) similarly described their experience with psychoeducational groups for HIV-positive psychiatric inpatients. Lyons et al. (1989) documented the extent to which AIDS patients utilize consultation-liaison psychiatry, social work, and discharge planning services disproportionately to their numbers in a general hospital setting. Wolcott (1986) offered a useful review of the ways in which the outpatient practitioner may be called on to provide support, for example, to a family attempting to reconcile themselves to a son's homosexuality as well as to his illness.

As improved retroviral and other treatments become available (Myers et al. 1993), AIDS patients may begin to live longer, causing a new kind of impact on patients, families, and medical and mental health providers. Suicide and depression rates for HIV-infected individuals may have started to diminish compared with those in the mid-1980s (Chesney and Folkman 1994; Rabkin et al. 1993). Such factors as age, route of HIV acquisition, gender, symptomatic status, and disclosure (or not) of seropositivity may all affect subjective or operationalized quality of life (Chesney and Folkman 1994). Race may not affect survival time if access to care is controlled for, but to the extent that black Americans may collectively have lower socioeconomic status and less access to care than do white Americans, their quality of life may be differentially affected (Curtis and Patrick 1993). (See Wallace et al. [1993] for a specific discussion of the impact of HIV infection on older patients.)

A final aspect of psychosocial treatment that deserves mention concerns the feelings of the therapist in working with AIDS patients and their loved ones. Wallack (1989) operationalized provider AIDS anxiety into a 79-item questionnaire. Perry and Markowitz (1986) described three common countertransference reactions in dealing with such patients: exaggerated fear of contagion, a tendency to stereotype patients who belong to high-risk groups, and difficulties in maintaining an empathic distance that is neither too uninvolved nor too overly identified. Adler and Beckett (1989) added therapist denial and intolerance of helplessness to this list. McKusick (1988) presented case illustrations of these and other issues and offered a starkly effective method of eliciting and dealing with these feelings: Clinicians are advised to assess their own AIDS risk and to imagine seeing themselves reacting to testing HIV positive.

Primary Prevention

A number of efforts toward primary prevention, chiefly in the form of risk reduction, have been undertaken in various centers. One area of risk reduction immediately relevant to community psychiatrists is that of AIDS education for patients with chronic mental illness. At least three groups (Brady and Carmen 1990; Goisman et al. 1991; Meyer et al. 1992) have described curricula involving psychoeducation, role playing, and instruction in condom use suitable for community mental health centers. Kelly et al. (1993) have comprehensively reviewed the literature in this area from a community perspective.

Another equally important area is that of substance abuse prevention, the effectiveness of which has been well documented by Hubbard et al. (1988). Valdiserri et al. (1988) have described the lack of AIDS education among incarcerated drug abusers, whereas Bakti et al. (1988) discussed the role of denial, anger, depression, and isolation in inhibiting effective substance abuse treatment in HIV-positive drug abusers. Flavin et al. (1986) have described similar problems in suicidal alcoholic homosexual men at high AIDS risk. Yet concrete interventions to decrease AIDS risk or ongoing substance abuse are both possible and effective; these include education in cleaning needles and not sharing them, providing needle exchanges, distribution of bleach for cleaning, and instruction in the use of condoms (Bakti 1990; Bing et al. 1990; Calsyn et al. 1992).

Many subcultures within American society have particular concerns regarding AIDS prevention and risk reduction, especially with the predominant belief that AIDS is a disease of homosexual white males (Bing et al. 1990). These may include, among others, strong prohibitions against acknowledgment of homosexuality among black or Hispanic men (Bing et al. 1990); the feeling, common among adolescents, that one is invulnerable to AIDS (Bowler et al. 1992); the belief that anal intercourse in the active position carries a low risk (Peterson and Marin 1988); and stigmatization of women who supply their partners with condoms as "loose" (Mays and Cochran 1988).

This last prejudice is especially ironic, as it punishes responsible risk reduction behavior in women, for whom sexual contact with intravenous drug users represents a major HIV risk factor (Mazzullo 1994). Women in general represent an understudied population in terms of AIDS risk, although 10% of all known AIDS cases in 1991 were in women (Wofsy et al. 1992). Female gender may be associated with more psychological symptoms and greater impairment of quality of life (Chesney and Folkman 1994).

Nonetheless, it is possible to develop risk reduction programs that are both culturally sensitive and effective, as long as group cultural norms are taken into account in the design of these programs (Mays and Cochran 1988; Peterson and Marin 1988; Stall et al. 1988). Programs specific to adolescents (Bowler et al. 1992; Nangle and Hansen 1993) and to women (Wofsy et al. 1992) have been developed as well. A previously underutilized resource in this area may be the family physician or other primary care provider; at least two articles have explored the importance of and technique for taking a sexual and drug history in a primary medical care setting (Gabel and Pearsol 1993; Lewis 1990).

Space limitations preclude detailed exploration of other areas of AIDS primary prevention. (See Krajeski [1990] for a synopsis of issues in HIV testing and to Carlson et al. [1989] and Wagner et al. [1993] regarding patients who present ongoing HIV risk to others. The excellent bibliography by Wallack et al. [1991] contains further references regarding these and other issues in primary prevention and risk reduction.)

Summary

In this chapter I have discussed a model of public health psychiatry applicable to the current AIDS epidemic in terms of primary, secondary, and tertiary prevention. I have outlined issues of psychiatric and neuropsychiatric differential diagnosis, including dementia and delirium, depression, anxiety, mania, psychosis, substance abuse, and AIDS-related psychopathology in HIV-negative individuals. I have described rational psychopharmacological treatment regimens for these indications, and I have discussed issues in the psychodynamic and cognitive-behavioral psychotherapy of AIDS patients. Finally, I have outlined a number of areas in which primary prevention efforts are called for and have met with some success.

Armed with all of this knowledge and more, the task confronting community psychiatry as it attempts to utilize its modicum of leverage to fight this epidemic still seems overwhelming. Yet it must be remembered that our profession does not have to "solve" this problem alone; our efforts have been fallible but helpful, and we thus have a limited role but a definite one. It is to be hoped that this chapter will be of assistance to those who are willing to step into that role.

References

Adler G, Beckett A: Psychotherapy of the patient with an HIV infection: some ethical and therapeutic dilemmas. Psychosomatics 30:203–208, 1989

American Psychiatric Association: Diagnostic and Statistical Manual of Mental Disorders, 4th Edition. Washington, DC, American Psychiatric Association, 1994

Baer JW, Hall JM, Holm K, et al: Challenges in developing an inpatient psychiatric program for patients with AIDS and ARC. Hosp Community Psychiatry 38:1299–1303, 1987

Bakti SL: Substance abuse and AIDS: the need for mental health services. New Dir Ment Health Serv 48:55–67, 1990

Bakti SL, Sorensen JL, Faltz B, et al: Psychiatric aspects of treatment of IV drug abusers with AIDS. Hosp Community Psychiatry 39:439–441, 1988

Beck AT, Rush AJ, Shaw BF, et al: Cognitive Therapy of Depression. New York, Guilford, 1979

Beckett A, Rutan JS: Treating persons with ARC and AIDS in group psychotherapy. Int J Group Psychother 40:19–29, 1990

Bialer PA, Wallack JJ: Mixed factitious disorder presenting as AIDS. Hosp Community Psychiatry 41:552–553, 1990

Bing EG, Nichols SE, Goldfinger SM, et al: The many faces of AIDS: opportunities for intervention. New Dir Ment Health Serv 48:69–81, 1990

Bowler S, Sheon AR, D'Angelo LJ, et al: HIV and AIDS among adolescents in the United States: increasing risk in the 1990s. J Adolesc 15:345–371, 1992

Brady SM, Carmen EH: AIDS risk in the chronically mentally ill: clinical strategies for prevention. New Dir Ment Health Serv 48:83–95, 1990

Brotman AW, Forstein M: AIDS obsessions in depressed heterosexuals. Psychosomatics 29:428–431, 1988

Calsyn DA, Meinecke C, Saxon AI, et al: Risk reduction in sexual behavior: a condom giveaway program in a drug abuse treatment clinic. Am J Public Health 82:1536–1538, 1992

Caplan G: Principles of Preventive Psychiatry. New York, Basic Books, 1964

Carlson GA, Greeman M, McClellan TA: Management of HIV-positive psychiatric patients who fail to reduce high-risk behaviors. Hosp Community Psychiatry 40:511–514, 1989

Catalan J: Psychosocial and neuropsychiatric aspects of HIV infection: review of their extent and implications for psychiatry. J Psychosom Res 32:237–248, 1988

Centers for Disease Control: Pneumocystis pneumonia—Los Angeles. MMWR Morb Mortal Wkly Rep 30:250–252, 1981a

Centers for Disease Control: Kaposi's sarcoma and Pneumocystis pneumonia among homosexual men—New York City and California. MMWR Morb Mortal Wkly Rep 30:350–358, 1981b

Centers for Disease Control and Prevention: HIV AIDS Surveill Rep 5(2):1–19, 1993

Chesney MA, Folkman S: Psychological impact of HIV disease and implications for intervention. Psychiatric Clin North Am 17:163–182, 1994

Curtis JR, Patrick DL: Race and survival time with AIDS: a synthesis of the literature. Am J Public Health 83:1425–1428, 1993

Empfield M, Weinstock A, Cournos F, et al: HIV seroprevalence study of involuntarily hospitalized mentally ill homeless from the streets of Manhattan, New York. Paper presented at the Fifth International Conference on AIDS, Montreal, Quebec, Canada, June 1989

Empfield M, Cournos F, Meyer I, et al: HIV seroprevalence among homeless patients admitted to a psychiatric inpatient unit. Am J Psychiatry 150:47–52, 1993

Faulstich ME: Psychiatric aspects of AIDS. Am J Psychiatry 144:551–556, 1987

Fenton TW: AIDS-related psychiatric disorder. Br J Psychiatry 151:579–588, 1987

Fernandez F: Psychiatric complications in HIV-related illnesses, in AIDS Primer. Edited by AIDS Education Project, American Psychiatric Association. Washington, DC, American Psychiatric Association, 1988

Fernandez F: Psychopharmacological interventions in HIV infections. New Dir Ment Health Serv 48:43–53, 1990

Field HL: Biopsychosocial aspects of AIDS. New Dir Ment Health Serv 53:51–60, 1993

Flavin DK, Franklin JE, Frances RJ: The acquired immune deficiency syndrome and suicidal behavior in alcohol-dependent homosexual men. Am J Psychiatry 143:1440–1442, 1986

Frierson RL, Lippmann SB: Suicide and AIDS. Psychosomatics 29:226–231, 1988

Gabel LL, Pearsol JA: Taking an effective sexual and drug history: a first step in HIV/AIDS prevention. J Fam Pract 37:185–187, 1993

Goisman RM, Kent AB, Montgomery EC, et al: AIDS education for patients with chronic mental illness. Community Ment Health J 27:189–197, 1991

Goldwurm GF, Zamparetti M, Caggese L, et al: Prevalence of HIV antibody tests (HIV ab+) among the patients of a psychiatric ward. Paper presented at the IV International Conference on AIDS, Stockholm, Sweden, June 1988

Halstead S, Riccio M, Harlow P, et al: Psychosis associated with HIV infection. Br J Psychiatry 153:618–623, 1988

Hintz S, Kuck J, Peterkin JJ, et al: Depression in the context of human immunodeficiency virus infection: implications for treatment. J Clin Psychiatry 51:497–501, 1990

Holland JC, Tross S: The psychosocial and neuropsychiatric sequelae of the acquired immunodeficiency syndrome and related disorders. Ann Intern Med 103:760–764, 1985

Hubbard RL, Marsden ME, Cavanaugh E, et al: Role of drug-abuse treatment in limiting the spread of AIDS. Rev Infect Dis 10:377–384, 1988

Katz MH: Effect of HIV treatment on cognition, behavior, and emotion. Psychiatric Clin North Am 17:227–230, 1994

Kelly JA, Murphy DA, Sikkema KJ, et al: Psychological interventions to prevent HIV infection are urgently needed. Am Psychologist 48:1023–1034, 1993

King MB: Psychosocial status of 192 out-patients with HIV infection and AIDS. Br J Psychiatry 154:237–242, 1989

Kokmen E, Naessens JM, Offord KP: A short test of mental status: description and preliminary results. Mayo Clin Proc 62:281–288, 1987

Krajeski JP: Legal, ethical, and public policy issues. New Dir Ment Health Serv 48:97–106, 1990

Lauer-Listhaus B, Watterson J: A psychoeducational group for HIV-positive patients on a psychiatric service. Hosp Community Psychiatry 39:776–777, 1988

Levine SH, Bystritsky A, Baron D, et al: Group psychotherapy for HIV-seropositive patients with major depression. Am J Psychother 45:413–424, 1991

Lewis CE: Sexual practices: are physicians addressing the issues? J Gen Intern Med 5 (suppl):S78–S81, 1990

Lippert GP: Excessive concern about AIDS in two bisexual men. Can J Psychiatry 31:63–65, 1986

Lyons JS, Larson DB, Anderson RL, et al: Psychosocial services for AIDS patients in the general hospital. Int J Psychiatry Med 19:385–392, 1989

Mahorney SL, Cavenar JO: A new and timely delusion: the complaint of having AIDS. Am J Psychiatry 145:1130–1132, 1988

Marzuk PM, Tierney H, Tardiff K, et al: Increased risk of suicide in persons with AIDS. JAMA 259:1333–1337, 1988

Mays VM, Cochran SD: Issues in the perception of AIDS risk and risk reduction activities by black and Hispanic/Latina women. Am Psychologist 43:949–957, 1988

Mazzullo J: HIV infection/viral hepatitis: update and treatment. Paper presented at the Fifth National Health Care for the Homeless Conference, Baltimore, MD, May 1994

McKusick L: The impact of AIDS on practitioner and client. Am Psychologist 43:935–940, 1988

Meyer I, Cournos F, Empfield M, et al: HIV prevention among psychiatric inpatients: a pilot risk reduction study. Psychiatr Q 63:187–197, 1992

Miller D, Riccio M: Non-organic psychiatric and psychosocial syndromes associated with HIV-1 infection and disease. AIDS 4:381–388, 1990

Myers SA, Prose NS, Bartlett JA: Progress in the understanding of HIV infection: an overview. J Am Acad Dermatol 29:1–21, 1993

Nangle DW, Hansen DJ: Relations between social skills and high-risk sexual interactions among adolescents. Behav Modif 17:113–135, 1993

Navia BA, Price RW: The acquired immunodeficiency syndrome dementia complex as the presenting or sole manifestation of human immunodeficiency virus infection. Arch Neurol 44:65–69, 1987

Nurnberg HG, Prudic J, Fiori M, et al: Psychopathology complicating acquired immune deficiency syndrome (AIDS). Am J Psychiatry 141:95–96, 1984

Ostrow D, Grant I, Atkinson H: Assessment and management of the AIDS patient with neuropsychiatric disturbances. J Clin Psychiatry 49 (5, suppl):14–22, 1988

Pepper B: The young adult chronic patient: population overview. J Clin Psychopharmacol 5 (suppl):3S–7S, 1985

Perry S: Psychosocial aspects of zidovudine treatment. HIV Frontline 3:1–6, 1991

Perry S, Jacobsberg LB, Fishman B, et al: Psychiatric diagnosis before serological testing for the human immunodeficiency virus. Am J Psychiatry 147:89–93, 1990

Perry SW: Organic mental disorders caused by HIV: update on early diagnosis and treatment. Am J Psychiatry 147:696–710, 1990

Perry SW, Markowitz J: Psychiatric interventions for AIDS-spectrum disorders. Hosp Community Psychiatry 37:1001–1006, 1986

Peterson JL, Marin G: Issues in the prevention of AIDS among black and Hispanic men. Am Psychologist 43:871–877, 1988

Rabkin JG, Remien R, Katoff L, et al: Resilience in adversity among long-term survivors of AIDS. Hosp Community Psychiatry 44:162–167, 1993

Rogers RR: Beyond morality: the need for psychodynamic understanding and treatment of responses to the AIDS crisis. Psychiatr J Univ Ott 14:456–459, 1989

Schaerf FW, Miller RR, Lipsey JR, et al: ECT for major depression in four patients infected with human immunodeficiency virus. Am J Psychiatry 146:782–784, 1989

Schaffner B: Psychotherapy with HIV-infected persons. New Dir Ment Health Serv 48:5–20, 1990

Schmaling KB, DiClementi JD: Cognitive therapy with the HIV seropositive patient. The Behavior Therapist 14:221–224, 1991

Shaw GM, Harper ME, Hahn BH, et al: HTLV-III infection in brains of children and adults with AIDS encephalopathy. Science 227:177–181, 1985

Sidtis JJ, Price RW: Early HIV-1 infection and the AIDS dementia complex. Neurology 40:323–326, 1990

Spivak B, Mester R, Babur I, et al: Prolonged fear of AIDS as an early symptom of schizophrenia. Psychopathology 23:181–184, 1990

Stall RD, Coates TJ, Hoff C: Behavioral risk reduction for HIV infection among gay and bisexual men. Am Psychologist 43:878–885, 1988

Starace F: Suicidal behaviour in people infected with human immunodeficiency virus: a literature review. Int J Soc Psychiatry 39:64–70, 1993

Stewart DL, Zuckerman CJ, Ingle JM: HIV seroprevalence in a chronically mentally ill population. J Natl Med Assoc 86:519–523, 1994

Torres RA, Mani S, Altholz J, et al: Human immunodeficiency virus infection among homeless men in a New York City shelter. Arch Intern Med 150:2030–2036, 1990

Valdiserri EV, Hartl AJ, Chambliss CA: Practices reported by incarcerated drug abusers to reduce risk of AIDS. Hosp Community Psychiatry 39:966–972, 1988

Wagner GJ, Rabkin JG, Rabkin R: Sexual activity among HIV-seropositive gay men seeking treatment for depression. J Clin Psychiatry 54:470-475, 1993

Wallace JI, Paauw DS, Spach DH: HIV infection in older patients: when to suspect the unexpected. Geriatrics 48:61–70, 1993

Wallack JJ: AIDS anxiety among health care professionals. Hosp Community Psychiatry 40:507–510, 1989

Wallack JJ, Snyder S, Bialer PA, et al: An AIDS bibliography for the general psychiatrist. Psychosomatics 32:243–254, 1991

Wiener PK, Schwartz MA, O'Connell RA: Characteristics of HIV-infected patients in an inpatient psychiatric setting. Psychosomatics 35:59–65, 1994

Wofsy CB, Padian NS, Cohen JB, et al: Management of HIV disease in women, in AIDS Clinical Review 1992. Edited by Volberding P, Jacobson MA. New York, Marcel Dekker, 1992, pp 301–328

Wolcott DL: Psychosocial aspects of acquired immune deficiency syndrome and the primary care physician. Ann Allergy 57:95–102, 1986

Chapter 14

Critical Time Points in the Clinical Care of Homeless Mentally Ill Individuals

Elie Valencia, J.D., M.A.
Ezra Susser, M.D., Dr.PH.
Hunter McQuistion, M.D.

In previous publications we have provided an overview of clinical care of homeless individuals (Breakey et al. 1992; Gounis and Susser 1990; McQuistion et al. 1991; Susser 1992; Susser et al. 1990, 1992). We have conceptualized the work of psychiatric programs for homeless people in terms of four stages: 1) the introduction of services into the community, 2) outreach, 3) provision of treatment and other services during the time that individuals remain homeless, and 4) support in the transition to housing (Susser et al. 1992). We have noted that in each stage there are features that differentiate work with homeless individuals from other types of outpatient health care.

In this chapter we restrict our attention to two of these four stages—namely, outreach and support in the transition to housing. We believe that there are some especially critical time periods in the course of treatment of

We thank the staff of the CTI Mental Health Program, Columbia Presbyterian Medical Center, at the Fort Washington Shelter for Men, New York City, for their contribution to this article. In particular, we would like to acknowledge the contribution of Alan Felix, M.D., Julio Torres, M.Div., and Sarah Conover, M.P.H. Support for this work was provided by National Institute of Mental Health Grant No. R18MH 48041.

homeless individuals. As in many forms of treatment, the initiation and the termination of clinical care are often the most challenging aspects. The initiation of care falls within the stage of outreach, while the termination of care ideally falls within the stage that we have termed *support in transition to housing*.

We expand on our previous discussions of outreach by describing some common principles that have emerged since the mid-1980s for the initiation of care. We illustrate these principles with examples from our clinical practice. By contrast, with respect to support in the transition to housing, we note the relative absence of consensus in the field. We present one model of care that has been developed for this stage and is presently being tested in the field.

Outreach

Early research on delivery of services to a subpopulation of chronically mentally ill, homeless people documented their sparing use of the mental health system (Goldfinger et al. 1984; Segal et al. 1977; Stickney et al. 1980). This was attributed to a combination of their clinical makeup and endemic service barriers, including inappropriate clinical expectations, patchwork health care planning, and administrative turf conflicts (Bachrach 1987). At the same time, the social epidemic of homelessness grew, creating increased visibility of the problem, often with a public perception that mental illness was a cardinal feature of the condition.

Realizing there was a necessity to find ways to engage those homeless people who were also mentally ill, program planners, particularly in the major urban centers, began to develop outreach initiatives (Putnam et al. 1986). These outreach programs grew rapidly in number and kind during the 1980s. By the end of the decade, outreach services had themselves become institutionalized as the entry point for homeless mentally ill people into housing, social benefits, and medical and psychiatric treatment systems.

Most outreach teams are assigned to public spaces such as parks, city blocks, and transportation terminals, where they approach people who appear to be homeless and mentally ill. The team offers food, clothing, or other assistance as a basis for the initial contacts, as well as the simple opportunity to talk as a relief from chronic isolation. Other outreach teams contact homeless mentally ill people as they pass through institutions such as drop-in centers, soup kitchens, shelters, and jails. For instance, in a good drop-in center, homeless people find a sort of sanctuary, a place to sit quietly or to talk and be heard out respectfully, and a place to form social ties safely. They are also offered food, access to showers, clothes, coffee, and the use of a telephone. Homeless people do not have to be enrolled in any treatment to use these services. Rather, the setting provides a meaningful context for the initial contact between clinician and client (Segal and Baumohl 1985; Gounis and Susser 1990).

The challenge to the clinician is to proceed from these various starting points to the introduction of comprehensive treatment. Just as outreach was invented as a novel response to the necessity of engaging a previously unreached clinical population, the outreach clinician's own technique must be inventive, too, even idiosyncratic. When working from the premise that conventional approaches have failed, there are few established precedents to follow.

There are also few precedents for the administrative structures to implement these programs, especially for the more creative outreach programs (Gounis and Susser 1990; Susser 1992). These programs vary widely in terms of professional staff, treatment philosophy, institutional connections, and other dimensions. For instance, some teams rely primarily on paraprofessional staff, whereas others rely mainly on highly trained clinicians and psychiatrists. Even within the same program, there may be substantial change in these features over time.

Thus, it can be difficult to discern common threads among the diverse forms of outreach that are practiced. As a clinical craft, outreach to homeless mentally ill persons is still in a formative stage, with a developing identity (McQuistion et al. 1991). Nonetheless, it is our impression that a distinctive body of shared principles and practices is emerging among outreach clinicians. Three principles appear to guide clinical practice in many outreach programs: 1) flexibility, 2) the creative use of incentives, and 3) persistence.

The fact that outreach clinicians have developed these principles is important. In the most immediate sense, this is significant because outreach represents the first line of contact to homeless mentally ill people and sets up expectations of treatment by the individual. Hence, in many ways the clinical orientation in outreach work shapes the behavior of subsequent providers to this population. It requires them, for example, to remain highly flexible.

Of equal importance is that none of these three principles are applicable only within programs for homeless people. The experience of engaging and treating this particularly hard-to-work-with group of chronically mentally ill individuals has been a crucial source for new ideas in the care of all people with severe and persistent mental illness. However, because these principles were conceived in programs for homeless persons, they have been applied with more vigor in these programs than in other settings.

Flexibility

In programs for homeless people, flexibility pervades the initial stages of the treatment process to an extent that is rarely seen in clinics and hospitals. These programs strive to recruit into treatment severely ill individuals who are not seeking help but may be persuaded to do so (Gounis and Susser 1990; Kass et al. 1992). Accommodations are made that would be unthinkable in most other settings. For example, medication in an ongoing way has been offered through street outreach programs to people who decline to attend any indoor program.

The pace of treatment is highly individualized. These programs generally allow for a gradual period of acquaintance before carrying out a full assessment. There may be a period of contact before treatment is even discussed. This can extend from weeks to even years. For instance, an outreach worker may hold regular conversations with a prospective patient, offer help with concrete daily needs such as food and clothing, and over time become familiar with the person's habits and social network. Formal treatment may be introduced only after a modicum of trust has been established.

The timing of interventions, be they verbal or concrete, is therefore crucial. This is perhaps even more critical in outreach than in other therapeutic endeavors, especially in the beginning stage of engagement when a relationship can be fragile and easily broken, with no subsequent opportunity for reestablishment. In our experience (Susser et al. 1992), as well as others' (Rosnow 1988), outreach clinicians struggle with the pace of interventions, often having to hold back from offering a referral, for example, until the person is truly ready to accept it.

Clinicians must be constantly aware of opportunities to intervene appropriately. They often present themselves at a time of relative stress for the homeless mentally ill person. Recognizing such an instance after having developed a solid relationship can make the difference. For example, a longtime street dweller who suffered from schizophrenia accepted a well-timed offer for a place at a specialized shelter during a particularly sweltering summer spell. There had been hot spells before, but this time his habitual train terminal location was "just too hot." At the same time, because of a major public event in the city that week, local police were more active in "sweeping" homeless people from the train terminal, and he was motivated to avoid them. Once he took the step of entering the specialized shelter, his anxiety about this unknown setting was relieved, and he was then able to use it as a resource.

It is not only paraprofessional staff who must adjust their pace. In one example, a psychiatrist played bingo with mentally ill women in a transitional hotel as a mean of establishing trust and familiarity before introducing treatment (Susser 1992). The game provided for a friendly and nonthreatening environment where these women could interact with the psychiatrist with no shame. This approach allowed the psychiatrist to become an accepted figure in the hotel and later to introduce treatment issues without being rejected.

In addition to adjusting the pace of treatment, clinicians make accommodations to an individual's idiosyncrasies that might be considered remarkable in other contexts. Patients differ in their requests for assistance, which can range from buying a pair of shoes to contacting a relative or settling a dispute with another person. They differ in patterns of use of services; some make appointments, others "drop in" every day, and still others appear episodically with a request for help and then are lost to contact until the next crisis. They differ in the type of contact that is possible. Some patients refuse any lengthy conversation with a clinician but will "hang out" and be observed over much of the day. Others want extended personal contact with a clinician and do not want to participate in any other type of care.

What is remarkable is not so much the variety found in these needs of homeless mentally ill people—after all, patients in any setting differ widely. Rather, it is the degree to which outreach clinicians have been willing to adjust to the distinct needs and expressed preferences of their patients. One patient known to us, a verbal and psychologically minded person with a narcissistic and dependent personality disorder, accepted a referral for supportive psychotherapy at a local clinic after his talents were validated by being a key member of a creative writing group at a drop-in center.

Creative Use of Incentives

Much of the art of clinical care in outreach consists of knowing when and how much to use incentives and mildly coercive approaches. The clinician has to identify an incentive that is particularly meaningful to an individual and then has to find a delicate way in which to interweave incentives into the treatment process without sacrificing the trust that is essential to its continued development.

In our view the strongest motivation for participation in treatment generally derives not from material incentives, but from the perception that one's sense of self-esteem and well-being will be strengthened. By simply listening to the patient when others do not, the clinician may create a strong incentive for attendance. Similarly, the program space itself may provide a warm atmosphere where a person feels accepted (Gounis and Susser 1990; Susser et al. 1992). Despite material deprivation, emotional needs remain a priority. In one example, a psychiatrist in a large men's shelter gave his old trumpet to a patient who was a jazz musician. This gift was significant not so much for its monetary value, but because it symbolized the psychiatrist's recognition of the patient's area of competency and of his deepest aspirations. It solidified the treatment relationship.

Although necessary, this type of motivation is often not sufficient for the treatment engagement of hard-to-reach patients, especially in this early phase. In many instances, clinicians attempt to connect the treatment process with the short-term or long-term goals of individual patients. The identification of these goals occurs in the course of outreach and is a demanding task that requires patience, insight, and compassion.

Some very ill patients may not directly express themselves. The clinician may have to observe these patients' daily activities to discern what is really of interest to them. In one case, an outreach team trying to contact a woman who had been living in bus terminals for years noticed that she had a fondness and talent for making clothing out of pieces of cloth. Although the woman refused to accept any food or clothing from the team, she was willing to accept the raw materials for her work—pieces of cloth—on a regular basis. This step not only constituted a form of personal recognition, as in the preceding example of the trumpet, but also created an incentive for continued contact with the team.

Less disturbed patients may reveal their goals more directly in a series of conversations. They may have some quite limited short-term goals that are felt very strongly. A patient's goal may be simply to play basketball with friends a few times a week, or to knit some piece of clothing for a relative. Once a goal that means something to the individual is clear, the clinician emphasizes the ways in which treatment of psychiatric problems will make it easier to reach the goal. He or she also interweaves into the treatment process concrete assistance in meeting the goal. This is de facto psychiatric rehabilitation (Anthony and Liberman 1986) and ultimately serves to enhance a person's independence while also providing a theoretical structure for the clinician's practice.

People may also express far broader aspirations. For instance, a patient may be preoccupied with reconciliation with his or her children. The person may respond only when treatment is framed as a step toward the fulfillment of this aspiration and when the clinician is seen to be helpful in this regard.

Programs can also use more concrete incentives such as money, small prizes, or cigarettes. These may be used to reward participation in groups, to reinforce compliance with medication treatment, or to enhance the probability of some specific critical step such as showing up for an appointment for a medical evaluation. In one program, in a group for patients with substance use as well as psychiatric disorders, monetary rewards were given to reward patients for drug-free urine tests.

In addition, patients may be given access to some special privilege only if they participate in some type of program activity or treatment. They may be required to take medications, attend groups, or stay off street drugs. For instance, patients in a program may from time to time receive a small payment in return for carrying out jobs that arise, such as running an errand. In an individual case, access to this work may be made contingent on compliance with medication treatment. On occasion patients are denied continued access to an activity in which they are already involved, unless they comply with a prescribed treatment. In this application the use of incentives may also be considered a form of mild coercion.

Neither concrete incentives nor coercion will achieve any useful purpose when they are applied in a nonindividualized manner and are used as the mainstay of treatment. They can be quite effective, however, when applied within a trusting relationship between patient and clinician that has been carefully developed over time.

For example, one anxious drop-in center member with posttraumatic stress disorder and borderline personality disorder realized he had a serious impulse control problem, often finding himself in physical confrontations with others, including his girlfriend. He eventually agreed to random urine testing, with negative urine tests linked to goals that were clear to him. This was accomplished after months of patient, supportive, and consistent engagement by staff concerning the role of his episodic drug use as a precipitant to his loss of control.

Persistence

As illustrated previously, clinical programs for homeless people can offer treatment to a mentally ill person on a daily basis over a period of months or longer. Clinicians may be rejected on every occasion, yet they must persist. They create new ways in which to frame the treatment option as they learn more about the individual; they seek opportunities to form a stronger relationship with the individual; and they continue to approach the person regularly, with offers of help, in the expectation that once sufficient trust has been built, the offer will be accepted.

Persistence may seem a heroic gesture. In fact, it is a pragmatic and effective treatment strategy. It can take much time, as well as trial and error, to persuade a person to enter psychiatric treatment. We are continually impressed at how persistent efforts to build trust tend to pay off eventually, even in the most difficult cases. Only in the most extreme cases, usually involving severe self-neglect, do outreach services need to resort to preemptive emergency hospitalization to engage a homeless mentally ill person into treatment.

It should be emphasized that persistence is not synonymous with repetition. A series of contacts may appear to be simply a repetition of a greeting or a casual conversation. Actually, the clinician is attempting to move gradually toward a stronger tie and toward treatment. He or she has to apply just the right amount of pressure to avoid losing the patient while moving ever closer to the introduction of treatment. Some of the most rewarding experiences in this field of clinical work are the fruits of this type of persistent effort.

One of the most moving experiences in the clinical careers of two of the authors was the result of just this type of persistence. A man with paranoid schizophrenia living in a large men's shelter had been homeless for more than a decade and seemingly unreceptive to any offers of treatment. He slept in the hallway of the shelter rather than on a bed. As a result of paranoid delusions, he never ventured outside the shelter into the street. Over many years, the on-site shelter psychiatry program presumed that this man represented one of the few who could not be engaged in treatment and housing placement. Rather than abandoning him, however, they maintained daily brief contacts and, when the need presented, assisted him in survival within the shelter environment. In the process, he gradually formed attachments to the outreach staff. After 5 years of outreach, he finally agreed to let the outreach team locate his family, and a sensational reunion was achieved. At the same time, he started medication treatment, and his delusions diminished. He was able to leave the shelter for initially short but increasingly longer periods of time until he was placed in a community residence, where he remains to date.

Support in the Transition to Housing

The foremost mission of many clinical programs for homeless mentally ill persons is generally to engage people in treatment. Thus, several renowned programs have been involved in refining our understanding of outreach to homeless mentally ill people. A literature on approaches to the initiation of care in this population has begun to emerge (Cohen and Tsemberis 1991; Gounis and Susser 1990; McQuistion et al. 1991; Segal and Baumohl 1985; Susser et al. 1992).

By contrast, relatively few programs have focused systematically on the termination of care by specialized programs for homeless people. We have termed this stage *support in the transition to housing* because it generally involves the transfer of care from programs for homeless persons to other community resources around the time of housing placement. It may be considered analogous to the transfer of care from hospital to community services at the time of hospital discharge. In the process of termination of clinical care, programs for homeless people seem less sophisticated. Moreover, such programs are far from a consensus as to how to proceed. However, in our impression, the termination and transfer of care are as critical and as difficult as the initiation of care in this population.

In this stage of care, clinicians may need to radically adjust their techniques. What was appropriate in earlier stages of care may not be so here. As patients proceed through outreach and on-site treatment, they increasingly depend on the clinical program to meet a wide range of needs. However, during the phase of termination, they must move toward greater autonomy. The proper timing and nature of the transfer of care are controversial. Many programs transfer care rather abruptly at the time of housing placement. This results in a discontinuity of care and a decrease in services for these patients. We disagree with this approach.

To improve on this practice, some programs have extended care into this critical transition period. In the text that follows, we present a model we have developed for clinical care during the stage of support in the transition to housing: the Critical Time Intervention (CTI) model for mentally ill individuals (Susser et al. 1992; Valencia et al. 1994). This model is being tested in a randomized clinical trial among homeless mentally ill men. This study which is near completion, has been conducted in the Columbia-Presbyterian CTI Mental Health Program for the Homeless, located at the Fort Washington Shelter for Men in New York City.

The Critical Time Intervention (CTI) Model

The CTI model aims to reduce the recurrence of homelessness among mentally ill individuals in the period of transition to community living. It is a time-limited intervention with a straightforward approach that could be replicated with ease (Valencia et al. 1994). The thrust of the intervention is to enhance the continuity of mental health services to mentally ill individuals at this time of transition. Thus, it is designed to bridge the gap between homeless and community services while complementing rather than paralleling the existing service system for the mentally ill.

CTI was motivated in large part by our clinical observation of a high recurrence of homelessness after community placement from a psychiatry program in a large New York City shelter (Gounis and Susser 1990). This impression was later confirmed in a follow-up study of patients placed into community housing from our psychiatry program for homeless mentally ill persons in the Fort Washington shelter. Following placement in the community, 16% had homeless episodes within the first 6 months (Caton et al. 1990) and were homeless again within 18 months (Caton et al. 1992).

We infer from our experience that the transition to community living is an especially vulnerable period for these individuals and that their need for support is at a peak at this time. In addition, the patterns of behavior and support systems required to maintain housing stability are not yet present. The adaptation to community living in this critical time of transition requires the establishment of an expanded support system. Therefore, an abrupt and complete transfer of care at such a time is perilous.

Creating linkages, both with formal service agencies and informal social supports, is a difficult task (Belcher and First 1987–1988; Gounis and Susser 1990; Mercier 1990; Morse et al. 1992). Negotiating such networks requires a high level of social skills, which many mentally ill individuals may not have. In addition, a significant proportion of these persons are struggling with other disabilities, including substance abuse (Drake et al. 1989; Susser et al. 1989, 1991) and human immunodeficiency virus (HIV) infection (Susser et al. 1993).

These difficulties are further exacerbated by the gaps existing in the delivery of community-based support services for mentally ill individuals. Services for homeless individuals and the community often operate independently of one another, particularly in large urban centers. These barriers limit the possibilities for the continuity of care that is essential for long-term community living among these patients (Harris and Bergman 1987; Stein and Test 1980; Witheridge and Dincin 1985).

We believe that continuity can be enhanced and recurrent homelessness minimized, however, by specialized support systems during a transition period. Too often these patients and community service providers are unable to find a way to accommodate one another. The patients tend to be difficult; they may come to appointments at the clinic only some of the time, get into fights or steal at the community residence, or spend their money on drugs. Service providers, for their part, may not know how to negotiate a treatment that the individual can tolerate and in a few cases may even be pleased if the patient drops out of care. A specialized intervention designed to foster collaboration between these patients and service providers can "cushion" the difficulties involved over a limited time period while they learn to work together and develop more durable ties.

We have also hypothesized that in the transition period we can reduce the frequency of severe disruptions in relationships between the patient and his family and social network. Patients may steal or cause trouble with neighbors. Family members frequently have not had any introduction to the patient's condition as a medical disorder or any guidance in problem-solving approaches. In a few cases family members are preoccupied by their own emotional or substance abuse problems. These relationships many times can be improved through the provision of a limited but focused intervention.

CTI is based on the premise that a well-timed intervention can influence the evolution of the relationships between the patient and the people on whom he or she must depend. For up to a maximum of 9 months after a patient leaves the shelter, the CTI team assists him or her in establishing durable systems of support. The assistance is highly focused. It focuses in one or two of four areas identified as crucial for stabilization in the transition by the CTI model: 1) medications, 2) money management, 3) substance abuse, and 4) housing-related crises. During the course of the CTI treatment, patients move toward greater autonomy, and community providers move toward more complete responsibility for care.

Implementation Phases of CTI

The implementation of the CTI model proceeds in four main phases in this transitional period: 1) support and assessment, 2) negotiation, 3) monitoring, and 4) transfer of care/termination.

Support and assessment.   The CTI intervention begins at the point when placement into community living has been arranged. The first stage focuses on providing intensive support and assessing the resources for the transition of care. In the first few weeks after placement in community living, the CTI team maintains a high level of contact with the patient. The team makes regular telephone calls to the patient at his or her new residence and some home visits. The patient is offered interim treatment by our psychiatry program until arrangements in the community are functioning (e.g., while the patient is awaiting results of an evaluation at a clinic or rehabilitation program). This assures the patient of some emotional support as well as treatment during the critical moment of transition.

In this first phase of the intervention, the patient is accompanied in person to some crucial appointments (e.g., to a medical clinic). The CTI worker in effect introduces the patient and the new providers at agencies such as mental health centers. We believe that these personal introductions by the CTI worker facilitate the development of a tie and a willingness to negotiate compromises when problems arise.

The team also meets with key figures in the patient's new residence. Key figures are most often the primary caretaker in a family home or staff in a supervised residence, but in some cases other people such as a hotel manager or a neighbor may be considered key figures. The CTI team offers support to these persons. Furthermore, the CTI team is prepared to intervene, when necessary, to mediate a compromise between them and the patient. Tensions tend to arise quickly as caretaker or staff and patient attempt to adjust to one another. Often a compromise worked out in the early phase of adjustment prevents eviction and also proves remarkably durable.

In these initial intensive contacts, the team also is gathering data that are needed for treatment planning in the transition period. They work together with patients and caretakers to detail proposed arrangements to ensure medication compliance, money management, or control of substance abuse. For instance, a system of medication compliance can involve, in addition to the patient, a clinician in an outpatient clinic, a family member, and a local pharmacist, each taking a limited role in monitoring and reinforcing compliance. The medication compliance system is then tested in vivo and modified if necessary during the transition period.

The CTI team makes detailed arrangements only in the one or two areas that are deemed most critical for the community survival of that individual (e.g., medication compliance). It is important not to be overambitious. There is also a strong emphasis on assessing the feasibility for the support systems that are established, because they are meant to last. In some cases a patient just will not visit a clinic with the recommended frequency, and the clinic, for its part, will not make any effort to encourage him to do so. In this circumstance, the clinician can recognize the limited possibilities and still have a significant impact, for instance, by ensuring that the patient continues to make some clinic visits and that the clinic maintains him or her in treatment on this basis.

Negotiation.   The second phase of CTI is devoted to testing and adjusting the systems of support. In the first month or so of operation of a support system, the CTI team is proactive: they identify potential crises, facilitate problem solving, and renegotiate systems as necessary. Unlike the previous phase, the provision of mental health services has moved to the community.

The CTI team identifies any problem areas that the patient may have in the transition to the community. However, priority will be given to one or two areas identified as crucial for stabilization in the transition to the community: medication and money management. Particular attention is directed to those issues that may lead to a housing crisis.

In this phase, the CTI team meets with the patient less frequently except when problems arise with his or her respective community support systems. Problem solving may take the form of a case conference or less formal meetings between the patient and those involved in the support system. The CTI worker acts as a primary resource for all the parties and assists them in setting up a system for resolving potential conflicts. For some patients, this period requires a renegotiation of treatment plans and a more active role of the CTI team in facilitating the implementation of these plans.

Monitoring.   The third phase of the intervention begins when the treatment plan for the transition has been implemented. At this point, providers in the community should have assumed primary responsibility for the provision of support services. This period focuses on assessing whether the support systems are functioning as planned. The emphasis is no longer on direct services but on monitoring.

The team encourages the patient and caretakers to handle problems that arise on their own. However, they maintain regular contact, continue to observe how the plan is working, and remain available to intervene when a crisis arises or when called on by a caretaker. In many cases the system turns out to need some adjustment to be viable in the long run.

Transfer of care/termination.   In the final phase, the focus of the intervention is on the completion of the transfer of care to community resources that will provide long-term support to the patient. Preliminary work leading up to termination has been done throughout the implementation of this transitional intervention.

The CTI team remains available for consultation throughout this period but does not engage in direct service. Its main function in this phase is to ensure that the most significant caretakers meet together and, along with the patient, reach some consensus as to the future system of care. Ideally, this occurs at least 1 or 2 months before the end of the 9-month transition period. Because snags can still be encountered, time must be allowed for adjustment.

The Role of the Psychiatrist in the CTI Model

The role of the psychiatrist in the CTI model is varied. However, its focus is on the coordination of the continuity of care and its comprehensiveness in this period of transition. In addition to his or her traditional role as a psychopharmacologist, the psychiatrist plays a vital role in establishing stability for the chronic mentally ill individual in the transition from institutional to community living. The psychiatrist must be familiar with the patient's past history, response to medications, and relationships to family and friends, as well as counterproductive behaviors in areas such as medication noncompliance, substance abuse, and criminal behavior. Within this context, the psychiatrist's recommendations and assessments shape the process for the continuity of treatment in the community to be implemented by the CTI team.

In addition to passing on information to new service providers, the psychiatrist negotiates on the patient's behalf. As a familiar figure, he or she is a source of stability for the patient and can also assuage many of the anxieties of the new housing and service providers. In the CTI model, it is important that the psychiatrist be flexible to continue to treat the patient following placement from the shelter, particularly in the earliest phase of the transitional period. This might include providing injections, writing out prescriptions, and providing counseling when needed. Much of this can be done on site at the discharging program, but occasionally it is necessary for the psychiatrist to go into the field.

Later, the psychiatrist plays a less central but not less important role as new service providers take over the patient's care in the community. During these phases, he or she may be called on occasionally to intervene if any crisis arises. In this period, the psychiatrist may engage in some family work to strengthen the new linkages and support systems developed in the community for the patient. He or she can assess the family's strengths and weaknesses to determine how much involvement the family, if willing, should have in the community system of the patient's care. For example, a family member may be effective in knowing whom to contact in the event of a crisis.

Moreover, throughout the implementation of CTI, the psychiatrist plays a unique role as a source of integration for the multiplicity of medical problems that often afflict this population, including substance abuse problems and HIV and tuberculosis infections (Susser et al. 1993, in press; Valencia et al. 1994). He or she supervises the CTI team's coordination of the various treatments that may occur at the same time. In this role the psychiatrist seeks to ensure the comprehensiveness of the new support system for the patient in the community.

CTI Versus Case Management

The CTI worker may on first impression appear to be a time-limited case manager. However, although the nature of the work shares much with case management, there are also fundamental differences. CTI aims to transfer care to other systems; the essence is creating, testing, and adjusting systems. There is no option or intention to assume responsibility oneself, as there is in clinical case management. A further distinguishing feature is that, because CTI is a time-limited intervention that seeks to have a durable effect, it must be more highly focused than clinical case management.

CTI is also different from "linkage" case management. The CTI worker carries a strong personal tie to the patient that is a result of the patient's prior intensive treatment in the program for homeless mentally ill people.

The preexisting tie serves as a springboard for effective intervention and especially for mediation between the patient and caretakers, including family members. The CTI worker's task is to gradually transfer this bond within 9 months to other service providers, who, when available, will include centralizing figures such a clinical case manager.

Effectiveness of CTI

Our clinical trial of this intervention is not yet complete. Therefore, we cannot document its effectiveness. However, if it does prove to be effective for patients in the men's shelter, we believe that the approach will have wide generalizability. It is designed to be feasible in a wide array of programs for homeless people. Moreover, the same approach could be used to enhance community stability for chronically ill psychiatric patients after discharge from other institutions such as hospitals or prisons.

Conclusion

We have discussed clinical strategies that relate to two critical time points in the care of homeless mentally ill individuals. The initiation of care with this population is currently highly developed. A broad consensus among clinicians on the usefulness of certain approaches, as well as a descriptive literature, have emerged.

Strategies for the transfer of care from specialized programs for this population to more long-term programs lag behind. There is neither a clinical consensus nor a literature. Indeed, only relatively recently has it been widely recognized that this stage of care is integral to the success of these programs. Some promising models are currently being tested, however, such as the CTI described in this chapter.

The uneven development of these different aspects of treatment of homeless mentally ill persons is a natural consequence of the way in these programs evolved. They were created in response to a social and public health crisis. They had, in addition to a clinical mission, a political one—namely, to show that government agencies were doing something to bring homeless mentally ill people into treatment. Outreach can be highly visible. What happens to patients after treatment by a homeless program tends to be forgotten in the political arena. However, allowing these patients to again "fall through the gaps" of uncoordinated systems of care will only turn their homelessness into another recurrent event in their lives; this can be avoided.

Difficulties at the point of transition are not specific to programs for homeless mentally ill persons. They are pervasive in the mental health system in the United States. Thus, strategies that are being developed for the transfer of care of homeless people may prove equally useful for other mentally ill populations.

References

Anthony WA, Liberman RP: The practice of psychiatric rehabilitation: historical, conceptual, and research base. Schizophr Bull 12(4):542–559, 1986

Bachrach LL: Issues in identifying and treating the homeless mentally ill. New Dir Ment Health Serv 35:43–62, 1987

Belcher JR, First RJ: The homeless mentally ill: barriers to effective service delivery. Journal of Applied Social Sciences 12:62–78, 1987–1988

Breakey W, Susser E, Timms P: Services for the homeless mentally ill, in Measuring Mental Health Needs. Edited by Thornicroft G, Brewin C, Wing J. London, England, Gaskell, 1992, pp 273–290

Caton CLM, Wyatt RJ, Grunberg J, et al: An evaluation of a mental health program for homeless men. Am J Psychiatry 147:286–289, 1990

Caton CLM, Wyatt RJ, Felix A, et al: Follow-up of chronically homeless mentally ill men. Am J Psychiatry 150:1639–1642, 1992

Cohen NL, Tsemberis S: Emergency psychiatric intervention on the street. New Dir Ment Health Serv 52:3–16, 1991

Colson P, Susser E, Valencia E: Improving adherence to TB chemoprophylaxis among homeless mentally ill. Psychosocial Rehabilitation Journal 17:157–160, 1994

Cournos F, Empfield M, Horwath E, et al: HIV infection in state hospitals: case reports and long-term management strategies. Hosp Community Psychiatry 41:163–166, 1990

Cournos F, Empfield M, Horwath E, et al: HIV seroprevalence among admissions at two psychiatric hospitals. Am J Psychiatry 148:1225–1230, 1991

Drake R, Wallach N, Hoffman JS: Housing instability and homelessness among aftercare patients of an urban state hospital. Hosp Community Psychiatry 40:46–51, 1989

Goldfinger SM, Hopkin JT, Surber RW: Treatment resistors or system resistors? toward a better service system for acute care recidivists. New Dir Ment Health Serv 21:17–27, 1984

Gounis K, Susser E: Shelterization and its implications for mental health services, in Psychiatry Takes to the Streets. Edited by Cohen N. New York, Guilford, 1990, pp 231–257

Harris M, Bergman HC: Case management with the chronically mentally ill: a clinical perspective. Am J Orthopsychiatry 57:296–299, 1987

Kass FI, Kahn D, Felix A: Day treatment in a shelter: a setting for assessment and treatment, in Treating the Homeless Mentally Ill. Edited by Lamb HR, Bachrach LL, Kass FI. Washington, DC, American Psychiatric Press, 1992, pp 263–277

McQuistion HL, D'Ercole A, Kopelson E: Urban Street outreach: using clinical principles to steer the system. New Dir Ment Health Serv 52:17–27, 1991

Mercier C: A three-year follow-up study of homeless women: methodological and programmatic issues. Paper presented at the American Evaluation Association Annual Meeting, Washington, DC, October 18–20, 1990

Putnam JF, Cohen NL, Sullivan AM: Innovative outreach services to the homeless mentally ill. International Journal of Mental Health 14(4):112–124, 1986

Rosnow M: Milwaukee's outreach to the homeless mentally ill: 1988, in Assisting the Homeless: State and Local Responses in an Era of Limited Resources. Washington, DC, Advisory Commission on Intergovernmental Relations, 1988, pp 111–119

Segal SP, Baumohl J: The community living room. Soc Casework, February, 1985, pp 111–116

Segal SP, Baumohl J, Johnson E: Falling through the cracks: mental disorder and social margin in a young vagrant population. Soc Probl 24:387–400, 1977

Stein LM, Test MA: Alternative to mental hospital treatment. Arch Gen Psychiatry 37:392–397, 1980

Stickney SK, Hall CW, Gardner ER: The effect of referral procedures on aftercare compliance. Hosp Community Psychiatry 31(8):567–569, 1980

Susser E: Working with people who are mentally ill and homeless: the role of a psychiatrist, in Homelessness: A Prevention-Oriented Approach. Edited by Jahiel RI. Baltimore, MD, Johns Hopkins University Press, 1992, pp 207–217

Susser E, Struening EL, Conover S: Psychiatric problems in homeless men: lifetime psychosis, substance abuse, and current distress in new arrivals at New York City shelters. Arch Gen Psychiatry 46:845–850, 1989

Susser E, White A, Goldfinger S: Some clinical approaches to the homeless mentally ill. Community Ment Health J 26:459–476, 1990

Susser E, Lin S, Conover S: Risk factors for homelessness in patients admitted to a state mental hospital. Am J Psychiatry 148:1659–1664, 1991

Susser E, Valencia E, Goldfinger SM: Clinical care of homeless mentally ill individuals: strategies and adaptations, in Treating the Homeless Mentally Ill. Edited by Lamb HR, Bachrach LL, Kass FI. Washington, DC, American Psychiatric Press, 1992, pp 127–140

Susser E, Valencia E, Conover S: Prevalence of HIV Infection among psychiatric patients in a New York City men's shelter. Am J Public Health 83:568–570, 1993

Susser E, Valencia E, Miller M, et al: Sexual behavior of homeless mentally ill men at risk for HIV. Am J Psychiatry 152:583–587, 1995

Valencia E, Susser E, Canon C, et al: The New York City Critical Time Intervention Study: making a difference guiding the transition to independent living. Interim Status Report of the McKinney Research Demonstration Program for Homeless Mentally Ill. Washington, DC, Adult Center for Mental Health Service, Substance Abuse and Mental Health Services Administration, U.S. Department of Health and Human Services, April 1994

Witheridge TF, Dincin J: The Bridge: an assertive outreach program in an urban setting. New Dir Ment Health Serv 26:65–76, 1985

Chapter 15

Violent Patients

Burr S. Eichelman, M.D., Ph.D.

The violent patient in community psychiatry is, to some extent, an enigma. There is no DSM-IV (American Psychiatric Association 1994) diagnosis of "violent patient." A schizophrenic patient with depression can receive two Axis I diagnoses: schizophrenia and depressive disorder not otherwise specified. A violent schizophrenic patient is not distinguished from a nonviolent schizophrenic patient by diagnosis. With the exception of DSM-III-R (American Psychiatric Association 1987) organic personality disorder or DSM-IV intermittent explosive disorder, the violent characteristics of community mental health patients are not delineated by diagnosis. Nevertheless, violent patients exist. Although the intellectual debate continues as to whether mentally ill patients are substantially more violent than other members of the community, clinicians clearly know that violent behavior is a characteristic of many of the mental health patients treated in the community. Violence is a frequent behavior preceding psychiatric admission (Binder and McNiel 1986). It is a significant event within inpatient treatment settings even if underestimated (Lion et al. 1981). It is a concern with regard to both clinician safety and legal liability issues. Most importantly, it is a focus central to the appropriate assessment and treatment of the mental health client in the community and central to the treatment of the victims of violent behavior.

This chapter is composed of five major clinical sections. These sections address 1) general techniques for working with violent patients, 2) the assessment of the violent patient, 3) treatment issues in the management of the violent patient, 4) clinician safety, and 5) intervention issues for the victims and potential victims of the violent patient. In the summary, the clinical areas are reviewed and some reflection is given to the future problems and opportunities for community psychiatry in the management of the violent patient.

General Techniques

One conceptualization for working with violent patients (Eichelman 1991) addresses some of the preparatory elements necessary for effective initial intervention and safety. These were initially articulated for the emergency department or ward and characterized under the rubric of "restraint" tools, but as principles, they extend to most facets of dealing with violent or potentially violent patients. These can be discussed under verbal, physical, and chemical topics.

Verbal interventions.   Conceptually, verbal interventions are most effective when they enhance the client's self-esteem, when they allow for some ventilation of affect in socially acceptable ways, when they reduce the level of emotional arousal, and when they are carried out with integrity and without deceit. Self-esteem issues for the client include such therapist behaviors as speaking with the client first, even if only in a brief manner, despite the presence of family or police or other parties who have brought the client in for treatment or evaluation. It includes seeing the client at the appointed time or, if called to see the client in an emergency department, responding in a timely manner (which also avoids the potential risk of escalating behavior to "get attention").

Verbal strategies include identifying oneself and one's role in the assessment or treatment process. When dealing with seriously disturbed, intoxicated, or demented patients, this can be enhanced with the use of a "white coat style" that clearly defines the clinician as part of the "medical team" and separate from police or other agency personnel. Body posture, distance, and tone are critical in conveying to the client a sense of neutrality in the interaction. Approaching from behind, standing above the seated patient, maintaining a "closed" (e.g., arms folded) or threatening posture (e.g., arms on hips) can escalate interactions with violent clients.

Verbal tone, marked by speed and emotional intensity, must meet the client's verbal tone ("active listening"). The clinician who addresses the agitated client with an analyst's detachment may find the interview escalating. However, just as a hypnotist "leads" the subject deeper into a trance induction, so, too, must a clinician "lead" the agitated client into a more controlled and less volatile emotional state. Technically this is accomplished by maintaining an emotional tone that is slightly below that of the client and continuing to recede as the client settles. With the agitated client, both what is said and how it is said are critical. Violent patients, particularly when agitated, may have limited verbal skills. It is imperative for the clinician to restate periodically to the client (paraphrasal) what he or she has been saying to affirm to the patient that he or she is being heard. However, for the agitated patient, a reasonable rule of thumb holds that the therapist should be active in the interview only, on average, 10 seconds out of every minute.

Physical interventions.   Physical strategies begin with a safe and minimally stimulating environment. We defeat our clinical purposes by trying to talk down an agitated patient in the middle of a busy urban emergency department corridor. Lighting, sound, and general tone of the interview room should be designed to reduce agitation: cool tones, muted but sufficient lighting, and a comfortable chair for the patient are helpful. As discussed in the section, "Clinician Safety," this does not mean a room "out of sight and out of mind" or one that is filled with hazardous "weapons" such as heavy ashtrays or razor sharp letter openers.

For the interviewer, such strategies encompass "a safe distance" from the client. "Two quick steps" has become a rule of thumb for some trainers, allowing the clinician the ability to avoid or intervene if the client escalates to overtly violent behavior. For the agitated, pacing patient, this requires a sideways stance, which reduces the chance of receiving a direct body assault. The body buffer zone work of Kinzel (1970) should alert the clinician that violent patients, compared with nonviolent patients, have a larger "body buffer zone" within which they feel threatened. Many clinicians suggest that the least threatening position to speak to clients is at a 45-degree angle facing them (but not directly). Physical interventions also include and overlap with clinician safety in the establishment of an emergency alarm system that can bring a full intervention team to the interview setting, a team trained in physical restraint, should it be necessary.

Chemical interventions.   Chemical interventions go beyond the scope of this chapter. They have been reviewed in other contexts (Eichelman 1988) and should not be overlooked, particularly if the client and his or her psychiatric condition is well known to the clinician. The "as needed" use of a slow-onset, short-acting benzodiazepine (e.g., oxazepam) or of an antipsychotic medication (for a schizophrenic or manic patient) may well serve as a psychological "coping strategy" and a moderate chemical restraint to decrease the potential for violence. However, the risk in medicating patients is medicating prematurely and missing a critical diagnosis.

Case 1

J.W., a 26-year-old male, was brought in by the police to the community hospital emergency department. He was placed in the psychiatric evaluation room, and the on-call mental health worker was asked to see him. Dr. R. arrived to do the assessment within 10 minutes. She was wearing her physician's coat and had dressed safely, without scarves, neck chain, dangling earrings, or pins. She made initial verbal contact with J.W. through the door, asking him whether she could safely enter and talk with him about what was going on. He agreed. She verified the safety of this with the police who had brought him and requested that they remain out of earshot but visible while she made her assessment. As J.W. was pacing about the room, she remained standing and listened to him as he told his story of discovery that his wife had been involved in an affair with his best friend. He told Dr. R. that he was so angry that he thought he could kill his friend. Dr. R. paraphrased his comments, gradually deescalating the tone of the interview until both of them could sit down to talk further. Although there was no need for physical intervention, the room had been prepared as a safe environment for dealing with violent patients. Dr. R. had access to a "panic button" that could be used to call a special intervention team. She also had kept the police within range of assistance for the initial stage of her evaluation. These and other principles are depicted in Table 15–1.

Assessment

The assessment of a violent patient encompasses mental status examination, diagnosis, assessment of behavioral risk factors, and assessment of the environment in which the client will be living. A more elaborate discussion of this assessment process can be found in Lion (1972), Tardiff (1989), and Reid and Balis (1987).

Table 15–1. Guidelines for general techniques

1. Control and stabilize the situation.
2. Work as a team.
3. Use verbal techniques, which include the following:
   • Informing the patient who you are (by words and attire)
   • Actively listening (nearly matching the patient's level of arousal initially and then deescalating the interview)
   • Using paraphrasal technique
   • Allowing the patient time to ventilate
4. Use physical techniques, which include
   • Maintaining a safe distance
   • Maintaining nonthreatening body posture
   • Conducting the interview in a safe environment
   • Having the ability to obtain assistance
   • Being trained in the use of physical restraint
5. Be willing and able to utilize medication to assist in de-escalating a situation if the patient is well known and responsive to such intervention.

Mental status examination and diagnosis are critical in the management of the violent patient. Community or emergency department clinicians will be called on to "manage the patient" when internal medicine or surgical colleagues exhaust their resources. However, premature transfer to psychiatry must be averted. For example, a violent demented 80-year-old man brought in by his spouse certainly has a dementia (well documented over the preceding 2 years), but the rapid onset of new violent behavior suggests a change that could be external (e.g., a transfer to new surroundings or care by a new nurse's aide) or internal (e.g., a urinary tract infection secondary to an enlarged prostate). The violence in an unruly, inebriated, homeless man can be related to an abrasion on the forehead and the missing Babinski reflex associated with a subdural hematoma.

An academic listing of these medical "zebras" has been enumerated by Reid and Balis (1987). I have encountered sepsis (bacterial and viral), malignant hypertension, hyponatremia, bromism, interictal confusion, drug withdrawal syndromes, intracerebral bleeding, and insecticide poisoning as instigators of violent behavior in patients sent for "psychiatric" evaluation. The assessment of an unknown violent patient must include a physical examination, vital signs, and often laboratory and imaging studies.

Once a medical etiology has been eliminated from the differential diagnosis, attention must be paid to the psychiatric diagnosis. While obtaining the requisite history of the patient and paying attention to risk factors, as enumerated later, the clinician must also assess the mental state of the client and make a formal psychiatric diagnosis. Much has been written about diagnosis as an indicator of violence potential (Tardiff 1992). Although patients who carry a diagnosis of paranoid schizophrenia have often been perceived to be at greatest risk for assault, it must be noted that patients within almost any diagnostic group can become violent. Diagnosis cannot be a reason to discount other risk factors for violent behavior.

Behavior continues to be the most reliable indicator for predicting future violence. This includes a history punctuated with assaults, particularly if associated with the elements of the present situation (e.g., psychosis, intoxication, family stress). In assessing the patient's imminent potential for violence, the clinician must attend to signs of emotional arousal: agitation, pacing, clenching of fists, explosive language, and gestures. Explicit threats and an identified target and plan increase the risk of violence, just as they do for suicide. Most clinicians weigh violent command hallucinations as increasing the risk of assault (although research data in this area are limited). As with suicide, the presence of a lethal weapon raises the risk. The patient with a loaded firearm in his or her car and a plan to use it must be taken seriously. Veiled threats, which may be associated with delusional thinking, should be fully explored to determine their strength and target.

States of intoxication of the client and his or her potential victim are critical. Approximately 50% of homicide perpetrators and victims are legally intoxicated at the time of killing. Alcohol leads all other drugs as a risk factor for violence. However, the paranoia induced by long-term cocaine or amphetamine abuse or the disinhibition induced with barbiturate or minor tranquilizer abuse can also raise the risk of assault. Similarly, the behavior associated with drug procurement (stealing to support a heroin habit or a cocaine habit) enhances the risk of violence.

Finally, although victims must never be assigned responsibility for violence, they nevertheless can contribute to increased risk. The spouse who dares her husband to hit her or shoot her in the middle of a verbal fight increases the risk of violence beyond that of the wife who leaves and, if necessary, obtains a restraining order against her husband.

Case 2

J.W., in relating his history (see Case 1), was noticeably intoxicated. No other psychiatric disorder, such as thought disorder, mania, or major depression, was evident. He did not give a history of any signs of a complicating medical illness. He proceeded to relate how he had gotten into an argument at home

Table 15–2. Guidelines for assessment

- Rule out any life-threatening medical conditions.
- Assess whether there is a likely medical etiology for the violent behavior.
- Make a psychiatric diagnosis, if appropriate.
- Make an assessment of dangerousness, which includes taking into account past violent behavior, a specific plan with elements that might include an identified victim and possession of a weapon, psychotic mentation that might affect the dangerousness, victim's behavior, ancillary stressors, and concomitant drug use.

---

with his wife about their finances and his drinking. She had compared him sexually to his best friend, awakening his realization that they had been sexually involved. He grabbed his hunting rifle and a box of shells, drove off, and stopped at a tavern, where he proceeded to drink and threaten until the police were called and he was brought to the emergency department. He related that he "could leave, get (his) truck with (his) rifle and drive to Chuck's house tonight and kill him" for this behavior. As the alcohol wore off, he refused to make a "nonviolence" contract with Dr. R. However, he was willing to be admitted to the inpatient unit to "cool down" and begin some problem solving, obviating the need to consider emergency detention. These guidelines are shown in Table 15–2.

Treatment

Simple and effective rules for treating the violent patient do not exist. These are most difficult patients with whom even the best clinicians are only modestly effective.

The first rule in the treatment of the violent patient is to treat the underlying disorder. Management of the violent schizophrenic or alcoholic patient hinges on adequate management of the primary disorder. Available interventions include outpatient psychiatric commitment to ensure medication compliance, the use of day hospital programs for the schizophrenic patient, or the use of disulfiram or Alcoholics Anonymous for the alcoholic patient.

"Systems" interventions can be designed to reduce a client's stress. Assistance in ensuring adequate housing and sustenance, or in buffering or resolving personal stressors (e.g., a sick child, being laid off from a job, dealing with a restraining order forcing the patient to move out of his house) will reduce general stress and the concomitant risk of violence.

Personal interventions can include educating the patient about the antecedents of his or her violent behavior so that the patient can identify the triggers of violence and work with the therapist to develop a behavioral response repertoire that lowers the probability that situations will escalate to violence (e.g., leaving the house during a fight with a spouse, calling a parenting hotline if feeling like hitting a child, calling the therapist if command hallucinations are becoming overbearing).

Particularly for the personality disorder client, anger management techniques that address relaxation and assertiveness as coping strategies (Alberti and Emmons 1990; Goldstein et al. 1987; Novaco 1975) are useful. Role playing with a cooperative and invested patient helps the patient learn nonviolent alternatives.

Many violent patients have poor self-esteem. Therapy that "plays to the client's strength" and enhances self-esteem will often assist in reducing the risk of violence. Treating the client with respect and integrity, searching and discovering the special talents and gifts of such a client (and praising him or her for them), and praising periods of nonviolent and successful coping all become powerful reinforcers of nonviolent behavior in the therapeutic setting. Associated with self-esteem is empowerment. The therapist may be able to teach the client to become empowered through more adept use of interpersonal skills, a greater understanding of the welfare system, or even a better understanding of the legal process. This, too, may lead to a substitution of such skills for previously unsuccessful, violent coping attempts.

The clinician should not overlook the innovative use of additional drugs in the psychopharmacology of treating violent psychiatric patients. In addition to the traditional psychotropic agents associated with the treatment of specific disorders, ancillary agents are showing some apparent efficacy. These include the use of mood-stabilizing anticonvulsants such as carbamazepine; beta-adrenergic antagonists such as propranolol and nadolol; serotonin active agents such as trazodone, fluoxetine, and buspirone; and slower onset benzodiazepines such as oxazepam or clonazepam.

Within the treatment structure, the therapist must be aware of his or her own treatment limitations. Failure to recognize and observe these limitations may lead to complications and additional crises in the ongoing therapy. Boundary issues of the therapist include the patient's disorder as an excusing legal condition, dealing with or overlooking of threats, possession of weapons, and compliance with treatment schedules or medication.

Clinicians have many styles of dealing with these boundaries. In working with the violent patient it is important to determine whether the patient is in treatment or not. If the patient is in treatment, then treatment is primary. To this end, for nonpsychotic patients in treatment for violence, it is often beneficial early on in the therapy to explain that they are legally responsible for their behavior, that this is charted in the medical record, and that the therapist would testify to this in a court of law. If the patient is in treatment, then the therapist can expect compliance with attendance at therapy sessions and with medication. Given the risks attendant in treating violent patients, I urge a fairly strict boundary in working with noncompliant patients. Patients who do not have a court order for treatment and who fail appointments or refuse appropriate interventions (antipsychotic medication for the psychotic patient) should be discharged from treatment, gently but firmly, with an invitation to return when their desire for and willingness to comply with treatment is greater. Otherwise the patient, the therapist, and the community believe the myth that the client is being effectively treated. This, of course, is not the case.

Often these limit-setting issues can be constructed for the patient in a way that does not assault the patient's self-esteem. For example, a patient keeping a weapon at home, which the therapist deems to be a high-risk situation, can be asked to sell the weapon or give it to a relative for safe keeping, not because the therapist "knows you will hurt somebody with it" (diminishing self-esteem), but "because I (the therapist) am so very anxious knowing you have a weapon at home, that I am not as effective a therapist for you as I would be if I knew you had placed it in safekeeping. Would you do me a favor and get rid of the gun?" (This empowers the patient to help the therapist. It accomplishes the same goal.) Limits can also be designed to empower the client. This can be accomplished by providing the client with two therapeutically acceptable choices: "Do you want to start Alcoholics Anonymous this week or next week?"; "Would you rather take the haloperidol by mouth or by injection?" Limits can often be affirmed while simultaneously enhancing or empowering the client.

Threats are also a boundary issue. Many clinicians seem to deal with threats and assaults with denial (Dubin et al. 1988). It is important for the clinician or treatment agency to make absolutely clear to the client that therapy cannot occur within an environment where the therapist feels intimidated and is afraid. Conditions must be altered so that threats are not an element of the "treatment." Again, this can be articulated as a condition of the clinician rather than a prohibition for the patient.

Finally, the successful treatment of the violent patient within the community setting requires an integration of mental health, legal, and social agencies. Failure of these agencies to work together and develop a systematic approach for the management of violent patients will allow clients not only to "fall through the cracks," but also to play one system against another as "responsible" for the violence of the individual. Within the mental health system, the individual treatment team must have a well-rehearsed relationship with the emergency care program. Ideally, this includes mobile mental health workers able to assess dangerousness on site should such a need arise. Admission criteria with an appropriate inpatient unit and operational criteria for emergency detention are also needed.

There should to be a solid relationship with law enforcement agencies, not only for the protection of the treatment facility, but also to avoid inappropriate criminalization of mentally ill individuals, disruption of treatment, and creation of an additional stressor when a return to an inpatient setting might be a more appropriate intervention then jail. The boundaries of patient confidentiality need to be worked out for community clinicians before they become an issue in a volatile situation. Staff need to know how much information can be shared with law enforcement officials with or, in some cases, without the consent of the client.

Social agencies also need to be part of this treatment and intervention loop. A timely social intervention to ensure general assistance resources or a temporary place to live may sufficiently reduce stress and reduce the risk of imminent violence.

Case 3

J.W. subsequently "cooled down" and made a nonviolence contract with his therapist. He has separated from his wife and is living with another male friend. He remains out of work. He is depressed, cries during therapy sessions, and complains of sleep difficulty. The community mental health center team is drawing up a treatment plan for him which includes attending Alcoholics Anonymous meetings. A psychiatrist on the team will follow him for possible antidepressant therapy, but this will not be initiated immediately. Social services have been utilized to assist him in obtaining some general assistance funds until his unemployment checks arrive. He has begun a job counseling program. Within the treatment program he is examining issues in his relationship with his wife and relates a history of spouse abuse associated with drinking. These episodes have occurred at times of verbal arguments with his wife in association with her demeaning him for his poor education and his drinking. The individual treatment plan targets the need to develop coping strategy techniques for management of his anger and assertiveness skills. His therapist is sensitive to his low self-esteem and attempts, through various positive compliments and reinforcers, to bolster it as well as treatment compliance. A supplemental treatment option is for J.W. to participate in a batterer's group for men. The foregoing issues are summarized in Table 15–3.

Table 15–3. Guidelines for treatment

- Treat the primary disorder first.
- A multisystem approach is necessary for dealing with clinical, social, and legal issues simultaneously.
- Individual therapy must address anger control, assertiveness in contrast to aggressiveness, and self-esteem.
- Treatment must include concrete coping strategies that the client can implement when faced with a situation that often is an antecedent to his or her violence.
- The therapist must maintain his or her boundaries with regard to compliance, weapons, threats, and responsibility when working with clients who test such boundaries.

Clinician Safety

Dealing with the violent patient carries risks for the clinician. Nearly 40% of psychiatrists (Madden et al. 1976) report being the target of patient assaults. Safety requires a safe environment and an intervention plan if violence occurs or is likely to occur. In the therapist-client interaction, the therapist must address both direct and veiled threats and potentially pathological transference situations to assess risk. She or he should have a mechanism of consulting with peers about potentially dangerous patients.

As indicated earlier, the assessment and treatment area should be safe. Offices should be sufficiently public to ensure assistance. Emergency department offices should have the ability to be visually or auditorially monitored. There should be some mechanism to signal for help. This includes the placement of "panic buttons" in an inconspicuous but accessible location; the telephone system, as prearranged with a receptionist, may be used to signal the need to call for outside help.

Whatever the emergency plan, it should be practiced, and there should be a response team. Within hospitals or mental health centers this can be a "Code Orange" team, which could include at least five members to enable the physical restraint of a client. Staff should be trained to distinguish between appropriate use of such a team with an agitated (but unarmed) client and one with a firearm (in which case additional people should not be brought onto the scene; only the police should respond).

Some agencies work with "ticklers" to advise staff that particular clients have a history of assaultive behavior. This may be a special process for coding the client's record or it can even make use of special messages within the computerized database of the clinic (Drummond et al. 1989).

Clinician safety depends on a safe interaction with the client. This includes clarifying ambiguous statements from the client that might be veiled threats or elements of a delusional belief system that, when followed, lead to dangerous conclusions and possible violence. Even elements of a psychosis not directly related to violence need to be clarified. The patient who believes the therapist can read his or her thoughts, who politely asks the therapist to stop asking "those questions," will become irritated and angry if the therapist persists. The clinician must find out early in the interview whether the patient feels the clinician can hear his or her thoughts and whether the patient believes the clinician can insert thoughts into his or her mind. Such beliefs can lead to misunderstandings during an interview, which in turn can lead to violence.

Direct threats must be addressed as they occur. The patient should understand that such threats can be frightening and intimidating and that they clearly decrease the efficacy of the clinician. Telling the patient that his or her threats are frightening is not the same as telling the client that he or she will be allowed to act on those threats or that the clinician would be unable to take action to control the situation. However, all clinicians should remember that in setting limits, it is imperative that the limits can be enforced. Situations where questionable limits are set are an "assault waiting to happen."

In working with psychotic patients, psychotic transference must also be paid special attention. In addition to the dangers of persecutory delusions that incorporate the therapist or treatment team, romantic delusions can also create a risk for the clinician and his or her family.

Even the experienced senior clinician can benefit from peer support and counsel in dealing with threatening patients who have psychotic transference. Difficult case conferences within the structure of a community psychiatric practice can allow for review of such situations. Under certain circumstances it becomes dangerous and inappropriate for the therapist to continue to treat the patient. Some patients who readily incorporate therapists into their delusional schema may require rotating therapists or participating in groups with more than one leader in order to diffuse the transference.

Case 4

J.W. arrives late at the community mental health center for his appointment. For the first time since being brought to treatment, he is intoxicated. He swaggers

Table 15–4.   Guidelines for clinician safety

- Maintain a safe environment.
- Maintain an alarm system coupled to a trained behavioral emergency response team.
- Consider marking the records of potentially violent patients.
- Always explore veiled or indirect threats.
- Always address threats directly.
- Monitor for psychotic or otherwise pathological transference.

into the treatment office, cursing that his unemployment check was stolen and cashed by someone else. He paces the room, picks up a textbook and throws it against the wall, directing his curses toward the therapist, whom he is "holding accountable" for the loss of his money. He does not respond to verbal redirection and deescalating techniques. The therapist pushes the office alarm at her desk, and a "code orange" team of five staff arrive swiftly. Their "show of force" is sufficient to quiet J.W., who sits down and breaks into tears. The foregoing guidelines are depicted in Table 15–4.

The Victims

The violent patient is violent toward someone or something. In addition to the clinician, the patient's parents, children, spouse, and friends may become targets for his or her violence. The therapist must obtain as clear a picture as possible of the potential victims. For example, state statutes must be understood and respected concerning the obligatory reporting of suspected child abuse. The boundaries of providing a *Tarasoff* warning to an identified individual whom the clinician believes is imminently at risk as a target for violence from the patient remain imprecisely defined. Again, the assistance of a clinical support network can be beneficial. (I recommend that whenever confidentiality is going to be broken, that such an action be explained, in advance, to the patient as an action of concern and an action to limit harm. It has been my experience that the negative reaction to such action has usually been overestimated.)

Therapists working with violent patients need information about victims' responses to violence, intervention programs in the community, and social resources for the victimized individual. A community treatment program for

Table 15–5.   Guidelines regarding victims

- Consider whether a duty to warn exists; if so, intervene.
- Know the state statutes for obligatory reporting of suspected child abuse.
- When dealing with potential victims, attempt to determine their role in the victimization and provide them access to clinical and social supports and information.
- When confidentiality must be breached, tell the patient directly that this is what you, as a therapist, must do to minimize harm to others and to the patient as a consequence of his or her planned, violent behavior.

violent patients should also include a treatment program for the victims of the violent patient (Table 15–5).

Case 5

Despite remaining sober for the next 5 weeks, J.W. calls the therapist's office, again intoxicated. He has just received the divorce papers from his wife. Although he has given up his gun to a friend for safekeeping, he shouts over the telephone that he is going to drive over to his wife's house and "beat the ___ out of her." He hangs up before the therapist is able to respond. After a very brief consultation with the associate clinic director, the therapist calls J.W.'s wife to warn her of his threat. Dr. R. also informs Mrs. W. of the possible use of a community safe house for battered women and of the resources available in the community for someone like herself. Dr. R. also calls the local police to alert them to J.W.'s threats and level of intoxication.

Summary

I have delineated some of the elements necessary for a community agency and its therapists to treat the violent patient. These include both individual and team techniques relating to verbal, physical, and medicinal interventions. They include the skills and techniques necessary to implement both a medical/psychiatric assessment and an assessment of dangerousness, which may need to be undertaken time and time again for such patients. They include an understanding of the principles of active treatment for such patients that address not only the primary mental illness, but also other special issues such as self-esteem and anger management. Finally, the safety of the clinical staff at both an institutional and individual level and the safety of the potential victims of the violent patient have been addressed.

One would hope that the future for dealing with the violent patient will include greater mental health resources to implement effective interventions. In addition, there must be an increased maturity in developing a nosology for clinically relevant, violent behavior that guides the clinician into specific treatment paradigms. Clinicians must test behavioral and pharmacological interventions to verify their efficacy and define the populations for which the intervention is effective.

At a broader level, society may well need to address violence as a public health issue that transcends the mental health patient population. This may affect our tolerance of the massive amount of violent behavior modeled on television and in other media. It may alter our willingness to allow such easy access to handguns and to tolerate our present levels of violence associated with alcohol (including vehicular violence). Even if our society, in general, adopts a greater abhorrence of violence, clinicians will remain involved with this group of behaviors in the community mental health patient. To this end, we must be trained and staffed adequately to intervene effectively.

References

Alberti RE, Emmons ML: Your Perfect Right—A Guide to Assertive Living, 6th Edition, Revised. San Luis Obispo, CA, Impact Publishers, 1990

American Psychiatric Association: Diagnostic and Statistical Manual of Mental Disorders, 3rd Edition, Revised. Washington, DC, American Psychiatric Association, 1987

American Psychiatric Association: Diagnostic and Statistical Manual of Mental Disorders, 4th Edition. Washington, DC, American Psychiatric Association, 1994

Binder RL, McNiel DE: Victims and families of violent psychiatric patients. Bull Am Acad Psychiatry Law 14:131–139, 1986

Drummond DJ, Sparr LF, Gordon GH: Hospital violence reduction among high-risk patients. JAMA 261:2531–2534, 1989

Dubin WR, Wilson SJ, Mercer C: Assaults against psychiatrists in outpatient settings. J Clin Psychiatry 49:338–345, 1988

Eichelman B: Toward a rational pharmacotherapy for aggressive behavior. Hosp Community Psychiatry 39:31–39, 1988

Eichelman B: Psychiatric mental health nursing with the violent patient, in Psychiatric Mental Health Nursing. Edited by Gary F, Kavanagh CK. Philadelphia, PA, JB Lippincott, 1991, pp 900–920

Goldstein AP, Glick B, Reiner S, et al: Aggression Replacement Training. Champaign, IL, Research Press, 1987

Kinzel AF: Body-buffer zone in violent prisoners. Am J Psychiatry 127:99–104, 1970

Lion JR: Evaluation and Management of the Violent Patient. Springfield, IL, Charles C Thomas, 1972

Lion JR, Snyder W, Merrill GL: Underreporting of assaults on staff in a state hospital. Hosp Community Psychiatry 32:497–498, 1981

Madden DJ, Lion JR, Penna MW: Assaults on psychiatrists by patients. Am J Psychiatry 133:422–425, 1976

Novaco RW: Anger Control: The Development and Evaluation of an Experimental Treatment. Lexington, MA, DC Heath, 1975

Reid WH, Balis EU: Evaluation of the violent patient, in American Psychiatric Press Review of Psychiatry, Vol 6. Edited by Hales RE, Frances AJ. Washington, DC, American Psychiatric Press, 1987, pp 491–509

Tardiff K: Assessment and Management of Violent Patients. Washington, DC, American Psychiatric Press, 1989

Tardiff K: The current state of psychiatry in the treatment of violent patients. Arch Gen Psychiatry 49:493–499, 1992

Chapter 16

Victims of Violence

Anne C. Hartwig, J.D., Ph.D.
Burr S. Eichelman, M.D., Ph.D.

Traditional psychiatry and mental health care have focused on classic "disorders" such as schizophrenia, depression, or anxiety. However, as mental health care has become increasingly based within the community, social problems, which are not clearly amenable to formal psychiatric diagnoses, have become increasingly more significant issues of concern. In particular, for community psychiatry in the United States, and indeed worldwide, issues of violence have become highly relevant. Although the victim and the perpetrator of violence are intertwined, they often present to the community psychiatrist or to other segments of public medicine quite separately. The clinician's intervention must be quite different in dealing with the victim and the perpetrator.

Effective intervention requires first an informed awareness of the magnitude of the problem of violence in North American culture. It necessitates the ability to develop a suspicion for its presence in certain clinical presentations. It requires an ability to elicit, sensitively and cautiously, the history of victimization. Finally, it obligates clinicians to be able to offer strategies that may reduce the risks of further victimization and of subsequent psychological morbidity in the traumatized victim.

With the introduction of posttraumatic stress disorder into psychiatric nosology, there has arisen a "treatable disorder" that has raised clinical awareness of the problems of victimization. Although research in this area is expanding, much of the effort in dealing with victimization rests with social agencies, which are often outside the experience of community psychiatry. Clinician awareness of these agencies and of their expertise in dealing with victimization is part of an effective clinical intervention strategy for community psychiatry.

In this chapter we discuss four victim areas: 1) domestic violence, 2) child and elder abuse, 3) rape and child sexual abuse, and 4) other victimizations (hostage events, witnessing violence, accident and natural disaster participation). Within each we delineate the incidence figures, characterize the manner in which such patients may present, and provide suggestions for therapeutic guidelines for the management and early stages of intervention and treatment. In a final section we address the community psychiatrist's opportunity to function as an educator for other mental health workers, emergency department physicians, and family practitioners and as cotrainer with other professional groups, such as law enforcement agencies; the legal system, including the courts; and community clergy. In the final section, additional research and resource issues are suggested.

Domestic Violence

Former Surgeon General C. Everett Koop has called domestic violence one of the major public health problems in American society today. Battering accounts for at least 20% of all medical visits by women and 30% of all emergency department visits (Stark and Flitcraft 1985). It is the single most common injury to women, more common than auto accidents, rape, and muggings combined (O'Reilly 1983). According to the Federal Bureau of Investigation, a battering incident occurs every 15 seconds in the United States. Medical costs from domestic violence total at least $3.85 billion annually. In 1980 it was estimated that one of every six women would be a victim of domestic violence during her lifetime (Gillespie 1989; Strauss et al. 1980). In 1994 this estimate was as high as one of three (Violence Against Women 1994).

Such staggering statistics mean that most clinics caring for women will have contact with substantial numbers of victims of domestic violence. How do such women present to the medical or mental health community? They may present with physical injury (e.g., contusions, fractures, diffuse abdominal pain, or miscarriage [25% of women who are beaten are pregnant, Zorza 1994]). They may present with diffuse somatic complaints (e.g., diffuse abdominal pain, muscle soreness, or headache). They may present with medical symptoms suggestive of stress (e.g., hypertension, headache, functional bowel symptoms, or psychosomatic disorders such as asthma). They may present with mood changes associated with posttraumatic stress disorder, including depression and anxiety (Cascardi et al. 1992). Twenty-five percent of all suicide attempts in women are preceded by a battering episode. They may present with gynecological complaints (marital rape is a correlate of domestic violence in 59% of cases in one survey [Cascardi et al. 1992]).

"Diagnosis" of domestic violence is not easily made by a clinical profile of the victim. Domestic violence is present at all socioeconomic levels, although it is reported most frequently by the lower socioeconomic groups. Women who have witnessed abuse as children or who have been in a previous abusive relationship may be at greater risk for subsequent abuse, but many women without such histories are abused, and the staggering statistics suggest that a prior exposure to violence is not at all a prerequisite to a violent episode.

Domestic violence often appears early in relationships. Physically violent relationships in college dating is reported to occur in 30%-40% of these relationships. In more than 30% of all abusive marriages, physical abuse was present in the year prior to the marriage. Tragically, abuse tends to escalate over the course of a marital relationship. Often it is marked by a "cycle of violence" characterized by a building of psychological tensions, followed by an episode of battery and then by a period of contrition and apology on the part of the abuser. Recidivism of the perpetrator is significant. Even with treatment (Saunders 1989), male recidivism approaches 50%. Safety is not necessarily achieved with escape. Approximately 75% of domestic assaults reported to law enforcement agencies occurred after the separation of the couple. Three of four female homicide victims are murdered by husbands or lovers.

Unfortunately, the community psychiatrist, as well as others, may find it enigmatic that women do not leave relationships at the initiation of battering. However, well-informed clinicians and others must be aware of the myriad and complicating factors that may account for a victim's "reluctance" or inability to leave an abusive relationship. Many factors are present in a sustained battering relationship. As noted earlier, the risk of more severe physical injury and even death increases after a decision to leave the relationship has been made and executed. Economic factors perpetuate the abuse. In many abusive dyads, the male abuser controls access to money, exit, communication, potential support systems (friends), and often children. The logistics involved in a woman leaving an abusive relationship, perhaps taking young children with her, without economic resources and with the threat of increased retaliation, is a powerful deterrent. In many communities it may take as long 90 days or more to provide economic public relief, if indeed any exists, for such a woman.

Psychological defenses also seem to impede escape from an abusive relationship. Ferraro and Johnson (1983) have listed examples of such defenses. The woman may appeal to a salvation ethic. She may deny the motives of the victimizer. She may deny or minimize the injury. She may deny that the behavior is abusive, denying the victimization. She may argue that she has no other options. She may appeal to "higher loyalties" (e.g., "til death do us part").

There is no clear identifying feature of the male batterer. He may present to the clinician as a most helpful, caring partner. However, more careful assessment of his behaviors can often uncover the hallmark of the abuser: the manifestation of controlling behaviors often associated with significant and unmerited possessiveness and jealousy. Nearly 50% have witnessed domestic violence as children (Rosenbaum and O'Leary 1981). Approximately 50% of abuse situations are associated with alcohol abuse. However, most clinicians working in the area of domestic violence view alcohol primarily as a "permissive lubricant" for the behavior, rather than the cause.

Witnessing children may also be the presenting patients in relation to domestic violence. They may manifest increased anxiety, poor school performance, increased aggressive behavior, and poor social problem-solving skills. If undiagnosed or interrupted, these children may proceed to behaviors with dire consequences.

Interventions

Initial interventions for the victim of domestic violence may be limited to helping the woman recognize and admit that she is being victimized. It may involve discussing with her the viable options for her, given her situation, and working with her to develop a way to communicate safely and, if necessary, a plan of escape for her and her children. Interventions must offer medical and psychiatric treatment for the physical injuries and the psychological trauma. Socially, the clinician can provide information regarding access to safe houses or shelters and access to women's referral networks and support groups. This information must be offered in absolute privacy, as divulging to the spouse that such material was provided not only may terminate the permission for medical or psychiatric attention, but also may increase the risk of subsequent battery.

Legal interventions are available. In some jurisdictions police are mandated to arrest the abuser once an assault has occurred. Mandatory arrests occur regardless of whether the woman denies the assault or refuses to press charges. Women also have the option in all states of filing and requesting a temporary restraining order (TRO) that provides them protection from the physical presence of the abusing spouse. In most jurisdictions this can be requested by the woman without the aid of an attorney. Numerous legal advocacy groups may provide help, but the process can be tedious and time consuming. Once a TRO has been obtained, the woman can request that police arrest the abuser if he violates the terms of the order. Unfortunately, enforcement of legal orders requires time, and such enforcement does not stop bullets.

Mrs. A. is a 39-year-old black Puerto Rican woman who presented to the emergency department with facial contusions and a possible maxillary fracture. She had been assessed previously for pelvic pain. At that time it was discovered that she was positive for the human immunodeficiency virus (HIV), apparently acquired from marital sexual relations with her drug-abusing spouse. Gentle questioning during this visit by a clinician willing to ask the "difficult" questions elicited that this injury had occurred during an episode of battery in punishment for her "revealing" to the medical hospital that she was HIV positive and that she had been infected by her husband.

The emergency department clinician discussed with her in private many of the issues of domestic violence, including its cyclical nature and escalating character and its origin in the abuser, not the abused. He provided her with various community options to interrupt the cycle, including information about shelters and restraining orders and how to reach such agencies. As a consequence of that conversation, she requested that he contact the police on her behalf. This led to her husband's arrest and the obtaining of a restraining order protecting her from his presence. Through resource contacts, she received support from the Hispanic community's program for domestic violence. She continues to receive both emotional and medical support from the clinician who dared to discuss this issue with her. Guidelines for intervention are given in Table 16–1.

Child and Elder Abuse

Victimization of dependent persons is another category for review. Child abuse reports totaled nearly one-half million in 1981 (O'Reilly 1983) with the expectation that there is significant underreporting. In the United States

Table 16–1.   Domestic violence: guidelines for intervention

- Maintain a high level of suspicion for domestic violence.
- Make available in a private area (e.g., the women's lavatory) information concerning domestic violence and community resources.
- Inquire about domestic violence only in absolute privacy.
- Assume that all nonprivate contacts are being monitored by the abuser.
- Assist the victim in developing a "safe plan" or escape strategy, even if she chooses not to leave the relationship initially.
- Provide informational and emotional support for the victim, but do not tell her what to do. You cannot guarantee her safety. Well-intentioned paternalism is yet another form of control, and may be viewed as abusive control.
- To be effective, learn about the domestic violence resources in your community—for both the perpetrator and the victim—and be familiar with the professionals working within these agencies.
- Assist in educating the family practitioners within the community about domestic violence.
- Educate mental health consumers about domestic violence through community workshops, school programs, prenatal clinics, and other public health programs.

it was not clearly recognized as a medical or public health issue until Kempe and colleagues coined the battered child syndrome (Kempe and Helfer 1972; Kempe et al. 1962). When first identified, the mortality rate for American children suspected of being physically abused was approximately one in eight. The seriousness of these mortality figures has prompted an obligatory reporting mandate for all caregivers, including physicians, who must inform a state's department of human services, if, on examination of a child, they suspect child abuse.

Child abuse occurs within all socioeconomic groups. Like domestic violence, however, it occurs more frequently in lower socioeconomic groups. Reasons given for this include the greater stressors within these classes (e.g., inadequate housing, overcrowding, lack of financial resources) that may contribute to the induction of violence, but there are other stressors that may similarly contribute to violence in middle and upper socioeconomic groups.

Clinicians must have a high index of suspicion for child abuse. In relation to childhood injury, the following are high-risk indicators (Schmitt 1978):

1. An unexplained injury or reluctance to explain an injury
2. A discrepancy between parents' and child's description of the incident that led to the injury
3. A discrepancy between the type of injury or wound the child has and the report of how it occurred
4. Suspicious injuries that are reported to be self-inflicted
5. Injuries reported to be caused by a third party
6. A history of suspicious injuries

Behaviorally, children who present to the clinician or teacher with excessive fearfulness or a marked stoicism; aggressive or depressed children; or children who behave inappropriately in certain situations (e.g., excessively panicked during an invasive medical procedure) should also be children for whom a suspicion of abuse is high.

Suspicion should also be raised in relation to either a male or female parent who is emotionally labile and impulsive and has a temper problem in other areas of his or her life. There is currently no reliable psychological profile of an abusing parent accepted by the medical community. However, many abusing parents have been described as expecting their child to behave "like a little adult." They often attribute "adult" motives to the child (e.g., "You are crying just to annoy me." "You soiled your pants just to make me late for work!"). These abusing parents often were abused themselves as children. They are often described as immature, having low self-esteem, and inexperienced in parenting. The child—as a target—may be marked as a "special child" as a result of a physical "difference" such as a physical handicap or chronic illness. It may also occur due to a psychological "difference," such as being the child from a previous marriage. Risk factors for child abuse are given in Table 16–2.

Interventions

The most successful intervention for child abuse is prevention. Parenting classes for inexperienced parents, respite for single mothers without extended family, and parental abuse telephone hotlines to provide immediate support for stressed parents offer prophylactic interventions. When abuse is directly suspected, state law requires reporting. Clinicians should do this in a matter-of-fact manner that is not further deprecating to a parent who already has low self-esteem. Suspicion should be based on the clinical presentation.

Table 16–2.   Child abuse: risk factors

- A young mother or father
- Inexperienced parents
- An unwanted pregnancy
- A difficult birth
- Other young children in the home
- A low-birth-weight infant
- Low education level of the parent(s)
- A mother with health problems
- A child with health problems
- A lack of respite from child care
- Social isolation
- An irritable or unresponsive infant
- Poverty (including a substandard environment; poor medical care; malnutrition, etc.)
- A history of domestic violence
- A father who has had a prior juvenile police record

Many abusing parents are personable individuals who appear to dearly love their children. This does not rule them out as abusing parents under situations of stress.

If abuse is substantiated, removal of the child to a safe environment may be obligatory. Work with the parents toward safer and supervised parenting may allow for the reintroduction of the child into the home or obviate the need for his or her removal.

Children who are physically abused may themselves need psychological therapy. They may feel responsible and guilty for bringing on the abuse. They may blame themselves for the abuse. Such blame may lead to self-defeating behaviors or even dangerous risk-taking behaviors, endangering the child still further. Intervention in such cases requires age-appropriate psychotherapy.

Two young graduate students brought their 6-month-old daughter to the hospital emergency department. The infant was listless and poorly responsive. The parents stated that earlier in the day she had fallen out of her baby chair from the kitchen table to the floor. She had appeared to cry normally but subsequently became more listless. Medical evaluation documented bilateral massive subdural hematomas and bilateral temporal skull fractures. Such injury could not be accounted for by a single fall to the floor. This child had to have been hit separately on both sides of her head. Forensic clinicians even raised the possibility that she had been thrown at a wall. Both parents adamantly denied abuse. After neurosurgical evacuation of the hematomas, the parents came every night to the intensive care unit. There were no more devoted-appearing parents on any of the pediatric floors. They never admitted to the abuse. However, on the basis of forensic pathological testimony, their daughter was placed in foster protective care.

The school gym teacher remarked to the school psychologist that one of his 8-year-old boys was refusing to put on his school T-shirt. Follow-up demonstrated that the boy had sharp abrasions across his back consistent with belt marks from a beating. Social work investigation revealed that he was being frequently beaten by his stepfather for trivial behavioral infractions. The child was allowed to remain in the home under close scrutiny from a community care worker. Both parents were required to participate in parenting classes at a community mental health facility. Subsequent abuse did not occur. Guidelines for interventions in child abuse are given in Table 16–3.

Elder Abuse

There is a less extensive literature related to the victimization of elderly individuals. The incidence of abuse can be expanded beyond physical abuse (estimated at 15%) to encompass neglect (74%), exploitation (10%), and abandonment (3%) (Pagelow 1984). In one early report (Lau and Kosberg 1979) nearly 10% of admissions to a chronic care facility were characterized as abuse cases, and approximately three-fourths of these patients showed signs of physical abuse.

In addition to the medical risks associated with such abuse, there may be concomitant psychological sequelae, including depression. Intervention can be successful simply by identifying the problem and monitoring for subsequent abuse while providing support for the caregiver. Elder abuse may be realistically perceived as a general symptom of family stress and its inadequate management. Tangible support may encompass respite care for the elderly individual as well as educative training for the abusive caregiver to develop more realistic expectations of the elderly person and to enhance the caregiving skills of the caregiver. Guidelines for intervention in elder abuse are given in Table 16–4.

Table 16–3.   Child abuse: guidelines for intervention

- Maintain a high index of suspicion for child abuse.
- Once there is a suspicion based on an evaluation of the child, obligatory public health reporting is generally required.
- Initial intervention must first ensure safety for the child.
- Not all abuse requires parental separation from the child; close supervision and access to abuse hotlines, parenting classes, and access to respite care may be sufficient to interrupt a pattern of abuse.
- Older children as victims may require individual psychotherapy dealing, in particular, with their sense of responsibility for the abuse.

Rape and Sexual Abuse

In 1985 approximately 138,000 rapes were reported in the National Crime Survey Data (Violence Against Women 1985). However, researchers estimate that only 1 rape in 10 is actually reported. More recently, forced and nonconsenting sexual behaviors within dating (date rape) and marriage (marital rape) have been identified. Although rape can happen to any person (man or woman, ranging in age from 5 months to 93 years), the highest risk group consists of females between the ages of 10 and 30. Most rapists are males younger than 25. Most reported rapes are perpetrated by someone of the same race as the victim. Approximately half of all rapes (not including marital rape) are perpetrated by someone known to the victim. Alcohol is frequently associated with the rape (in approximately 30% of the cases). As noted earlier, marital rape may be a component of more broadly occurring domestic violence.

Table 16–4.   Elder abuse: guidelines for intervention

- Maintain a high index of suspicion for abuse.
- Provide medical and psychological support for the abused elderly person.
- Provide monitoring, respite resources, and skill training for the elderly person's caregiver, including the necessity of adding formal community resources.

Victims of rape manifest consistent patterns of behavior described by Burgess and Holmstrom (1974) as the *rape-trauma syndrome*. The syndrome is divided into an acute phase marked by the following:

- An overcontrolled—or, alternatively, an overly expressed—emotion
- Manifestation of physical symptoms and concern for those body parts affected by the assault
- A disturbance in sleeping and eating
- Other elements of an acute posttraumatic stress disorder

The victim may have feelings of disbelief, shock, guilt, shame, embarrassment, self-blame, anger, and a desire for revenge.

After several days to weeks, the victim may psychologically move into a reorganization phase. This phase may be marked by a return to some level of functioning, often more dependent on a family support system. There may be recurrent nightmares or the development of fears and phobic behavior specific to the assault. There may be a pseudo-adjustment to the situation utilizing defenses such as denial, rationalization, or suppression. From this point, a healthy reintegration of the trauma may occur, or the victim may proceed to develop a full-blown posttraumatic stress disorder. In addition to such psychological symptoms, there may be increased risk-taking behavior subsequently by the victim. Caregivers should be aware that a rape victim has a four-fold greater risk of being raped a second time than does someone who has never been raped.

S.E. was a 23-year-old female jogger who was accosted while running alone through a nature preserve. She was raped and severely beaten during the attack, subsequently discovered by other runners, and taken to a hospital emergency department. This emergency department had a special rape protocol that included the use of a female rape counselor who provided emotional support for the victim and buffered S.E. from the demands of the police and emergency department physicians. She encouraged S.E. to use her parents for support and to attend a rape therapy group. She made sure that she remained with S.E. until her medical treatment was completed and S.E.'s family took her home. In addition, she recontacted S.E. to ascertain what symptoms were developing and whether S.E. was following up with the therapy group.

Despite these "textbook" interventions, S.E. began to develop traumatic nightmares. She became phobic about being alone and stopped her running, remaining isolated at home. Clinically, she was both anxious and depressed. The rape group therapists referred her to specialized behavioral treatment for posttraumatic stress disorder. In addition, she was symptomatically treated with medication for her depressive and anxious symptoms. Over several months of treatment, her symptoms remitted. However, for several years she would become symptomatic on experiencing similar settings (being in a nature preserve, being ap-

proached by a male runner) or on the anniversary date of the rape. Guidelines
for intervention in rape are given in Table 16–5 (McCombie 1980).

Child Sexual Abuse

Precise incidence figures for child sexual abuse do not exist. Estimates can
range as high as 50% in various selected populations (Finkelhor 1983). Such
estimates currently are further confounded by assertions of a "false memory
syndrome" or of iatrogenic or therapist-suggested memory recall of abuse.
Nevertheless, it is clear that the majority of victims are women, and the
majority of perpetrators are men. Victimization can occur early (e.g., 3 years
of age) and can extend into adolescence.

Abuse may be discovered in childhood through medical findings such as
vaginal tears or the development of a sexually transmitted disease (e.g., gon-
orrhea). It may become suspected on the basis of the onset of behavioral
change, including clinging, fear of specific individuals, sleep disturbance, anxiety, appetite disturbance, problems in school performance, and the development of physical complaints. Adult patients, particularly those with borderline
personality traits or dissociative disorders, should be evaluated for a history of
childhood sexual abuse (but such abuse should not be "suggested").

Table 16–5.   Rape: guidelines for intervention

- Understand that rape is a violent act that takes control away from the
  victim.
- Even though forensic and medical attention is necessary, mental health
  staff can oversee its provision and allow the victim some control, privacy,
  and protection so as to not be further victimized during the "treatment."
- Recognize that both successful and pathological coping with rape progress
  through phases, and the clinician should follow up, watching for maladaptive behaviors suggestive of a more chronic posttraumatic stress disorder.
- Intervention should include assisting in the mobilization of a supportive
  and protective environment.
- Intervention should include encouragement for therapy, such as a rape
  support group.
- Should signs of a more severe posttraumatic stress disorder develop, the
  mental health worker should refer the victim to more intensive treatment
  for the disorder.

A.B. was a 28-year-old college student who presented for therapy with symptoms of a major depression, some episodes of bingeing and purging, and bouts of excessive drinking. In addition to current relationship problems with a boyfriend and a dissolving parental marriage, she related a history of incest by her older brother. She described how she was made to participate in vaginal intercourse periodically from age 8 until age 12. She related how this had been kept a secret under threat of injury, but it had been so disturbing for her that she became regularly enuretic at night and did increasingly poorly in school. However, no discovery or intervention occurred. As an adult, she confided this occurrence to her younger anorexic sister, an "overachiever" who also confirmed that she had been briefly abused by the brother, but to a lesser extent. Therapy, in relation to the abuse, focused on helping her to understand that the abuse was not her fault, that as a young child she had limited abilities to prevent the behavior. She also had to address her anger at her parents' blindness to the situation and their denial of problems despite the enuresis and school performance failures. Guidelines for intervention in child sexual abuse are given in Table 16–6.

Victimization of Other Types

The psychological sequelae of traumatic events can develop from many situations. The community mental health worker should be aware of the breadth of such traumatic events. These can include interpersonal events such as being taken hostage, the assault of a co-worker by a client, being the victim of a natural disaster such as a tornado, and feeling victimized by a medical illness such as cancer.

Symonds (1983) described a sequence of events that appears to apply generally to all traumatic events. The acute phase has two components. The initial component is one of denial, marked by shock and disbelief. This is followed by a second phase in which denial is overwhelmed by the reality of the situation. At this time the victim's behavior may include such responses as "frozen fright," clinging or compulsive talking. Then follows a third phase, the subacute phase, which may continue and become chronic. This period is marked by traumatic depression and self-recrimination. The depression may be marked by apathy and resignation, irritability, a sleep disturbance, exaggerated startle responses or flashbacks, and a continual replay of the traumatic events. Excessive dependency and phobic behaviors may develop. Hopefully, the victim moves into a fourth phase of resolution and integra-

Table 16–6.   Child sexual abuse: guidelines for intervention

- Maintain a high level of awareness of the problem.
- If abuse is suspected in a young child, reporting to protective services is required, and if abuse is confirmed, the child must be afforded a safe environment.
- Abused children need psychotherapy to deal with their sense of responsibility and guilt for the behaviors.
- Older children will benefit from therapy in dealing with the reestablishment of a sense of trust for mature sexual and loving relationships.
- Adults with a history of abuse may need therapeutic interventions to deal with elements of a posttraumatic stress disorder or associated mental disorders, which can include borderline personality disorder and various dissociative disorders.

tion. In this phase the victim develops defense mechanisms and responses to minimize or prevent future victimization. There may evolve a change in values and attitudes toward people and material possessions. This period entails an integration of the traumatic event into the victim's life history. Interestingly, Symmonds commented that successful coping with a traumatic event involves the incorporation of the event into the person's total life experience, with the final healthy outcome of "having won" by virtue of "having survived."

Intervention for such traumatic events therapeutically begins with a replacement of protective denial by a recognition of the traumatic event. The emotional weight of the event can often be lightened through a group process in which other individuals, similarly victimized, share their feelings of a common event, feelings that may include an acknowledgment of terror, helplessness, guilt (even survivor guilt), and anger. Such group or individual therapeutic interventions can then move to the development and implementation of subsequent coping strategies. These may include the implementation of behaviors to prevent a repetition of the traumatic event or retributive actions. They may also include individuals "going on with their lives" to protect ongoing jobs or personal relationships. The greater the alacrity of the mental health intervention, the less morbidity is associated with the traumatic event.

Late one Friday afternoon, the sheriff's department of a local county decided to stage a hostage takeover of the courthouse to practice hostage intervention tactics. Police cadets from another county were enlisted. They broke into the courthouse, threatening the employees with visible handguns, forcing them into a basement room, shouting, and demeaning them. Approximately 10 employees, men and women ages 23 to the late 50s, were the victims. However, more than 2 hours into the event, the sheriff's team "discovered" that the employees had never been told that this was a practice exercise. Subsequently, the victims were released and debriefed. One of the hostages contacted a local lawyer. The attorney requested the immediate involvement of a clinical psychologist for those who were willing to participate. The psychologist initiated several group therapy sessions during which the victims shared their feelings of terror, helplessness, and anger.

Despite the initial manifestation of an acute posttraumatic stress disorder for several of the hostages, with continued therapy most of the symptoms subsided. Behavioral techniques were utilized to assist the employees to return to work, managing their anxiety linked to the work environment. The group then joined together to bring legal action against the county for their experience. This provided a response to overcome the helplessness they had felt. Unfortunately, at the time the case came to trial, most of the plaintiffs appeared nearly symptom free. They "won" their lawsuit, but because the psychological interventions had been so timely and effective, the damages to the victims were minimal. Guidelines for intervention in victimization are given in Table 16–7.

Roles of the Community Psychiatrist or Mental Health Worker

As the preceding cases indicate, many victims may only secondarily make their way to a community mental health setting for evaluation and treatment. Certainly, under such conditions the role of the clinician is relatively straightforward. It generally involves attempting to maximize safety for the victim and then to treat the symptoms of a traumatic stress disorder, if present.

However, for those victims who do not present initially to the community mental health worker, there are still other substantial areas of intervention. These areas include education. The community psychiatrist can become an educator and co-trainer for the emergency department staff who, as front-line clinicians, may be the medical staff who will either detect or miss the cases of domestic violence or child abuse. Active mental health education regarding incidence, detection, and intervention strategies will clearly be beneficial to the emergency department environment. Similarly, such education can be extended to family practitioners, the other front-line medical personnel.

Table 16–7.   Victimization: guidelines for intervention

- Intervention for a traumatic event should be immediate.
- Intervention should be tailored to the stage of resolution in which the individual appears to be as a consequence of the event.
- Intervention is often more effective when it includes a group format so that victims can affirm that they are not alone in being a victim and in experiencing the various feelings that occur with victimization.
- Although successful therapy often involves moving the victims from a position of helplessness to one of coping and action, successful coping often concludes with a psychological reintegration, the "bottom line" of which is simply "I survived."
- Such successful therapy continually returns to living and coping in the present, avoiding a fixation on the traumatic event and a psychological freezing, developmentally, at the time of the trauma.

Beyond the medical community there remain still additional groups that may participate in training by the community mental health professional. Preventive training in awareness of dating violence, conflict resolution, and parenting and information programs regarding resources for victims of traumatic events can be greatly beneficial. Other professional groups may also want to share in and learn about clinical problems. Both law enforcement agencies and the court system may need and seek additional training concerning the psychological stress on victims of abuse. The opportunity for clinicians to participate as a co-trainers and educators has not yet been exercised fully.

Summary and Conclusions

In this chapter we have reviewed aspects of victimization as related to the child and adult population who present to community mental health workers. We underscore the widespread nature of victimization in our society and review various community mental health interventions. Some of the interventions are proactive and of a preventive nature. They include, for example, the treatment of posttraumatic stress disorder and the suggestion for training and educating the community at large in relation to the identifying issues of violence. Awareness about the problems related to violence and knowledge of the resources available to minimize both physical and psychological trauma from victimization are critical to the clinician's effectiveness.

The field of community psychiatry in relation to victimology requires continued effort in obtaining better and more reliable incidence figures. Additional research is necessary to follow the long-term psychological consequences of victims in terms of psychological and physical well-being; better-designed research treatment protocols are needed to validate or modify the currently accepted methods of treating posttraumatic stress disorders. In the broader picture, the community mental health clinician must be a social advocate, speaking out against cultural acceptance of violence within our society, demonstrating the extraordinary psychological costs such violence exerts on our culture, and teaching the mental health consumer by participating with others in society in developing techniques to reduce violent behavior and reduce the pathological effects of victimization.

References

Burgess AW, Holmstrom LL: Rape: Victims of Crisis. Bowie, MD, Robert J Brady, 1974

Cascardi M, Langhinrichesen J, Vivian D: Marital aggression: impact, injury, and health correlates of husbands and wives. Arch Intern Med 152:1178–1184, 1992

Ferraro KJ, Johnson JM: How women experience battering: the process of victimization. Soc Probl 30:325–339, 1983

Finkelhor D: Child Sexual Abuse: New Theory and Research, New York, The Free Press, 1983

Gelles RJ: Family Violence, 2nd Edition. Newbury Park, CA, Sage, 1987

Gillespie C: Justifiable Homicide: Battered Women, Self Defense, and the Law. Columbus, OH, Ohio State University Press, 1989

Kempe CH, Silverman FN, Steele BF, et al: The battered child syndrome. JAMA 181:17–24, 1962

Kempe CH, Helfer RE (eds): Helping the Battered Child and His Family. Philadelphia, PA, JB Lippincott, 1972

Lau E, Kosberg J: Abuse of the elderly by informal care providers. Aging September/October:10–15, 1979

McCombie SL (ed): The Rape Crisis Intervention Handbook. New York, Plenum, 1980

O'Reilly J: Wife beating: the silent crime. Time, September 5, 1983, pp 23–26

Pagelow M: Family Violence. New York, Praeger, 1984

Rosenbaum A, O'Leary KD: Children: the unintended victims of marital violence. Am J Orthopsychiatry 51:692–699, 1981

Saunders DG: Cognitive and behavioral interventions with men who batter: application and outcome, in Treating Men Who Batter: Theory, Practice, and Programs. Edited by Caesar PL, Hamberger LK. New York, Springer, 1989

Schmitt BD: The physician's evaluation, in the Child Protection Team Handbook. New York, Garland STPM Press, 1978, pp 39–57

Stark E, Flitcraft A: Spousal abuse. Surgeon General's Workshop on Violence. Presented at Surgeon General Meeting on Violence and Public Health, Leesburg, VA, October 1985, p 2

Straus M, Gelles R, Steinmetz S (eds): Behind Closed Doors: Violence in the American Family. New York, Anchor Press. 1980

Symonds M: Victimization and rehabilitative treatment, in Terrorism: Interdisciplinary Perspectives. Edited by Eichelman B, Soskis D, Reid W. Washington, DC, American Psychiatric Association, 1983, pp 69–81

Violence Against Women: a National Crime Victimization Report. Washington, DC, U.S. Department of Justice, 1985

Violence Against Women: a National Crime Victimization Report. Washington, DC, U.S. Department of Justice, January 1994

Zorza J: Women battering: high cost and the state of the law. Clearinghouse Review 28:383–395, 1994 (Special issue)

Chapter 17

Community Treatment of Older Adults

Lynn Verger, M.D.
Timothy Howell, M.D., M.A.

T he challenges facing the psychiatric clinician working with elderly patients in the community are both formidable and exciting. The numbers are daunting: about 12% of all Americans are currently 65 years of age or
older, but over the next 30 years, that figure is anticipated to rise to 15%.
Already, the "old-old" (85 and older) are the fastest growing segment of the
U.S. population, and as the "baby boom" generation enters late life, the absolute numbers of older adults are expected to double, from approximately
30 million in 1990 to 60 million during the first quarter of the 21st century
(Coffey and Cummings 1994).

At present, older adults make up only about 4% of those served by
community mental health services, probably because of a combination of
individual and structural barriers, including the stigma of mental illness,
transportation, cost, lack of geriatric-oriented services, and difficulties in
the coordination of multiple services required for those who are needy
(Goldstrom et al. 1987). The demand for such services, however, is likely
to mushroom in the coming decades.

Providing psychiatric services to the older segment of the population
can be quite satisfying, as there is much that can be accomplished in ameliorating the lives of elderly patients with mental illnesses. In this chapter we

try to share with the reader some of the concepts that we have found to be useful in doing geriatric psychiatry. We first review the principles of geropsychiatric evaluation and psychopharmacology and then look more specifically at selected areas of psychopathology (i.e., depression, anxiety, schizophrenia, and dementia), highlighting key notions. It is beyond the scope of this chapter to provide much detail, but there are a number of useful geropsychiatric texts to which we refer.

Geropsychiatric Evaluation

Psychiatric evaluations of elderly persons need to be more thorough to be of maximum benefit. Geropsychiatric evaluations are often quite lengthy and complex and may require multiple visits to complete. Although labor intensive, such comprehensive geropsychiatric assessments can pay lasting dividends. In this section we will review the basic parts of such evaluations, with special emphasis on their application to the elderly patient.

The referral process is often a difficult first step. There is much stigma and embarrassment associated with mental illness for many older persons, so a psychiatric referral may be met with reluctance and resistance. The process can go more smoothly if the referral source prepares the patient. Often a trusting relationship with those working with older adults (e.g., outreach workers associated with an aging coalition, primary physicians) must be established before the patient will agree to see a psychiatrist. Making initial contacts in more familiar or neutral places such as a senior center or patient's home can be helpful.

Several factors can help the initial interview proceed smoothly. Inquire how the patient prefers to be addressed. Note and address any vision, hearing, or speech impairments. Ask if the patient usually wears glasses or a hearing aid and if these are functional. Inquire about dentures (poor fitting or absent) if the patient's articulation is impaired. Position the patient and the interviewer so that they can look and speak directly to each other. Assess whether the patient can manage a lengthy interview or if patient comfort, cooperation, and information gathering would be enhanced by a number of shorter sessions. Touch can sometimes be reassuring and can be done in the context of checking pulse and blood pressure.

Eliciting a chief complaint and history can be difficult. For various reasons an elderly person may hide or minimize symptoms. Important parts of the history may be forgotten. Therefore, collateral sources are vital in obtaining a complete history and assuring that specific concerns are addressed. In addition, caregivers can provide a day-to-day history, with information on premorbid functioning and psychiatric history.

Obtaining a complete as possible medical history is very important in assessing geriatric patients. A complete list of medications, including nonprescription medications and any shared medications, should be obtained. Having patients bring in all their medication bottles or check their medicine cabinet can provide a sometimes surprising picture of what they are really taking. Information regarding current medical problems is best obtained directly from the patient's primary care physician and ideally before the psychiatric evaluation. Although at times embarrassing, questions about the patient's use of caffeine, tobacco, alcohol, street drugs, and human immunodeficiency virus risk factors should not be avoided.

The social history provides the context in which psychiatric signs and symptoms are manifested. The patient's living situation, supports, contacts, mobility, ability to do activities of daily living (i.e., functional abilities), family structure, finances, etc., all can impact on physical and emotional health. Any changes or losses, such as retirement, divorce, moves, and deaths of loved ones (including pets), may be significant stressors for older adults. Assessing the social situation is instrumental in planning psychosocial interventions. Home visits, if feasible, can be extremely enlightening.

Including a standardized cognitive screen such as the Mini-Mental State Exam (MMSE) is essential (Folstein et al. 1975). Even if the individual appears cognitively intact, such a screen can provide a helpful baseline in the future. Rather than the standard judgment questions (e.g., "What would you do if you found a stamped addressed letter on the street?"), practical judgment questions (e.g., "What would you do if you were home alone, fell, and broke a leg?') provide more useful information about the patient's ability to exercise sound judgment.

In the geriatric population, "Occam's razor" does not apply: the simplest hypothesis that explains the most is usually misleading. The etiologies of psychiatric problems in older individuals are almost invariably multifactorial. Concurrent acute and chronic medical problems, medication effects and interactions, psychodynamic issues, psychosocial stressors, and premorbid personality traits can all coexist with psychiatric disorders, interact, and change over time. However, with thorough geropsychiatric evaluation, the clinician can unravel these intertwining factors and thereby more adequately address them.

Geriatric Physiology and Psychopharmacology

Mental health professionals working with older persons must be well informed as to how normal physiological changes that occur with aging can affect drug metabolism, distribution, and excretion, and sensitivity to medication (Maletta et al. 1991a, 1991b). This section will review these changes and how they affect the use of various psychotropic medications.

The major physiological changes associated with aging that have pharmacological impact include the following (Salzman 1992):

- Decreased total body water decreases the volume of distribution for water-soluble drugs (e.g., lithium), thereby increasing the potency of a given dose.
- Increased body fat and fat-to-lean muscle ratio increases the volume of distribution of lipid-soluble drugs (i.e., most psychotropic medications), so that they tend to accumulate.
- Decreased liver perfusion and enzyme activity results in decreased drug metabolism (especially oxidation), thereby prolonging drug half-lives. An exception are the short-acting benzodiazepines oxazepam and lorazepam, which are primarily glucuronidated and much less affected by decreased liver metabolism.
- Decreased renal perfusion and glomerular filtration rate reduce excretion of drugs through the kidneys, which prolongs half-lives and can raise serum drug levels.
- Decreased serum albumin reduces protein binding, thereby increasing the free fraction of protein-bound drugs. (The free fraction is usually the active component of the drug.)
- Decreased number of neurons and changes in metabolism cause the older brain to be more sensitive to psychotropic drugs.

These changes vary from individual to individual and even within an individual over time, making the geriatric population a quite heterogeneous group. To the extent that psychotropic medications in elderly persons tend to stay in their systems longer, lower doses and medications with shorter half-lives are preferable. Because of the increased heterogeneity among older persons, however, some individuals may require substantial doses. In light of this, a useful rule is to start low (one-fourth to one-half the usual starting dose for a younger adult); go slow, but keep titrating the dosage as long as the target symptoms keep improving and the patient is able to tolerate the medication. For example, we have seen patients benefit from as little as 12.5 mg or as much as 600 mg per day of trazodone.

Antidepressant selection for elderly individuals is based in large part on the side effect profile. Anticholinergic side effects are poorly tolerated by older persons. Dry mouth is not only bothersome but can accelerate the development of dental caries, cause dentures to be ill fitting, and interfere with the absorption of sublingual medications (e.g., nitroglycerin for angina). Urinary retention can be problematic, especially for older men with prostatic hypertrophy. Blurring of vision can impair functioning and increase the risk of falls. Constipation can result in fecal impaction. Elderly individuals are also more susceptible to sedation, confusion, and anticholinergic delirium. Orthostatic hypotension may contribute to falls. Hip fractures and head trauma associated with falls can cause considerable morbidity in elderly individuals. The hypotensive effect of monoamine oxidase inhibitors may not show up for 6 to 8 weeks after initiating treatment. Preexisting cardiac conduction delays can be worsened by tricyclic antidepressants. Decreased appetite associated with selective serotonin reuptake inhibitors can lead to malnutrition (Potter et al. 1991).

There are several reasonable antidepressants to use in older persons. Nortriptyline is probably least likely to cause orthostatic hypotension (Davidson 1989), and desipramine causes the fewest anticholinergic effects of the tricyclic antidepressants and can be started in doses as low as 10 mg. Trazodone has few anticholinergic effects and its sedating effects may be useful in those with insomnia. The selective serotonin reuptake inhibitors have considerably fewer, if any, anticholinergic effects (Potter et al. 1991). Sertraline has a shorter half-life than fluoxetine and so can clear the system more quickly if intolerable side effects develop.

Stimulants (e.g., methylphenidate) may have some usefulness in medically ill depressed patients, withdrawn postoperative patients, patients with poststroke depression, and patients whose rehabilitation and recovery are impaired by depression. The response to stimulants is rapid, usually 1 to 3 days. Stimulants are generally well tolerated. If doses are taken no later than early afternoon, insomnia is rarely a problem (Davidson 1989; Roccaforte and Burke 1990).

The side effect profile is also a major consideration in prescribing antipsychotic agents for older persons. Essentially all antipsychotic agents have extrapyramidal, anticholinergic, sedative, and orthostatic hypotensive side effects, to varying degrees. Low-potency antipsychotic agents are much more sedating, have more anticholinergic effects, and are more likely to cause orthostatic hypotension. Higher potency antipsychotic agents are less anticholinergic but more likely to cause extrapyramidal side effects (Jenike 1989). Because both ends of the antipsychotic potency spectrum may be associated with significant side effects for older patients, using a medium-potency antipsychotic may minimize these side effects to a certain extent. We have found such antipsychotic agents (e.g., molindone, loxapine) to work well. The clinician must be also mindful that with increasing age, a patient may become more sensitive to his or her usual dose of antipsychotic and therefore require dosage adjustments.

Tardive dyskinesia (TD) can be a significant side effect of antipsychotic agents in elderly individuals. Older persons are more at risk for TD: Approximately 40% of those on long-term antipsychotic agents develop TD, and approximately two-thirds of these cases are irreversible. Thus, restraint should be used in prescribing antipsychotic agents. Because about 5% of elderly persons who have never been exposed to antipsychotics develop TD-like symptoms (senile dyskinesias), a baseline Abnormal Involuntary Movement Screen should be performed prior to instituting antipsychotic medication (Jeste et al. 1990).

Antiparkinsonian medications such as benztropine, trihexylphenidate, and diphenhydramine have often been used to ameliorate the extrapyramidal side effects of antipsychotic agents. However, these medications also have substantial anticholinergic effects that often create significant problems for older persons. If extrapyramidal side effects develop the clinician can try to decrease the dose of the antipsychotic or switch to a somewhat less potent one, avoiding anticholinergic agents if possible. Amantadine, a dopaminergic antiparkinsonian agent, may be a reasonable alternative treatment for extrapyramidal side effects for some (Jenike 1989).

The use of benzodiazepines in older persons can be associated with sedation, cognitive impairment, and ataxia with falls. Hence the longer acting benzodiazepines (e.g., diazepam) should be avoided, and the shorter acting benzodiazepines (e.g., lorazepam, oxazepam) are preferable. Alternatives to benzodiazepines should be considered (Salzman 1992).

The use of lithium in elderly patients requires careful monitoring. Serum creatinine levels may misleadingly appear to be in the normal range, because a reduced renal clearance of creatinine may be balanced by decreased production of creatinine (because muscle mass decreases with age). Age-associated reduction in total body water and volume of distribution can lead to elevated lithium levels. Concurrent medication, such as thiazide diuretics or nonsteroidal antiinflammatory drugs, can increase lithium levels. Elderly persons can experience toxic side effects even at ostensibly therapeutic serum lithium levels. Of all the side effects of lithium, cognitive impairment and ataxia appear to be more likely to develop (Jefferson et al. 1987).

Starting doses of lithium in an elderly person can range from 75 mg to 300 mg a day. Therapeutic and maintenance levels of 0.4–0.7 mg/ml are usually effective. Lithium levels should be checked frequently in elderly individuals (Jefferson et al. 1987).

Depression in Late Life

Although depressive symptoms are common in elderly individuals, depression is not a normal part of the aging process. Approximately 15% of community residents over 65 years of age suffer from depressive symptoms (NIH Consensus Development Panel 1992). Overall, about 1% suffer from major depression, and another 2% develop dysthymia (Blazer 1989). The rate is even higher in nursing home residents (25%–35%). Widowed elderly men are in the highest risk group for suicide.

Depression in older adults tends to be underdiagnosed, in part because it is difficult to diagnose. Diagnostic dilemmas occur for many reasons. Many older individuals will not complain of feeling depressed but present instead with somatic symptoms. Some will not seek treatment or will deny symptoms for fear of stigma. Many have concurrent medical problems to which neurovegetative symptoms such as fatigue, sleep disturbance, and poor appetite can be attributed. Coexistent dementia can complicate the picture. Often elderly depressed patients do not meet the DSM-IV criteria for a major depressive episode, yet still are significantly depressed (American Psychiatric Association 1994).

Given this often confusing picture, the clinician is well served to be broad minded when assessing depression in older adults. In this section we will review and discuss the differential diagnoses of depression in elderly individuals and address treatment modalities.

In diagnosing major depression in geriatric population, the presence of some of the classic neurovegetative symptoms can sometimes be difficult to interpret. Medical problems can cause weight change, fatigue, and sleep disturbances. Also, age-related changes in sleep patterns (e.g., more shallow sleep with more frequent awakenings) can result in complaints of insomnia. Therefore, it can be helpful to solicit psychological symptoms of depression. Inquiring about anhedonia can be a key component in ascertaining the presence of depression. Feelings of helplessness, hopelessness, worthlessness, and guilt may also indicate depression. Suicidal ideation must be addressed, as the risk of suicide increases with age, although a wish to be dead, by itself, is not necessarily abnormal in older individuals.

Some elderly patients may have a "minor depression," with a several-month history of being unhappy and some neurovegetative symptoms, but not enough to meet the DSM-IV criteria for a major depressive episode or dysthymia. If symptoms are distressing or interfere with the ability to function in usual activities, then treatment is indicated.

Other psychiatric diagnoses to consider are dysthymia, adjustment disorder with depressed mood, and organic affective disorder. Dysthymia in an older person is similar to that in a younger person. Adjustment disorders can persist longer than 6 months in elderly individuals and develop into a minor depression or dysthymic picture.

Symptoms of depression are seen during bereavement. Death of a spouse, child, or pet may be especially difficult. Crying spells, poor concentration, poor appetite with weight loss, and insomnia are commonly experienced. Feelings of guilt over things not said or done prior to the time of death, thoughts that the survivor should have died instead of the deceased, and brief episodes of seeing or hearing the deceased are not uncommon and are within the range of normal. Excessive and inappropriate guilt, suicidal ideations, feelings of worthlessness, prolonged and marked functional impairment, and psychomotor retardation suggest a bereavement complicated by depression.

In working with elderly individuals, the clinician must be aware of the many medical problems and medications that can either cause an organic mood disorder or exacerbate some other depressive disorder. These include cardiac and pulmonary diseases, metabolic and endocrine disorders, neurological problems, nutritional deficiencies, drugs, and medications. To rule out the more common medical problems causing depression, routine screening laboratory tests for an elderly person with depressive symptoms include a complete blood cell count, thyroid function tests, chemistry panel, and determination of vitamin B_{12} and folate levels. In consultation with the patient's primary physician, physical examination and other clinically indicated tests (e.g., chest radiograph, electrocardiogram, neuroimaging) can be considered (Jenike 1988).

Psychosocial factors often contribute to depression in older persons. Retirement, relocation, physical decline or impairments, loss of ability to drive, relocation of adult children, and deaths of friends or family members all can have an adverse impact on emotional well-being.

There are many modalities that are useful in treating geriatric depression. Psychosocial interventions to increase activity and social contact include senior center activities, volunteer opportunities to enable the person to feel productive, exercise groups, meal sites, friendly visitors, and telephone contacts. Acquiring a pet can be helpful, especially if the person has a history of having pets. Psychotherapy in its various forms, including supportive, insight-oriented, cognitive, family, and support groups, can be effective.

Pharmacotherapy with antidepressants has been discussed previously. As with younger patients, adequate doses and duration of treatment are important. In some cases an adequate trial of an antidepressant in an older person may require 8 weeks or more on a therapeutic dose (Salzman 1992).

Anxiety

The prevalence of generalized anxiety disorder in community dwelling elderly individuals (65 and older) is about 2% (Salzman 1992). When elderly patients complain of anxiety or nervousness, most are reporting a subjective state of internal distress, worry, or apprehension that may or may not be associated with physical symptoms (Pies 1986). Many factors can contribute to anxiety in older persons (Pies 1986). In this section we will review the diagnosis of anxiety in geriatric patients and then outline treatment strategies.

The differential diagnosis of geriatric anxiety is extremely long and includes psychosocial factors; psychiatric disorders; medications; substance abuse; and medical problems, especially cardiac, pulmonary, endocrine, and neurological disorders (Jenike 1983).

Changes associated with aging can cause significant stress and anxiety. Psychosocial stressors in older adults include failing health in self or spouse, relocation of self or adult children, financial concerns, retirement, increased dependency, deaths of friends and family members, upcoming medical or surgical procedures in self or family, and caring for an ill spouse or family member.

The patient should be assessed for any psychiatric illness; depression often presents as anxiety in the geriatric population. Awareness of memory problems in early dementia can be anxiety provoking. Other psychiatric diagnosis to consider include adjustment disorder with anxious mood, phobias, panic disorder, obsessive-compulsive disorder, and generalized anxiety disorder.

Anxiety can be a side effect of many substances, prescription medications, and nonprescription drugs. Caffeine, nicotine, and stimulants in nonprescription drugs such as ephedrine can cause anxiety. If the patient is consuming caffeine, a slow taper is recommended to lessen any withdrawal symptoms. Other medications that can cause anxiety include anticholinergic drugs; antihypertensives; and, when at too high levels, digoxin and lithium. Akathisia from antipsychotic medications can mimic anxiety. Alcohol and sedative withdrawal are also associated with anxiety.

Anxiety is often seen in association with many acute and chronic medical problems. Because so many medical problems—some potentially serious—can present with anxiety, a medical evaluation is indicated. In the office the psychiatrist can obtain a brief review of systems; check pulse, blood pressure, and respiration rate; and order routine laboratory tests. Referral to an internist or geriatrician may be indicated.

Treatment of anxiety consists of addressing the contributing factors. Usually there are more than one. Psychosocial interventions may include supportive psychotherapy, grief counseling, involvement in support groups, stress management, relaxation techniques, and provision and coordination of supportive services. Medication adjustments may include tapering of caffeine and nicotine and dose reductions of medications likely to contribute to anxiety (e.g., bronchodilators) if possible. Any acute or chronic medical problems require treatment (Greist et al. 1986).

If symptoms of anxiety persist and interfere with functioning after underlying problems have been addressed, then pharmacological treatment can be considered. Benzodiazepines are the mainstay of anxiety treatment. However, because of the side effects to which older adults are especially sensitive (i.e., sedation, falls, and impaired concentration and memory), they require judicious use (Salzman 1990). Shorter-acting benzodiazepines are preferred, as discussed earlier. Other medications used to treat anxiety include buspirone (Rickels 1990), beta-blockers, antidepressants, and antihistamines. However, beta-blockers must be avoided in patients with diabetes, congestive heart failure, bradycardia, or bronchospastic disease. Antihistamines likewise tend to be quite anticholinergic and hence should be avoided.

Schizophrenia

It is estimated that about 1% of noninstitutionalized persons age 65 and older have schizophrenia (Lazarus et al. 1988). These patients face new sets of problems as they age, and clinicians must adjust treatment plans accordingly. These include not only the psychopharmacological changes discussed earlier, but also the effects on chronic mental illnesses of concurrent medical problems, dementia, and changes in social support systems.

Elderly persons in general are more likely to suffer from acute and chronic medical problems. These can exacerbate psychotic symptoms and hence should be considered when an elderly schizophrenic patient decompensates. Obtaining adequate medical care can be problematic for the patient with schizophrenia.

He or she may need help in deciding when to seek medical care for an illness or injury and assistance in arranging medical follow-up. Often mentally ill patients need an advocate when dealing with the medical system so that their complaints will be addressed and not simply attributed to their mental illness. For example, a 68-year-old man with schizophrenia slipped on ice and fell down a flight of stairs, fracturing a leg and hitting his head, but not losing consciousness. While he was hospitalized on an orthopedic surgery service, subsequent mental status changes mandated a neurological evaluation and cranial computed tomography scan (e.g., to rule out a subdural hematoma), rather than being assumed to be secondary to his schizophrenia.

Dementia or organic personality syndrome can be another complicating factor in schizophrenia. It is often difficult to pick up early organic symptoms, but these should be considered when elderly patients with schizophrenia seem to have increased difficulty coping or changes in their usual psychotic symptoms or when response to usual medication decreases.

Social support systems can change as a patient with schizophrenia ages. The patient's caregivers (e.g., parents, spouse, or children) may be aging as well and no longer able to provide the previous level of support. Such changes need to be anticipated and planned for.

Late-onset schizophrenia often presents with the positive symptoms of schizophrenia, but without the negative symptoms. Previously well-functioning older persons may develop delusions or hallucinations usually focused on some aspect of their social environment (Jeste et al. 1988). They often manage quite well in the community and only come to psychiatric attention when their psychotic symptoms lead to disruptive behavior such as repeated calls to the police.

These patients can be extremely distressed and fearful. For example, an 82-year-old retired man was afraid that his neighbor was taking pictures of him while he slept. He began sleeping on a cot in the basement, boarded up his windows, and eventually spent his night awake huddled in a basement closet to escape this "torture."

Most patients with late-onset schizophrenia have normal premorbid functioning but may have been considered eccentric or odd (Post 1987). Risk factors associated with late-onset schizophrenia include living alone; social isolation; and sensory impairment, especially hearing loss and poor vision, which can interfere with reality testing (Pearlson and Rabins 1988).

Treatment of late-onset schizophrenia includes addressing any sensory impairment, increasing community support and social contacts, and prescribing antipsychotic medications. Attempts to talk the patient out of his or her delusion are futile and may hamper rapport. Most patients do not feel they need medication. The use of medication can be presented to the patient as something to help the nervousness associated with their unusual experiences. The delusions associated with late-onset schizophrenia usually do not remit but can lessen in intensity. A reasonable goal of treatment is for such patients to be less distressed and less impaired by their symptoms.

Dementia

By DSM-IV criteria, dementia consists of impairment in short- and long-term memory plus impaired executive function (e.g., planning, organizing, thinking abstractly) or a disturbance in higher cortical functioning (apraxia, aphasia, or agnosia). Such impairment must result in significant psychosocial dysfunction and must represent a significant decline from the patient's premorbid level of functioning. Complications often associated with dementia include delusions, hallucinations, mood changes, anxiety, agitation, catastrophic reactions, wandering, sundowning, and sexually inappropriate behavior. Premorbid personality traits are often accentuated in dementia. The prevalence of dementia increases with age. Of those age 65 and older, about 5% are severely affected by dementia, and 10% are mildly to moderately affected. By age 80, approximately 20% are severely affected by dementia. About half of all cases of dementia are due to Alzheimer's disease (Coffey and Cummings 1994). Although there is still no cure for most dementias, much can be done to improve patients' quality of life during the course of the illness and to help both patients and caregivers cope with its consequences.

The concept of excess morbidity is a very useful notion in this context. To the extent that elderly patients in general, and dementia patients in particular, have diminished coping reserves, they can be more easily "tipped over" by a medical or psychosocial stressor. They may thus appear to be more impaired than their actual baseline level. The exciting challenge in working with dementia patients is then to identify and remedy the sources of excess morbidity and restore the patient to his or her baseline level of functioning.

When evaluating a patient for dementia, the clinician must assess cognitive and functional abilities. There are a number of cognitive screening tools available. The most commonly used is the Folstein MMSE (Folstein et al. 1975). It has a maximum of 30 points; takes about 10 minutes to administer; and covers immediate recall, orientation, short-term memory, attention, calculation, naming, reading, writing, and constructional abilities. Because these tools are just screening tests, they may miss patients with early dementia, especially those who are well educated. Collateral sources can provide information about changes in cognitive or functional abilities. Family may be the first to notice the patient's forgetfulness or difficulty with usual tasks, such as balancing a checkbook, cooking, driving, or dressing.

The causes of dementia are legion and include endocrine and metabolic disorders, infections, drugs and toxins, alcohol, brain injury, brain tumors, normal pressure hydrocephalus, neurodegenerative disease (e.g., Alzheimer's disease, Parkinson's disease), cerebrovascular disease, nutritional deficiencies, and depression.

Because up to 12% of cases of dementia are potentially reversible (Clarfield 1988), in part or full, it is important to do a complete workup on any patient suspected of having dementia. The usual workup includes, in addition to a physical and neurological examination, a complete blood cell count, tests for vitamin B_{12} and folate deficiency, chemistry panel, thyroid function tests, tests to determine the presence of a sexually transmitted disease, chest radiograph, and an electrocardiogram. Neuroimaging (computed tomography or magnetic resonance imaging) is helpful with new cases of dementia. A lumbar puncture, electroencephalogram, tests to determine drug levels, and other more specific tests may be clinically indicated. Neuropsychological testing can be helpful in clarifying early or ambiguous cases.

Management of patients with progressive dementing illness requires a comprehensive approach addressing current difficulties and planning for future complications (Jarvik and Wiseman 1991). Patients newly diagnosed with dementia and their families may need encouragement to get their affairs in order while patients are still competent to make important decisions. Such issues as making a will, deciding advance directives, and obtaining a durable power of attorney for health care as well as a power of attorney for finances can make life easier for the patient, family, and health care providers later in the course of the illness. Safety issues such as the ability to drive and live independently must be periodically assessed. Caregiver stress is a significant complication of dementia. Education about dementia, support groups, respite services, and day care can be vital to the caregiver's—and hence the patient's—well-being. *The 36-Hour Day* (Mace and Rabins 1991) is one example of a very useful manual for family members and professionals alike to acquire familiarity with the multiple aspects of caring.

In managing the behavioral complications of dementia, first consider any underlying medical problem that might be contributing to an increase in symptoms or change in behavior (Knopman and Sawyer-DeMaris 1990). Acute illnesses (e.g., urinary tract infections and pneumonia), exacerbations of chronic illnesses, pain, constipation, medication side effects, and drug interactions can all present in dementia patients with only behavioral signs and symptoms. Neuroleptic-induced akathisia may mimic the agitation being treated. Environmental factors should also be considered. These include relocation, change in supports, noise level, and interpersonal difficulties. Psychiatric problems such as concurrent agitated depression, delirium, or psychosis can contribute to behavioral problems. Precipitants of aggressive behavior should be noted. Bathing, toileting, or other cares may precipitate catastrophic reactions. Remember, more often than not there is more than one contributing factor involved. Only after causes of excess morbidity have been addressed can the clinician more confidently attribute behavioral complications to progression of the dementia (Howell and Watts 1990).

Once medical and psychiatric problems have been addressed, environmental and behavioral interventions can be devised depending on the nature of the problem and its precipitants (Teri and Gallagher-Thompson 1991). Enlisting caregivers as detectives in discovering patterns of agitation can serve more than one purpose. It can help to determine precipitating factors and potentially useful interventions. It can also help build a therapeutic alliance and allay caregiver feelings of helplessness. Modifying environmental stimulation, redirection, foreshadowing, distraction, and developing caregiver tolerance for nonharmful behaviors can all be employed as indicated.

Pharmacological interventions should be employed judiciously, given the generally increased sensitivity of dementia patients to psychotropic medications. Any psychiatric disturbance should be treated appropriately. Although not well studied, many psychotropic medications have been used in managing agitated and aggressive behavior. In addition, neuroleptics, trazodone, beta-blockers, carbamazepine, and lithium have been shown to be sometimes effective (Tariot et al. 1995). The use of antipsychotics, long the first choice in these clinical situations, has come under increasing scrutiny, given their potential for significant side effects. They are perhaps effective only one-third to one-half of the time at best (Schneider et al. 1990), and their use in nursing homes is now subject to federally mandated regulations (Omnibus Budget Reconciliation Act 1987). Hence, increasing research is currently being conducted to determine safer, more effective treatments.

Legal Issues

Legal issues in geriatric psychiatry often arise in the areas of competency, informed consent, guardianship, critical care planning, durable power of attorney, and protective payeeship. These arise most prominently in older patients with dementia. Although the technical points of the law and its implementation vary from state to state, some general principles apply.

Competency is a legal determination. The court decides whether a person is competent. The role of the psychiatrist is to assist the court by giving an opinion regarding a person's competency (Kern 1987). It is important to be aware that competency is not necessarily a global characteristic of a person. Thus, an individual may be incompetent is some areas, but competent in others. For example, a patient with early vascular dementia may have lost the ability to manage financial affairs or to vote, but may still have the ability to participate in making a more concrete decision regarding whether efforts should be made to restart his or her heart (i.e., cardiopulmonary resuscitation) if it were to stop beating. In some jurisdictions it is possible, and even required, that a psychiatrist assessing someone's competency may make recommendations to the court as to which areas the patient retains the ability to make competent decisions. In this manner, limited guardianships can be established, with provisions for periodic review as the situation changes.

Steps taken while a patient with dementia retains some competency can facilitate future care and decision making. With advance directives individuals can delineate wishes regarding critical care (e.g., cardiopulmonary resuscitation, ventilators, antibiotics, feeding tubes, and other medical interventions). Durable power of attorney for health care provides for the designation of other individuals to make medical decisions for them when they become incompetent to do so.

Long-Term Care

Psychiatric practice in long-term care facilities such as nursing homes, group homes, and community-based residential facilities is becoming more widespread. The roles a psychiatrist can assume in such settings are multiple. Most commonly, the psychiatrist works as a consultant, assessing and treating those residents who have psychiatric problems. It is usually better to accomplish this in the facility rather than requiring the patient to be transported to an office or clinic. Nursing home patients, for example, may clinically present in a different, misleading manner out of their usual milieu. To see them in their usual setting, where relevant records and familiar staff are readily available, can help ensure more accurate evaluations and monitoring of treatment.

A psychiatric consultant to a long-term care facility can also provide informal and formal education services, teaching residents, families, and staff about psychiatric problems, either on an ad hoc basis or through inservice education programs. Educational activities such as these may help to improve and maintain the quality of mental health services in the facility. Occasionally, psychiatrists may even become nursing home medical directors, thereby facilitating their work as members of interdisciplinary teams and further enhancing the psychiatric component of the residents' care. Whatever their role, however, it is important that psychiatrists working in long-term care facilities advocate for their patients and the staff who serve those patients.

Summary

Because the treatment of elderly patients requires a comprehensive biopsychosocial approach, it behooves psychiatrists working with them in community setting to familiarize themselves with the principles of geriatric psychiatry. To the extent they can enhance their medical diagnostic skills, locate medical and nursing colleagues with whom they can work in tandem, and learn and enlist the sometimes diverse social and psychological resources available for older adults, they can accomplish much to improve the lives of their geriatric patients. With experience, and a growing tolerance for diagnostic and prognostic ambiguity, the initially bewildering complexity of interfacing psychiatric, medical, and social problems commonly encountered with older mental health patients becomes instead an exciting diagnostic and therapeutic challenge.

Looking to the future of community geriatric psychiatry on another level, one encounters the already arriving crisis of how to allocate increasingly limited resources in the face of demographically expanding needs. We hope that a new intergenerational consensus can help to transform this growing dilemma into an ultimately satisfiable challenge.

References

American Psychiatric Association: Diagnostic and Statistical Manual of Mental Disorders, 4th Edition. Washington, DC, American Psychiatric Association, 1994

Blazer D: Affective disorders in late life, in Geriatric Psychiatry. Edited by Busse EW, Blazer DG. Washington, DC, American Psychiatric Press, 1989

Clarfield AM: The reversible dementias: do they reverse? Ann Intern Med 109:476–486, 1988

Coffey CE, Cummings JL (eds): Textbook of Geriatric Neuropsychiatry. Washington, DC, American Psychiatric Press, 1994

Davidson J: The pharmacologic treatment of psychiatric disorders in the elderly, in Geriatric Psychiatry. Edited by Busse EW, Blazer DG. Washington, DC, American Psychiatric Press, 1989

Folstein MF, Folstein SE, McHugh PR: Meni-Mental State: a practical method for grading the cognitive state of patients for the clinician. J Psychiatr Res 12:189–198, 1975

Goldstrom I, Burns B, Kessler L, et al: Mental health services use by elderly adults in a primary care setting. J Gerontol 42:147–153, 1987

Griest J, Jefferson J, Marks I: Anxiety and Its Treatment. New York, Warner Books, 1986

Howell T, Watts D: Behavioral complications of dementia: a clinical approach for the general internist. J Gen Intern Med 5:431–437, 1990

Jarvik L, Wiseman E: A checklist for managing the dementia patient. Geriatrics 46:31–40, 1991

Jefferson J, Griest J, Ackerman L, et al: Lithium Encyclopedia for Clinical Practice, 2nd Edition. Washington, DC, American Psychiatric Press, 1987

Jenike M: Treating anxiety in elderly patients. Geriatrics 38:115–119, 1983

Jenike M: Assessment and treatment of affective illness in the elderly. J Geriatr Psychiatry Neurol 1:89–107, 1988

Jenike M: Geriatric Psychiatry and Psychopharmacology: A Clinical Approach. Chicago, IL, Year Book Medical, 1989

Jeste D, Harris J, Pearlson G, et al: Late-onset schizophrenia: studying clinical validity. Psychiatr Clin North Am 11:1–13, 1988

Jeste D, Krull AJ, Kilbourn K: Tardive dyskinesia: managing a common neuroleptic side effect. Geriatrics 45:49–58, 1990

Kern S: Issues of competency in the aged. Psychiatric Annals 17:336–339, 1987

Knopman D, Sawyer-DeMaris S: Practical approach to managing behavioral problems in dementia patients. Geriatrics 45:27–35, 1990

Lazarus LW, Jarvik LF, Foster JR, et al: Essentials of Geriatric Psychiatry. New York, Springer, 1988

Mace N, Rabins P: The 36-Hour Day, Revised Edition. New York, Warner Books, 1991

Maletta G, Mattox K, Dysken M: Guidelines for prescribing psychoactive drugs in the elderly: part 1. Geriatrics 46:40–47, 1991a

Maletta G, Mattox K, Dysken M: Guidelines for prescribing psychoactive drugs in the elderly: part 2. Geriatrics 46:52–60, 1991b

NIH Consensus Development Panel on Depression in Late Life: Diagnosis and treatment of depression in late life. JAMA 268:1018–1024, 1992

Omnibus Budget Reconciliation Act: P.L. 100-203, 101 stat. 1330, 1987

Pearlson G, Rabins P: Late-onset psychoses: possible risk factors. Psychiatr Clin North Am 11:15–32, 1988

Pies R: Differential diagnosis of anxiety in the elderly. Geriatric Medicine Today 5:94–104, 1986

Post F: Paranoid and schizophrenic disorders among the aging, in Handbook of Clinical Gerontology. Edited by Carstensen LL, Edelstein BA. New York, Pergamon, 1987

Potter W, Rudorfer M, Manji H: The pharmacologic treatment of depression. N Engl J Med 325:633–642, 1991

Rickels K: Buspirone in clinical practice. J Clin Psychiatry 51 (suppl):51–54, 1990

Roccaforte W, Burke W: Use of psychostimulants for the elderly. Hosp Community Psychiatry 41:1330–1333, 1990

Salzman C: Anxiety in the elderly: treatment strategies. J Clin Psychiatry 51 (suppl):18–21, 1990

Salzman C: Clinical Geriatric Psychopharmacology, 2nd Edition. Baltimore, MD, Williams & Wilkins, 1992

Schneider L, Pollock V, Lyness S: A metaanalysis of controlled trials of neuroleptic treatment in dementia. J Am Geriatr Soc 38:553–563, 1990

Tariot PN, Schneider LS, Katz IR: Anticonvulsant and other non-neuroleptic treatment of agitation in dementia. J Geriatric Psychiatry Neurol 8 (suppl 1):S28–S39, 1995

Teri L, Gallagher-Thompson D: Cognitive-behavioral interventions for treatment of depression in Alzheimer's patients. Gerontologist 31:413–416, 1991

Section IV

Special Topics

Chapter 18

Guidelines for Community Psychiatric Practice

Alexander S. Young, M.D.
Gordon H. Clark, Jr., M.D., M.Div.

Since the 1980s health care spending has continued to rise, and governments and businesses have increased their efforts to contain these expenditures. The federal government has provided little direction for this cost containment, allowing many different strategies to emerge in the public and private sectors (Sharfstein et al. 1993). Psychiatry, along with other medical specialties, has felt the effect of these new cost containment strategies. In the private sector, cost containment is best understood by examining the market forces felt by insurance companies. Private health insurance companies have encountered a dramatic rise in psychiatric costs, led by chemical dependency treatment. These insurers have simultaneously been under increasing pressure from their various customers to limit their charges. This combination has resulted in the development of managed care paradigms that use utilization management and other techniques to control costs (Tischler 1990). These approaches attempt to assess the appropriateness of treatment and encourage the least costly effective treatment.

Unfortunately for psychiatrists, and presumably psychiatric patients, much of the psychiatric care currently being delivered is vulnerable to charges that it is neither efficient nor effective. Specifically, there is little research to justify the expense of providing long-term psychotherapy using psychiatrists instead of less expensive psychotherapists, or of allowing prolonged inpatient hospitalization. In fact, few of the many psychiatric treatments in widespread use have been systematically defined and evaluated to determine their effect on patient outcome. There is also limited agreement among mental health disciplines about what psychiatric care should be and who should do it. Managed care companies have made use of these uncertainties to dramatically reduce reimbursement for psychiatric care. This has been accomplished by limiting access to care and by shifting necessary care to outpatient venues, primary care physicians, the least expensive provider, and public mental health agencies. Insurance companies have also successfully negotiated contracts with psychiatrists for lower reimbursement rates. Although managed care has not yet affected all psychiatric reimbursement, psychiatrists should anticipate that the movement in this direction will continue, and that it will soon extend to nearly all reimbursement sources. Any national health care reform is likely to increase the use of managed care techniques.

Physicians' efforts to define appropriate practice can be seen as a healthy response to the increasing tendency of insurers and regulators to intervene in the physician-patient relationship. Indeed, the American Psychiatric Association (APA) and other professional organizations have responded by developing practice policies that define the nature of psychiatric care. A practice policy defines the appropriate treatment of a specific disorder (Eddy 1990a). Practice policies can be divided into three types: standards, guidelines, and options (Eddy 1990b). These differ according to the flexibility with which they are meant to be applied. *Standards* are intended to be rigidly applied: they must be followed in almost all cases. Practice standards for psychiatric disorders are generally not advisable, given the limitations in our understanding of appropriate psychiatric treatment. *Guidelines* are meant to be more flexible and are appropriate for much of current psychiatric practice. They should be followed in most cases, but exceptions can be justified based on individual needs. *Options* merely specify the different possible treatments, without specifying which should be used.

The APA has begun to establish practice guidelines for psychiatric disorders as defined in DSM-IV (American Psychiatric Association 1994). The establishment of these guidelines has involved a complex interaction among research, clinical lore, and political consensus building. The APA practice policies so far completed are the *Practice Guideline for Eating Disorders, Practice Guideline for Major Depressive Disorder in Adults, Practice Guideline for Treatment of Patients With Bipolar Disorder, Practice Guideline for Psychiatric Evaluation of Adults,* and *Practice Guideline for Treatment of Patients With Substance Use Disorders: Alcohol, Cocaine, Opioids.* Other guidelines are being developed (as of the writing of this chapter). Hopefully, these practice guidelines will be used to raise the usual quality of psychiatric treatment, increase the consistency of treatment between providers, encourage aggressive treatment of severe psychiatric disorders, and provide justification for reimbursement. However, many groups in the public and private sector have developed practice policies, and it remains to be seen which, if any, of these will have a substantial impact on treatment and reimbursement.

Psychiatric Practice in the Public Sector

The traditional distinction between public and private mental health care has been increasingly blurred by efforts to privatize public sector treatment and by legislation preventing private insurance companies from excluding people with severe or chronic psychiatric illness. This chapter, however, will focus on psychiatric practice in community mental health centers (CMHCs), as this is likely to remain the preeminent model for community-based psychiatric care.

Like their private sector counterparts, federal, state, and local agencies have been forced to contain the rise in health care expenditures during a period of limited reimbursement. Public mental health agencies have responded to this challenge in different ways. One common approach has been to close programs, cut clinical staff, and make access to care more difficult. This has renewed concern about the availability of mental health services for the poor and refocused attention on long-standing concerns about the quality of care delivered in these public systems.

The diminished role of psychiatrists at CMHCs has been identified as an important factor related to poorer quality of care (Clark 1990). Although there is little research addressing this issue, numerous authors and organizations have concluded that the care delivered to seriously mentally ill individuals has deteriorated significantly since the 1970s (Mechanic and Aiken 1987). This viewpoint is supported by the failure of many CMHCs to adopt important new clinical technologies, such as clozapine therapy (Young and Vaccaro 1994), assertive clinical case management, and behavioral family management (Vaccaro et al. 1993). This deterioration of CMHC care has occurred over a period when the number of high-quality psychiatrists practicing at CMHCs has steadily decreased. This decrease is remarkably similar to one previously seen at state hospitals, when professional involvement was reduced or eliminated and the quality of care deteriorated (Fink and Weinstein 1979).

Many CMHCs currently function with little clinical care or leadership from psychiatrists. Psychiatrists are often used only to sign prescriptions and insurance forms and usually do not supervise or interact with other practitioners involved in the patient's care. Indeed, the clinical care provided by psychiatrists is frequently limited to 5- to 15-minute medication visits. This diminished role has resulted both from administrative changes at CMHCs and also from a reduction in the number of competent psychiatrists willing to work in these settings.

Several factors have contributed to these trends (Talbot 1979). First, reductions in mental health budgets have often led to a reduction in the money spent on clinical care, without a concurrent reduction in administrative bureaucracy. In fact, public systems have often responded to shrinking budgets by increasing the paperwork necessary to justify clinical care and creating targeted or model programs requiring significant administrative effort. Some programs, such as Medicare, spend relatively little money on administration; however, these are the exception. A second significant factor has been the expense of psychiatrists relative to other providers. In the short run, substituting for psychiatrists appears to save money. Third, the traditional orientation of psychiatrists has contributed to their exodus. Many psychiatrists prefer to practice as independent professionals and to use individual psychotherapy. This style of practice is inherently more expensive than group and team approaches and hence is less available at CMHCs. There have also been strong financial incentives for psychiatrists to enter private practice, where they command higher salaries. Finally, academic institutions have decreased their involvement with CMHCs (Faulkner et al. 1982).

The abandonment of CMHCs by competent psychiatrists has made the situation more difficult for those who have chosen to remain. Without conscientious psychiatric leadership at CMHCs, policies are often decided on without regard for their effect on clinical care or the psychiatrist's ethical and legal concerns. Psychiatrists are therefore placed in positions where they are repeatedly directed to deliver substandard care. They are held responsible for the quality of their patients' care without being given the authority necessary to ensure this quality. This generates a significant level of stress for psychiatrists at CMHCs (Vaccaro and Clark 1987). Indeed, many conscientious psychiatrists have chosen to withdraw rather then work in this system. Although this may solve a personal dilemma, it generates an ethical one by contributing to the overall deterioration of community psychiatric care.

Practice Policies and the Public Sector

Despite the gloomy state of psychiatric practice in many CMHCs, there are some programs that have had remarkable success (Olfson 1990). There also appears to be a resurgent movement within psychiatry to improve CMHC practice. This movement has occurred, in part, because solo practice has become less financially viable for many psychiatrists. Increased competition from nonphysician psychotherapists and higher levels of intrusion from managed care companies have caused many psychiatrists to look seriously at practice in public mental health settings. Also, psychiatrists practicing in CMHCs have begun to organize in an effort to improve their situation. This organization has led, for instance, to the recent founding of a new professional organization, the American Association of Community Psychiatrists (AACP).

The AACP and other psychiatric organizations have worked to convince policymakers that improving the role of psychiatrists at CMHCs and improving quality of care are inextricably linked. Most would agree that good mental health care involves careful, expert oversight by the most experienced clinicians to ensure that each patient's problem is correctly evaluated and treated (Borus 1978). Because of budget cuts, many CMHCs no longer have the luxury of treating the worried well. They have, therefore, increasingly been called on to treat serious, chronic mental illnesses. The clinical treatment of patients with serious mental illness is uniquely suited to psychiatrists, because psychiatrists are usually the only professionals trained in the use of medication and rehabilitation for disorders such as schizophrenia (Berlin et al. 1981; Liberman et al. 1994). The seriously mentally ill also have a high rate of concurrent medical problems, requiring a physician comfortable with the treatment of medical illnesses.

The AACP and APA have advocated for the establishment of CMHC practice guidelines as a mechanism to improve both psychiatric practice and quality of care in these settings. Toward this end, the APA issued the *Guidelines for Psychiatric Practice in CMHCs* in July 1991 after consultation with the AACP and the National Council of CMHCs (American Psychiatric Association 1991). This document clearly describes the appropriate role of the psychiatrist at CMHCs and offers model job descriptions for the medical director and staff psychiatrist positions. These descriptions address the role of the psychiatrist in ensuring quality of care, performing clinical supervision, and directing clinical policy. Authority and responsibility are clearly linked. Guidelines were also issued for emergency services, multidisciplinary team work, psychiatric signatures, and psychiatric staffing. Every psychiatrist practicing at a CMHC should be familiar with these guidelines (Table 18–1). The guidelines describe a minimum expected level of quality and provide the basis for negotiating a position description and for refusing to collude with a harmful system.

Ultimately, clinical agencies such as CMHCs succeed or fail based on the quality of the clinical care they deliver (Astrachan 1980). Indeed, we can

Table 18–1.   The medical director model job description

Medical Director

Responsibilities

Unless the Chief Executive Officer (CEO) is properly trained and qualified to serve this purpose, the medical director has the ultimate authority and responsibility for the medical/psychiatric services of the center.

Specifically, this includes responsibility for:

(1)   Assuring that all center patients receive appropriate evaluation, diagnosis, treatment, medical screening, and medical/psychiatric evaluation whenever indicated.

(2)   Assuring that clinical staff receive appropriate clinical supervision.

(3)   Overseeing the work of all physicians, including residents assigned for training.

(4)   Assuring the appropriate implementation of clinical staff development and staff training activities.

(5)   Assuring, through a multidisciplinary process, the appropriate privileging and regular performance review of all clinical staff.

(6)   Providing direct psychiatric services.

(7)   Advising the CEO regarding the development and review of the center's programs, positions, and budgets that impact clinical services.

(8)   Assisting the CEO by participating in a clearly defined and regular relationship with the Board of Directors.

(9)   Participating, in cooperation with the CEO, in regular and direct communications with the state mental health program director's office, where appropriate, regarding psychiatric issues.

(10)   Providing liaison for the community mental health center with community physicians, hospital staff, and other professionals and agencies with regard to psychiatric services.

(11)   Developing and maintaining, whenever possible, all educational programs in concert with various medical schools and educational programs.

(12)   Assuring the quality of treatment and related services provided by the center's professional staff, through participation (directly or by designee) in the center's ongoing quality assurance and audit processes.

The Medical Director, by licensure, training, and prior clinical/administrative experience, shall be qualified to carry out these functions. He or she should be employed full time, and at least half of his or her time should be allocated to direct clinical care and clinical oversight functions.

Source.   American Psychiatric Association Official Action: *Guidelines for Psychiatric Practice in Community Mental Health Centers* (approved by the Board of Trustees of the APA, December 1988). Used with permission.

expect that CMHCs will be replaced by managed care companies or other mental health systems if they fail to deliver cost-effective, quality care. Many states have been exploring alternative organizational structures for managing their mental health care (Lehman 1989). Fiscal changes have included, for instance, turning over part or all of their Medicaid mental health programs to managed care companies. CMHCs will need to prove that they deliver efficient, quality care or they risk losing public funds over the next decade. Unfortunately, this fact alone will probably not be enough to cause most CMHCs to make appropriate changes. In fact, it is unclear how many CMHCs possess the expertise necessary to improve the efficiency and quality of their care.

There have long been arguments for formal accreditation of CMHCs based on genuine monitoring of quality of care (Kubie 1968); however, this has not yet come to pass. Although CMHCs often have utilization review and quality assurance committees, they often focus on meeting the various reimbursement requirements rather than actual quality of care. Efforts have been made to change this. The Joint Commission on Accreditation of Healthcare Organizations (JCAHO) has produced "Principles for Accreditation of Community Mental Health Service Programs" that addresses privileging and quality assurance. The Commission on Accreditation of Rehabilitation Facilities (CARF) has also developed principles for accrediting CMHCs. Although the value of these accreditation processes is controversial, it is clear that there is generally little or no connection between accreditation and reimbursement for CMHCs. Therefore, the JCAHO and CARF guidelines have had little or no impact. Direct linkage of quality of care and accreditation with reimbursement will be necessary if psychiatric practice guidelines are to improve care significantly at CMHCs. Accurate assessment of quality of care requires objectively measuring the process of care and the outcomes that result from treating people with serious mental illness. This will require strong ties between CMHCs and academic institutions that can develop valid and reliable measurements of quality of care.

Strategies for CMHC Practice

Given the political and economic forces described above, we can expect significant change in community psychiatric practice during the next few years. While this change unfolds, there remains much that can be done by individual community psychiatrists to improve their job satisfaction and the quality of care they deliver. There are some CMHCs that have retained academic affiliations, who respect the role of the psychiatrist, and that deliver modern and efficient care. Most community psychiatrists do not have an opportunity to work at such a CMHC. Instead, psychiatrists often encounter systems that suffer from many of the faults discussed above. Although it is sometimes possible to work well in suboptimal settings, this can only be achieved through advocacy, careful negotiation, and continued vigilance.

The community psychiatrists must be prepared to define his or her role with a CMHC through negotiation of an appropriate position description. This negotiation begins with a thorough understanding of the CMHC's organizational structure. Whether through personal experience or personal contacts, the psychiatrist needs to understand the system's administrative and economic functioning. Certain administrative questions will often arise: Is there a medical director, and if so, what standard does he or she set for the psychiatric role at the CMHC? Who is the chief executive officer (CEO), and how effectively do the medical director and CEO interact? What functions do psychiatrists perform at the CMHC? Whom do they report to administratively: the medical director, the CEO, or a middle-level bureaucrat? Does the CMHC have a strong academic affiliation? Economic questions should also be raised: How does the CMHC get its money? If the CMHC has multiple separate contracts, how are psychiatrists involved in the negotiation and administration of these contracts? These sorts of questions will reveal whether the psychiatrist is likely to be able to negotiate an appropriate position. It also can direct the psychiatrist toward certain clinical areas that are more in need of psychiatric staffing. Getting answers to these questions can actually be the most difficult part of the negotiating process, as administrators often guard this information to ensure their power and position. Contacts for obtaining this information can include psychiatrists and other clinicians in present or past practice at the CMHC and individuals working at the public mental health authority. As many sources as possible should be consulted. The psychiatrist may even want to take a limited role at the CMHC, such as a part-time, short-term consultant, to obtain this information. This can also be helpful to establish goodwill with CMHC staff and to demonstrate one's clinical and administrative expertise.

Once one knows the present system, the next stage is to draft and negotiate a position description. This should begin with one of the model position descriptions from the APA *Guidelines for Psychiatric Practice in CMHCs*. There are several issues to which one should pay close attention. First, authority must follow legal and fiscal responsibility. Specifically, the psychiatrist must have clinical authority over the system within which he or she practices. If, for instance, he or she will be the primary psychiatrist for a day treatment program, then he or she should be designated as medical director of this program. Second, one must pay careful attention to the administrative hierarchy of the system. A staff psychiatrist should not report solely to an administrator. An administrator's concern is often with financial and structural imperatives, not clinical realities. Reporting to an administrator creates, therefore, a situation where the administrator may instruct the psychiatrist to act without regard for quality clinical care. The psychiatrist is also unable to receive appropriate clinical direction or guidance in the event of a difficult clinical situation. The staff psychiatrist should be sure that he or she reports to another psychiatrist. Third, how will the psychiatrist communicate with other professionals involved in the care of patients? What time and forum will be necessary, for instance, to collaborate with and supervise social workers and case managers?

The CMHC psychiatrist should also be ready for attempts to encroach on previously negotiated issues. It is not uncommon, for instance, for a CMHC to pressure a psychiatrist to inappropriately sign reimbursement-related documents. Steadfastness regarding this and other pressures to compromise professional values must be maintained. Finally, maintaining affiliations with other CMHC physicians can be helpful for support. Maintaining ties with local academic institutions and national societies, such as the AACP, go a long way toward making CMHC work rewarding.

Conclusions

The rising cost of health care has led private and governmental agencies to increase efforts to control the physician-patient relationship in an attempt to minimize cost. The most effective defense psychiatry can use against these intrusions is to define clearly the effectiveness and efficiency of psychiatric treatment and to make this definition known to policy makers. Careful studies of a treatment's structure, outcome, and cost are imperative if psychiatrists expect to use that treatment modality over the long term. In the meantime, establishment of practice guidelines, based on available research and clinical experience, can help define quality care. Toward this end, the APA has established *Guidelines for Psychiatric Practice in CMHCs*. Quality of care assessment could also be a useful tool in improving the quality of care delivered at CMHCs. Unfortunately, neither guidelines nor meaningful measurements of quality are presently in widespread use.

Changes in public policy that create a link between quality, cost-effective care and reimbursement could improve patient care at many

CMHCs. Individual psychiatrists can also improve the quality of care at their CMHCs by carefully negotiating their positions in these organizations. They can use available practice guidelines and gain a knowledge of mental health organization and financing to combat the tendency of CMHCs to minimize psychiatric participation. Although much remains to be done before high-quality care is delivered consistently in community systems, the active involvement of conscientious psychiatrists can make a significant difference.

References

American Psychiatric Association: Guidelines for psychiatric practice in community mental health centers. Am J Psychiatry 148:965–966, 1991

American Psychiatric Association: Diagnostic and Statistical Manual of Mental Disorders, 4th Edition. Washington, DC, American Psychiatric Association, 1994

Astrachan BM: Regulation, adaptation, and leadership in psychiatric facilities. Hosp Community Psychiatry 31:169–174, 1980

Berlin RM, Kales JD, Humphrey FJ, et al: The patient care crisis in community mental health centers: a need for more psychiatric involvement. Am J Psychiatry 138:450–454, 1981

Borus JF: Issues critical to the survival of community mental health. Am J Psychiatry 135:1029–1035, 1978

Clark GH: Assuring quality in community mental health centers. Psychiatr Clin North Am 13:113–125, 1990

Eddy DM: Practice policies—what are they? JAMA 263:877–880, 1990a

Eddy DM: Designing a practice policy: standards, guidelines, and options. JAMA 263:3077–3084, 1990b

Faulkner LR, Eaton JS, Bloom JD, et al: The CMHC as a setting for residency education. Community Ment Health J 18:3–10, 1982

Fink PJ, Weinstein SP: Whatever happened to psychiatry? the deprofessionalization of community mental health centers. Am J Psychiatry 136:406–409, 1979

Kubie LS: Pitfalls of community psychiatry. Arch Gen Psychiatry 18:257–266, 1968

Lehman AF: Strategies for improving services for the chronic mentally ill. Hosp Community Psychiatry 40:916–920, 1989

Liberman RP, Kopelowicz A, Young AS: Biobehavioral treatment and rehabilitation of schizophrenia. Behav Ther 25:89–107, 1994

Mechanic D, Aiken LH: Improving the care of patients with chronic mental illness. N Engl J Med 317:1634–1638, 1987

Olfson M: Assertive community treatment: an evaluation of the experimental evidence. Hosp Community Psychiatry 41:634–641, 1990

Sharfstein SS, Stoline AM, Goldman HH: Psychiatric care and health insurance reform. Am J Psychiatry 150:7–18, 1993

Talbot JA: Why psychiatrists leave the public sector. Hosp Community Psychiatry 30:779–780, 1979

Tischler GL: Utilization management of mental health services by private third parties. Am J Psychiatry 147:967–973, 1990

Vaccaro JV, Clark GH: A profile of community mental health center psychiatrists: results of a national survey. Community Ment Health J 23:48–55, 1987

Vaccaro JV, Young AS, Glynn S: Community-based care of individuals with schizophrenia: combining psychosocial and pharmacologic therapies. Psychiatr Clin North Am 16:387–399, 1993

Young AS, Vaccaro JV: Making clozapine available. Hosp Community Psychiatry 45:831–832, 1994

Chapter 19

Multidisciplinary Teamwork

Ronald J. Diamond, M.D.

T he use of multidisciplinary teams is critically important for the effective treatment of persons with serious mental illness. In many cases people with serious mental illness need a larger variety of different kinds of supports and skills than can be provided by any one clinician, including housing and vocational supports, crisis intervention, psychological supports, and medical/psychiatric treatment. In addition, many people with serious mental illness need more availability than can be provided by any single clinician, no matter how dedicated. Crises often occur outside of normal business hours, and even some scheduled services such as medication monitoring must to be available 7 days a week. Finally, the sharing of clinical responsibility among several people can decrease the burden associated with working with taxing clients and thus reduce subsequent burnout.

The psychiatrist and primary clinician often function as a team, regardless of whether this is formally acknowledged, and case management usually involves some level of shared or team responsibility. Some teams are set up to function as true shared case managers with shared responsibility and

Special thanks are extended to Dr. Len Stein, Dr. Michael Bohn, and Terry Pelliterri for reading early drafts of this chapter.

decision making. At the other extreme are those teams where each clinician has sole responsibility for his or her own clients, with little shared responsibility. Intermediate degrees of shared responsibility can also develop. For example, in some teams each clinician may take responsibility for specific and well-delineated areas such as housing or vocational training. Clinicians working in such a team may refer clients to each other but may have little sense of shared responsibility for clinical decisions.

In this chapter I begin with a general discussion of multidisciplinary teams but focus primarily on teams with case management responsibility. The chapter will concentrate on the relationship between the case management team and the psychiatrist. For reasons that will be discussed later, this relationship is often complicated, as both share overall responsibility for the client's treatment. Some of the potential problems and possible solutions of working within a multidisciplinary team will be addressed.

Multidisciplinary Teams

Multidisciplinary teams exist within the mental health system whenever a group of clinicians or staff regularly works together to meet the needs of persons with mental illness. The teams that exist on a formal organizational chart may be quite different from the informal teams that develop spontaneously when clinicians or other staff work together to meet the needs of a shared client. Teams often include people from different disciplines and may include people from different agencies. The defining characteristics of the team are its purpose, composition, size, and working relationships, including both formal and informal structure. Each of these component parts affects how the team will operate.

Purpose

Teams often define themselves by their purpose. The more specific the purpose of the team and the more all members of the team understand and agree to that purpose, the more likely the team is to be effective. For example, one treatment team in the mental health center of Dane County has responsibility to provide ongoing community-based treatment and rehabilitation for 140 clients who have a serious and persistent mental illness. Another treatment team has the responsibility to provide a 24-hour mobile crisis response, with the specific goal of decreasing the need for hospitalization by providing a range of community options. Other teams can be set up to provide services to a clearly defined geographical area or a population otherwise defined.

Without a clearly defined mandate, different people are likely to interpret the job of the team in very different ways, leading to confusion about who should be served and how staff should be spending their time. For example, some time ago, one of the teams in Dane County was set up to provide day treatment services to persons with serious mental illness. There was ongoing, energy-draining debate both about the purpose of the program and which clients should be served. The program was supposed to provide rehabilitation services, but without a clear definition of what this meant, outcome criteria for the program could not be designed. Without a clear definition of the purpose of the program, it was difficult to agree on the design of the program. The lack of clarity over the purpose of the program made it difficult for the staff to agree on such basic clinical decisions as how much responsibility they should take for clients who stopped coming into the program.

The defining mandate of many teams is too vague to provide a clear focus and direction. For example, when teams are established to provide mental health services to a geographical area, there is often disagreement about whether the team should prioritize people who are most ill, most motivated, most likely to be helped by traditional psychotherapeutic and psychopharmacological approaches, or most visible to other elements of the community. Without a clearly defined purpose, it is more difficult to assess the effectiveness of the team or justify to funding agencies that the team is performing as intended.

Composition

In many treatment systems the formal treatment team that exists on an administrative chart is composed of clinicians who have professional degrees. The functional team, however, may be quite different from this. Often a secretary, clinicians from a variety of different agencies, and staff from a variety of nonclinical backgrounds all actively work together on a regular basis, sharing information and responsibility for common clients, and informally constitute a "team." In some systems a minister, a police officer, or even a very involved landlord may all be part of the functional team, sharing information and acting as part of a cohesive unit.

At the mental health center of Dane County, for example, the program secretaries are seen as integral members of their respective teams. Team secretaries answer the telephone, deal with clients and other outside professionals, and help the teams interface with the outside world. How clients feel about a treatment team may be strongly influenced by the initial reception provided by the secretary. Often these secretaries have important information about clients and other matters that is unknown to other team members. It is important to ensure that the secretaries' behavior with clients is consistent with the rest of the treatment plan, and that the information that they have is made available to the rest of the clinical team. These program secretaries participate in treatment planning meetings and are involved in a variety of decision-making activities. They are trained and supervised to increase their clinical skills, and their interfacing with the outside world is considered a core clinical function. Most clerical staff who interact with clients have useful information unavailable to clinical staff, and it is a mistake to exclude them from some kind of participation with the rest of the clinical team.

Psychiatrists can either be included or excluded from the multidisciplinary team. Psychiatrists can be included in team discussions and share information with other team members or alternatively can work in relative isolation from the rest of the treatment team. Decisions about medications, like decisions about housing or other aspects of treatment, can be discussed by the entire team or kept as the sole province of a single clinician. There are many factors that influence how the psychiatrist will work with other team members. The interests and skills of the psychiatrist certainly play a major role. Psychiatrists can be interested and knowledgeable about all aspects of a client's treatment or can see their roles as restricted to a narrower focus such as medication. The job description also plays a major role. Psychiatrists may have the time to participate in team discussions or be so busy with medication reviews that any expanded participation is impossible. Even geographical proximity influences the role of the psychiatrist. The psychiatrist who shares office space with the other clinicians on the team will have a different relationship the team members than the psychiatrist who has an office in a separate building.

Size

Groups of 8 to 10 people seem to function better than groups that are much larger. It is difficult in larger groups for individuals to feel that what they do matters much to the group as a whole. Larger groups tend to split off into smaller subgroups. "Teams" of 20 to 30 clinicians are actually an organizational structure that is not likely to act as a coherent team. A common problem is that teams start with a workable number of clinicians, but over time the number of clients and clinicians involved grows beyond a workable number. In this instance, it is often difficult to split a team that has gotten used to working together and sees itself as one unit, even after the realities of growth make the increasing size less efficient. On the other hand, small size is less of a problem. Teams may be quite small and still be effective. In small programs, two or three colleagues working together can form a team with many of the same advantages as larger ones.

Team Process

There are many ways to describe the internal processes of teams. There are three areas that seem particularly important to team functioning:

1. The degree to which the team is more hierarchical or more egalitarian
2. The degree to which responsibility for decisions is shared by all members of the team or divided with each team member having specific areas of responsibility
3. The degree to which a team functions as a single social cluster or multiple clusters

Each of these is discussed below.

Hierarchical Versus Egalitarian Team Structure

Teams can be organized hierarchically with direction coming from a supervisor or senior clinicians to junior staff and aides. An example would be a team in which case managers developed treatment plans and supervised psychiatric aides in implementing these plans. Alternatively, the team can be organized so that different members of the team are clearly identified as having different expertise and information, but each member of the team functions as a full participant. For example, a social worker, nurse, and technician could all work with the client to develop a treatment plan with the understanding that the social worker might be most expert about dynamic issues in the relationship with the client, although the technician might have the most information about how the client actually functions in the community.

The degree to which a particular team functions hierarchically often depends as much on informal as formal structures. A team leader may encourage the entire team to share in clinical decisions. A social worker may encourage a psychiatric aide to function as a professional colleague and support him or her to make independent decisions. Alternatively, a team member with no formal authority might have a dominant role in decision making, either by force of character or by expertise. Psychiatrists, as high status members of the team, often have considerable influence over team relations. The psychiatrist who engages other team members as equals will model egalitarian behavior for other members of the team; alternatively, psychiatrists who assert the presumed perquisites of their profession influence hierarchical behavior by the rest of the team.

Shared Versus Delineated Responsibility

Some teams are structured so that the team assumes responsibility for most decisions, even decisions where a staff person has focal expertise. Other teams assume that specialists will be responsible for decisions within their areas of expertise. For example, the housing specialist on the team may get information about the client's preferences, develop a list of housing options, do a functional assessment of required supports, and then facilitate a decision about where the client should live. Alternatively, the housing specialist can provide information to the team so that the entire team can be actively involved in working with the client to make the decision.

Similarly, the psychiatrist can make decisions about a client's medication and then inform the rest of the staff about that decision. Alternatively, the psychiatrist can actively involve other staff in medication decisions by seeking staff input about what is going on in the client's life and by involving other staff in weighing the pros and cons of possible medication changes. In all cases the psychiatrist continues to be the expert on psychopharmacology and is ultimately responsible for all medication decisions, but the involvement of the rest of the team can vary enormously.

Single Versus Multiple Clusters Within the Team

In a single cluster team, all staff working with a client function as an integrated unit, freely sharing information and diffusing the decision making across the entire team. A large team can functionally divide into several smaller teams for more efficient functioning, but each would include all of the staff who need to work together to develop an integrated plan. Alternatively, separate clusters can evolve that cut across functional lines. When this occurs, the psychiatrist and nurse are often in one cluster and communicate with each other over medication decisions, whereas other team members form a second cluster that addresses work, housing, and other rehabilitation issues. Often there is relatively little communication among the clusters and still less shared planning or shared decision making.

Although the problems are obvious, solutions are often difficult to devise. There must be coordination among the different components of a treatment system. Staff responsible for developing housing or vocational options for a person with serious mental illness must coordinate with staff who will provide ongoing support, which in turn requires a coordinated treatment planning process, communicating with the prescribing psychiatrist, and involving whatever staff working with the person's family. Especially when working with clients with serious mental illness and extensive needs, case management must be a function of the entire team rather than the responsibility of a single individual. A significant problem is the integration the psychiatrist within the team and, in particular, how the psychiatrist and case management team can develop complementary roles.

The Psychiatrist and the Multidisciplinary Team

There are many sources of potential conflict between the psychiatrist and other members of the multidisciplinary team, including role conflict, ideological differences, and the special problem of medical expertise and responsibility. There are ways of minimizing these potential problems areas, each of which will be discussed below.

Role Conflict: Who Is Responsible for What?

There are inherent conflicts in the roles and responsibilities of the case manager, other clinicians, and the psychiatrist. The nature of the conflict depends on the specific model of case management being considered. Most discussions about clinical case management assume that the case manager will be in a central position in the client's treatment. With access to all relevant information, the clinical case manager has the presumed authority to organize an integrated and coherent treatment plan. Other clinicians, having their own agenda and sense of parochialism, may resist giving up their own sense of primacy to the case manager.

Such conflicts become particularly problematic when one of the involved clinicians is a psychiatrist (Arce and Vergare 1985). Psychiatrists tend to think of themselves in a central position with many of the same attributes as case managers—that is, they tend to see themselves as responsible for the client's entire treatment. The training of psychiatrists in medical school, internship, and psychiatric residency socializes them to assume overall responsibility for the treatment of their clients. The literature on the role of the psychiatrist considers a variety of clinical roles but almost never considers the case manager's central position or the need for the psychiatrist to acknowledge, come to terms with, and support this central role (Langley and Barter 1983).

In turn, the case management literature ignores the reality of having a psychiatrist involved. The psychiatrist not only has special expertise, but also inevitably has legal liability for decisions even if responsibility for those decisions has been delegated to a nonmedical mental health professional. This confusion over who is ultimately responsible is further heightened by administrative policies that require that the psychiatrist supervise and "sign off" on services provided by other clinicians.

There Are No Easy Answers

Many of the conflicts are caused by ambiguity over who is responsible for what. Resolution depends on developing complementary roles for the case manager and psychiatrist. One extreme position is to make the psychiatrist the team leader and clinical supervisor of all of the other professionals (Leong 1982). Conflict is avoided by putting the psychiatrist in charge and making the case manager subordinate. However, there are multiple problems with this approach. The psychiatrist may be with the team part time or, by virtue of skills or personality, may not be the best team leader. Other clinicians may not agree that the psychiatrist should lead the team, and furthermore, it may not be the best use of the psychiatrist's expertise to lead the team (Tucker 1987). An alternative but equally extreme position is to limit the job of the psychiatrist to prescribing medication and other, strictly medical, tasks. In this case, conflict is avoided by limiting the role of the psychiatrist to a well-defined set of tasks. Unfortunately, this limits the usefulness of psychiatrists and allows only part of their expertise to be utilized. More importantly, it enforces an artificial separation between "medical" and "nonmedical" parts of the client's treatment.

Regrettably, there is ongoing disagreement about the appropriate roles and the relative responsibilities of case managers, psychiatrists, and other team members (Clark 1987). Whereas the roles of various professionals are complementary at some agencies, in other agencies there appears to be continuous friction over who is responsible for what. There are, however, some general principles that seem useful in minimizing these conflicts and increasing the chance for fruitful collaboration and effective treatment planning.

The Client Comes First

It is important for the needs of the client to override personal or guild issues. Unfortunately, in the exegeses of operating in the real world, clinicians often forget to follow this precept. We work in imperfect systems and at times get annoyed with our colleagues—sometimes for good reason. It is difficult to work with another clinician who does not return telephone calls or refuses to collaborate in a shared treatment plan, and a natural tendency is to stop trying. Unfortunately, it is the client who is most often harmed when this happens.

Clinicians need to start by thinking about what their client needs. Then they need to act to get those needs met. This may require that they do things counter to their own preferences. Ideally, a psychiatrist should be an active member of the team, participate in treatment planning meetings, and be part of the informal information net of well-functioning teams. When information needs to be exchanged, the psychiatrist should work as hard to contact the case manager and other members of the team as the case manager does to contact the psychiatrist. Unfortunately, this does not always happen. Part of the difficulty may be structural. The psychiatrist's job description may preclude participation in team meetings, and an office at a site separate from the team will interfere with informal "touching base" with other team members.

At times, however, the problem is one of attitude. For example, a case manager may keep "forgetting" to give a psychiatrist adequate notice of treatment planning meetings, or a psychiatrist may delay returning calls the case manager initiated. These behaviors are often irritating and are perceived by the injured party as a mark of disrespect or rejection of that party's potential usefulness. Although the behavior may be irritating, the needs of the client must take precedence. The psychiatrist may have to keep pushing for participation in the planning process, even if the scheduled meeting needs to be rearranged, and the case manager may have to pursue the psychiatrist so that necessary information gets exchanged and medications are appropriately prescribed.

It is easier to get consensus on a specific treatment plan for a specific client than it is to come up with an agreed-on treatment philosophy. For example, different professionals, with different views on the role of the hospital, can have endless arguments about whether hospitalization should be used more or less and whether it is useful or injurious. However, when a specific client comes into the office with increasing suicidal ideation, and the historical information, treatment successes, current supports, and stressors are reviewed and discussed by the treatment team, the role of hospitalization usually becomes clearer. Even where there is philosophical disagreement, the specific issues facing a "real client" shape a treatment plan that all involved clinicians can support.

Look for areas of agreement, rather than concentrating on areas of disagreement. Frequently clinicians are so drawn to areas of disagreement that they fail to recognize that areas of conflict may be a fairly minor part of the entire picture. A negotiated team decision usually leads to a better outcome than an imposed decision.

It is important for all members of the treatment team to support the client's relationship with other members. Team members may differ in their approach to treatment, but embroiling the client in this conflict runs the risk of increasing the client's stress and symptoms (Stanton and Schwartz 1954). Supporting a consistent treatment plan is almost always more beneficial to the client than feuding over whose approach should be followed. As there is often no "right" answer in treatment, the different team members can usually discuss and offer the client a range of options. Presenting options is very different from having professionals, on whom the client is dependent, fighting over the "correct" course of action.

Team members must be willing to gather and present the data for their respective positions, rather than falling back on authority, familiarity, or unexamined feelings. The psychiatrist, case manager, and other team members should support their positions with information or expertise that can be shared and considered by the other clinicians. For example, it is not very useful for the psychiatrist to issue the edict, "I am the physician, and I feel that John should be on more medication." Similarly, the case manager cannot justify his or her decision by relying on the assumption that "I know the client best!" A much more useful approach is demonstrated in the following two vignettes.

A case manager was concerned about the side effects caused by raising a client's medication. The psychiatrist explained that she felt the increase was necessary because the client seemed more disorganized and bothered by intrusive, auditory hallucinations. The psychiatrist also referred to the client's similar exacerbation the year before and improvement after the medication was increased. Given the history, the case manager was able to support the decision to increase temporarily the dose of antipsychotic medication. At the same time, the discussion increased the psychiatrist's sensitivity to the problems caused by the side effects and led to a decision to add another medication to treat them. The case manager worked with the client to develop a set of target symptoms to monitor both exacerbation of symptoms and side effects, which provided the psychiatrist with better information for future medication adjustments.

A psychiatrist believed that a particular client needed the supervision of a group home, whereas the case manager wanted to support the client's request for a supported apartment. The case manager pointed out that the client would live alone, but would have staff dropping by several times a week to monitor the client's functioning and to assist with shopping, budgeting, and other realities of living. An inventory of the client's specific skills (he made friends easily and could ask for help) and specific deficits (he was unable to budget money, cook, or organize any complicated task) led to a discussion of the client's previous trials in independent living and group homes. This shared information made planning the client's independent living trial easier and more success oriented than previous trials. The discussion also led to a clearer understanding of the risks involved (he might cause a disturbance and get himself evicted, but he was unlikely to be dangerous or get himself into serious trouble). By the end of the treatment planning process, the psychiatrist, case manager, housing consultant, and client were able to agree on a plan that was different from any that each of them would have come up with independently. The client was supported in living in his own apartment and in turn was willing to accept closer supervision than he might have preferred.

A critical element in developing a shared treatment approach is shared responsibility. It is rarely useful to criticize a plan if a better one cannot be derived. For example, when there is disagreement on the need for hospitalization, the clinician who believes that hospitalization is unnecessary has the responsibility to develop ideas for an alternative that can be discussed and examined by the other clinicians working with the client. On the other hand, the clinician who thinks that hospitalization is needed has the responsibility to develop specific goals for the hospitalization and an idea of what is going to happen after discharge.

It is equally ineffective to come up with a plan requiring another clinician to do more work or take more responsibility than he or she is willing to assume. For example, a psychiatrist suggested that a decompensating client should be treated in the community rather than with a hospital admission. After some discussion about the specific needs and behavior of the client, the team involved in treatment planning quickly agreed that treating this client in the community would require several home visits a day for the next few days. It also became clear that the case manager did not have the time to do this, and although other staff could help, the staffing needs of the proposed treatment plan could not be met. Instead, a 2-day hospitalization was arranged that helped to stabilize the client and give staff time to organize better coverage for when the client was discharged.

The clinician can often achieve a good outcome by continuing to be reasonable, even when other clinicians seem unreasonable. Although this is often hard to do, it is surprisingly effective when achieved. If another clinician becomes dogmatic, authoritarian, or avoids a shared decision, there is a complementary pull to become equally unreasonable. There may also be a pull just to avoid working with this other clinician. Either way, the client typically loses. If, in the face of this dilemma, the responsible clinician continues to look for areas of common agreement, consider seriously the view of the other clinician, and examine the available client data, there will be a strong reciprocal pull for that other clinician to respond in turn and thus look for areas of compromise and potential agreement.

Consider the Needs of the Other Clinicians

It is important to consider what the other clinicians need to adequately perform their jobs. For example, an emergency department at a nearby hospital had an administrative rule that required discharge clearance by a psychiatrist whenever a client was seen following a suicide attempt. Even if an experienced case manager assessed the client and recommended discharge, there was a need for at least telephone clearance from a psychiatrist. The case managers were annoyed that they were required to review each case with the on-call psychiatrist and felt as though the psychiatrist was "second guessing" their professional assessment. In discussing this annoyance, case managers were asked what kind of information they would want if they were placed in the role of the psychiatrist and had to take responsibility for releasing a client from the emergency department. Considering the psychiatrist's needs and responsibility helped the case managers understand and accept the detailed questioning.

Familiarity Breeds Solutions

Knowing each other helps. All too often, informal networks of community support staff do not include the psychiatrist. The case managers and other staff meet to discuss joint clients, visit agencies, and thus know each other as real people. The psychiatrist, on the other hand, exists only as a voice on the telephone or as a set of cryptic medication notes. This lack of familiarity is unfortunate and often discourages integrated treatment. To counter this, psychiatrists should attempt to establish personal relationships with other members of the team. Psychiatrists should regularly invite other team members to confer about shared clients and to participate in joint meetings. Although the initial relationship building requires face-to-face contact, much of the communication, including conference treatment planning calls, can be done over the telephone after these personal ties are formed.

Developing these personal ties is often difficult and may even seem risky. Clinicians are busy, and it is awkward to begin a connection with a stranger. Moreover, there is always the risk that attempts at closer collaboration will expose hidden conflicts and make the working relationship more difficult rather than easier. These anxieties often lead the involved clinicians to believe there will be less conflict if the relationship between the psychiatrist and the case manager is allowed to remain more distant, even though this is clearly not in the client's best interest.

Different Ideologies

Just as potential problems are caused by conflicting roles, there are potential problems caused by different ideologies. The psychiatrist and the other team members often talk different languages and have different ideologies. This goes beyond the previously discussed conflict over who is responsible for what. It has more to do with different ways of viewing the world, different ways of conceptualizing problems, and different kinds of goals. These differences are most evident when the treatment team is part of a rehabilitation program and the psychiatrist is part of a treatment program. Rehabilitation programs have generally stressed the differences between rehabilitation and treatment (Anthony et al. 1984; Cnaan et al. 1988). Such programs have typically been based on the belief that treatment services (including psychiatric services and medication monitoring) are important but should be clearly separated, or at least put at some distance and not allowed to "contaminate" rehabilitation. It is all too easy for case managers working in such programs to feel that psychiatrists are trying to impose a traditional, paternalistic, and illness-based orientation. Psychiatrists, in turn, are often uninformed about rehabilitation programs and do not understand the importance of maintaining a rehabilitative perspective.

Even case managers working from a more traditional treatment orientation often see themselves as having a different focus from that of psychiatrists. Regardless of whether this focus is truly different, the perception of difference and the use of a different language sets up barriers that accentuate professional rivalries, concern about dominance, and turf issues. The decision about whether to use the word *consumer, client,* or *patient,* and the underlying view that each represents have led to monumental struggles in some mental health systems.

These ideological conflicts are accentuated in journal articles and academic discussions and appear less relevant at the level of direct service workers. This seems particularly true in those settings where psychiatrists and case managers have good working relationships. Just as there are general principles that can help resolve role conflicts, the following principles can help resolve conflicts resulting from ideological differences.

Concentrate on Common Goals

The clinical interventions involved in making a diagnosis, prescribing medication, meeting with families, and helping clients to handle stress or obtain a job are all interrelated. All of these interventions are aimed at helping the client improve his or her quality of life. For the most part, getting a client to come for an appointment or to take medications are not ends in and of themselves; they are designed to decrease symptoms, increase functional capacity, and improve overall quality of life. These are goals that practitioners from all disciplines and community programs can share. Once we realize that our long-term goals are shared, it becomes easier to question ourselves about whether a particular intervention helps.

Become Informed About the Ideology of the Other Clinicians

It is important for the psychiatrist and the case manager to learn about, listen to, and understand the ideology of one another. Many arguments over alternative ideologies are caused by having a simplistic view of the alternative point of view or by confusing bad practice with a particular orientation. Nonmedical professionals often rail against a "medical model." In fact, a sophisticated medical model stresses a holistic approach that includes consideration of psychological and social factors along with biological ones. What is generally criticized in these discussions is not this kind of comprehensive medical model, but rather medical dominance or attempts to limit consideration of the client to biology. Psychiatrists, in turn, sometimes stereotype nonmedical mental health professionals as being unable to make accurate assessments or appreciate the importance of medication. Although this is certainly true for some nonmedical clinicians, it is no more representative of many social workers or psychologists than is the representation that psychiatrists prescribe medications and do nothing else.

At times disagreement is based on an accurate appraisal of having different tasks. A rehabilitation expert might not pay much attention to a DSM-IV diagnosis or even be concerned as to whether someone is mentally ill (American Psychiatric Association 1994). The expert's focus of concern is on a functional assessment and a plan to overcome functional limitations. This does not mean that the rehabilitation expert dismisses the reality of mental illness or the importance of another professional taking an alternative treatment approach to the client, but only that the rehabilitation professional approaches the client's problems from a different perspective.

Psychopharmacology and Other "Medical Topics"

The psychiatrist's exclusive expertise regarding medication and other medical topics can be a source of significant role conflict between the psychiatrist and nonmedical members of the treatment team. Often team members who are actively involved in most other major issues in their clients' lives abdicate involvement in medication decisions. There are many reasons for this. One is the mental health system itself. It is often unclear what role, if any, the nonmedical members of the case management team should have in decisions about psychotropic medication.

Other reasons why nonmedical clinicians are removed from medication decisions involve knowledge and responsibility. Many case managers are not particularly knowledgeable about such medical topics as psychopharmacology. Involvement in medication issues is particularly intimidating if the psychiatrists are not in the practice of working collaboratively with other clinicians. Perhaps more importantly, many case managers do not see "medical" decisions as part of their responsibility and do not feel an obligation to become knowledgeable in this area.

Psychiatrists often participate in keeping case managers and other team members out of medication decisions (Samuelly 1986). Some psychiatrists feel that all of the responsibility for medication management, including assessment, prescribing, and monitoring, should be left entirely to physicians. Many of these psychiatrists have defined their role so narrowly and rigidly that they prescribe medication without thinking through the repercussions of those medications on the overall treatment plan or on others involved in the client's care. Other psychiatrists would be willing to use case managers in some way but do not know the system well enough to know how to include the case manager in this aspect of care, or they believe that case managers and other nonphysicians can inform the psychiatrist about how the client is doing, but should have no direct input in any medication decisions, thus putting the case manager in a distinctly peripheral role.

This lack of integration continues despite the reality that other team members are often in a better position than psychiatrists to evaluate the effect of medication changes on a client's functional ability. The case manager and other team members usually see a client more often and in a wider variety of settings. Therefore, they are in a better position to recognize subtle medication side effects and early signs of decompensation. In addition, other team members are often in a good position to monitor whether their client is taking prescribed medication. Clients often have a close relationship with their clinical case manager and may tell them about noncompliance. Lastly, the case manager has contact with the client's support system and can utilize this to help monitor medication when clinically appropriate.

All team members have a professional obligation to be concerned with medication, just as they should be concerned with other major aspects of the client's life. They need to know what medications might be useful for their clients, what prescribed medications their clients have, what medications their clients are actually taking (which is often different from what is prescribed), and what impact and side effects those medications may have. Although this might seem like an intimidating prospect, it is actually less difficult than it would seem on the surface.

Psychiatrists have an obligation to inform team members (and the client) about psychotropic medications, their indications, and their side effects and to enlist the aid of the team in monitoring the effects of medication. Psychiatrists should teach their nonmedical colleagues about medication, not for the purpose of prescribing, but to monitor beneficial and side effects appropriately. This teaching can involve formal minicourses or lectures. An even more important aspect of the learning process occurs when the psychiatrist involves the team in the decision-making process. Team members learn nothing about the effects and side effects of a medication if the only involvement is being told that a client started a particular medication at a particular dose. Much more information is transmitted and remembered when the psychiatrist and the rest of the team jointly consider the pattern of the client's symptoms, look at the therapeutic indications for different medications, and discuss the pros and cons of each.

Case managers and psychiatrists must work together to connect medication issues to the rest of the client's life and to the client's own goals and agendas (Diamond 1983, 1985). All too often, medication prescription is something that is done "to" clients instead of "with" clients. Clients almost always have their own goals and agendas. One client may miss playing basketball but be too paranoid to leave his apartment. Another client may want to get a job but be too disorganized and too bothered by voices to follow through. Still another client may want to keep his own apartment, but his late night yelling and talking to himself may lead to threats of eviction. In each case medication can be presented as something that will help the client achieve what he or she wants. For example, it is often more effective to present medication as something that might help the client become less afraid so that he can play basketball again rather than as something that will help with the more abstract concept of decreasing symptoms. Making concrete connections requires considerable information about clients, their needs, and their own goals.

Lower medication doses can be used when the entire treatment team is involved in the monitoring process. In most public mental health systems, clients meet with their psychiatrist for a brief session at relatively infrequent intervals. The psychiatrist cannot monitor day-to-day or even week-to-week fluctuations. Moreover, the psychiatrist typically observes the client in one setting: the office. The other members of the team, on the other hand, have information from a variety of settings. With careful monitoring, prodromal relapse symptoms can be identified at an early stage, thus allowing medications to be increased before hospitalization is needed. In addition, careful monitoring can allow some clients to be maintained on a targeted medication strategy in which medication is only used for relatively short, targeted periods when symptoms reemerge. All of this becomes much more difficult when the psychiatrist and the rest of the treatment team work in isolation from one another.

Information Sharing

A conscious effort is required by the psychiatrist, case manager, and other caregivers to ensure that the psychiatrist has enough information about the client's life and treatment to prescribe and monitor medication effectively and to resolve crises. Too often the psychiatrist ends up outside the information net. To facilitate the inclusion of the psychiatrist in the information net, the case manager and the psychiatrist must decide what kind of information they need to share and how this will occur.

Summary

Treatment of persons with serious mental illness requires that many clinicians work together. This is true whether treatment takes place in the hospital or in the community. The hospital, however, has a long tradition of teams with a clear role for each of the team members. There is much more ambiguity in roles and responsibilities in community settings. In the community, clinicians may have different goals and different treatment ideologies and may operate out of different settings. The potential for role conflict is increased because of poorly defined and overlapping responsibilities. These problems are usually most evident in the relationship between the psychiatrist and other members of the treatment team, but the potential for conflict and communication breakdown is present throughout the team.

These problems can be resolved. It is possible for the psychiatrist to be a fully integrated member of the multidisciplinary team and to work with other team members to develop a comprehensive approach to treatment. It is important for all members of the team to understand the need for an integrated approach to treatment. In doing so, all members of the team must understand the role of the other members and must define their complementary roles. This is actually not difficult once all team members recognize they are involved in the shared task of improving the clients' quality of life.

References

Adler DA: The medical model and psychiatry's tasks. Hosp Community Psychiatry 32(6):387–392, 1981

American Psychiatric Association: Diagnostic and Statistical Manual of Mental Disorders, 4th Edition. Washington, DC, American Psychiatric Association, 1994

Anthony WA, Cohen MR, Cohen BF: Psychiatric rehabilitation, in The Chronic Mental Patient: Five Years Later. Edited by Talbott JA. New York, Grune & Stratton, 1984, pp 137–157

Arce AA, Vergare MJ: Psychiatrists and interprofessional role conflicts in community mental health centers, in Community Mental Health Centers and Psychiatrists. Washington, DC, American Psychiatric Association, 1985, pp 51–68

Beigel A: The remedicalization of community mental health. Hosp Community Psychiatry 35(11):1114–1117, 1984

Cnaan RA, Blankertz L, Messinger KW, et al: Psychosocial rehabilitation: toward a definition. Psychosoc Rehab J 11(4):61–77, 1988

Clark GH: CMHCs and psychiatrists: a necessarily polemical review. Presented at the annual meeting of the American Association of Community Psychiatrists, Denver, CO, 1987

Diamond RJ: Enhancing medication use in schizophrenic patients. J Clin Psychiatry 44(6, sec 2):7–14, 1983

Diamond RJ: Antipsychotic drugs and the quality of life: the patient's point of view. J Clin Psychiatry 46(5 sec 2):239–241, 1985

Kanter J: Clinical case management: definition, principles, components. Hosp Community Psychiatry 40(4):361–368, 1989

Lamb HR: Therapist–case managers: more then brokers of services. Hosp Community Psychiatry 31(11):762–764, 1980

Langley DG, Barter JT: Psychiatric roles in the community mental health center. Hosp Community Psychiatry 34(8):729–733, 1983

Leong GB: Psychiatrists and community mental health centers: can their relationship be salvaged? Hosp Community Psychiatry 33(4):309–310, 1982

Samuelly I: Dual treatment by psychiatrists—beware. The Psychiatric Times, September 1986, pp 8–9

Stanton AH, Schwartz MS: The Mental Hospital. New York, Basic Books, 1954

Tucker C: Turf issues in CMHCs (letter). Hosp Community Psychiatry 38(11):1225–1226, 1987

Chapter 20

Working With Advocacy, Support, and Self-Help Groups

Charles R. Goldman, M.D.
Harriet P. Lefley, Ph.D.

E stimates indicate that from 9 to 12 million adult Americans utilize self-help groups (Lieberman 1990). Sharfstein and Beigel (1988) have recommended "expansion of community involvement and relations with self-help groups" as a survival strategy for psychiatrists in private practice, a tactical suggestion earlier offered by Panzetta (1985) for private sector practitioners. Ironically, community psychiatrists have long considered this "strategy" to be an integral part of their role. Despite the importance of this activity, relatively little has appeared in the psychiatric literature to guide our efforts. Most recent works on the treatment and rehabilitation of persons with serious mental illness emphasize that professionals form collaborative relationships with patients and their families. Some offer specific conceptual models and techniques for collaborating with them, typically with respect to treatment issues (Bernheim 1989; Diamond 1985; Gruenbaum and Friedman 1988; Hahn et al. 1988; Hatfield and Lefley 1987; Hyde and Goldman 1989; Yee 1989). In addition, consumers themselves have contributed to the professional literature and have made very helpful suggestions from the patient's perspective (Blaska 1990; F. Frese, unpublished manuscript, 1992; Leete 1987; Ruocchio 1989).

Few authors, however, have addressed the specific issue of psychiatrists working on an organizational and mutual referral level with advocacy, support, and/or self-help groups. Mosher and Burti (1989) made several references to the value of mutual help groups and the importance of working with them. Imber-Black's (1988) book, *Families and Larger Systems,* provides a very thorough conceptual model but does not directly address the issue of psychiatrists' roles in working with advocacy groups within these systems. A few articles have directly addressed the self-help issue and have offered some tentative recommendations (Lieberman 1990; Toro et al. 1987; Toseland et al. 1989) but have not spoken to the specific issues confronting community psychiatrists.

In this chapter we address the role of community psychiatrists in working with groups that have unitary or mixed agendas of advocacy, support, and mutual self-help. *Advocacy groups* are generally oriented toward social and legal remedies to improve the lives of mentally ill individuals. *Support groups* focus on personal relief and learning through experiential sharing, unburdening, and information exchange. *Self-help groups* aim toward therapeutic growth and skills development for oneself and one's peers through mutual efforts rather than through professional interventions. In many groups these functions tend to be mixed. Self-help groups have larger agendas than simple support groups, but they almost always offer the same types of experiential sharing and learning. Some of the larger advocacy organizations offer all three channels of activity.

Self-help groups, by definition, tend to avoid involvement by professionals (except for those who share the problem and participate as knowledgeable peers). In some cases or under certain circumstances, however, the groups may welcome consultation, education, resource information, or other types of expertise in effecting their goals. Spontaneously organized support groups tend to be localized and in some cases self-limiting unless they become part of a larger organization. They may solicit professional participation as the need arises, but for the most part they tend to rely on their own resources. Some support groups are organized by a mental health facility as a service for patients and families, whereas others are ongoing adjunctive activities of an advocacy organization. In both cases they tend to welcome psychiatric input, particularly in answering questions about medications and other medical concerns. Citizen and family organizations tend to welcome psychiatric participation as educational resources and in shared advocacy efforts, and consumer advocacy organizations will sometimes affiliate with professionals who share their views.

In this chapter we focus primarily on linkages between community psychiatrists and organizations that deal with serious and persistent mental illnesses or addictions. Self-help groups are increasingly being incorporated as important components of the treatment system for these populations and are beginning to have a significant role in rehabilitation and community reintegration. In discussing the interrelationships of self-help, support, and advocacy groups and community psychiatry, we focus on reciprocity—that is, on how community psychiatrists can be helpful and collaborate effectively with these organizations and how persons who have experienced mental illness and their advocates can contribute to psychiatric training and practice. We also note in passing the rise of advocacy organizations that tend to have antipsychiatry views of the nature of mental disorders and their appropriate treatments, and suggest ways in which community psychiatrists may educate their memberships.

Overview of Citizen, Family, and Consumer Advocacy Movements

Self-help groups for recovering psychiatric patients (e.g., Recovery Inc.) and for persons with addictions (e.g., Alcoholics Anonymous) have existed for many years. It is primarily since the 1980s that we have seen the development of family and consumer organizations that not only offer mutual support but also have political agendas for social and legal change. Together with attorneys and citizens concerned with mental health law, these organizations have also generated new types of protection and advocacy legislation reinforcing patients' rights to adequate resources as well as to humane and effective treatment. These movements have affected the operations of service delivery systems, added new dimensions to clinical training, and altered traditional relationships between mental health professionals and recipients of their services.

Prior to 1979, the major advocacy group for persons with serious mental disorders was the National Mental Health Association (NMHA). Despite its founding by a former mental patient, Clifford Beers, the NMHA has had a limited emphasis on serious mental illness and a broad-based mission to improve mental health in the population at large. In most areas local MHA branches became the major umbrella organization linking professionals with citizens interested in psychological issues. Such branches developed a range of projects such as providing adult volunteers to befriend troubled schoolchildren, training police to deal with interethnic conflict, and running support groups for widowed or other bereaved persons. Legislative advocacy and other efforts on behalf of persons with major psychiatric problems were just one component of a multifaceted program that was targeted toward alleviating the impact of multiple life stressors in the general population. However, at both state and national levels, the MHA has almost always joined with the American Psychiatric Association (APA) and with other advocacy groups, such as the ones described later, in lobbying for legislation to improve services for persons with serious mental or developmental disabilities.

Most local MHAs have tried to attract psychiatrists to their governance and advisory boards and to use them as educators and group leaders. There are often friendly affiliative relationships between local psychiatric societies and the local MHA. In the main, however, there has been greater participation from those in other disciplines, such as psychologists and social workers.

On the legal front, the Mental Health Law Project (1991), now the Judge David L. Bazelon Center for Mental Health Law, was organized in 1972 by lawyers and professionals in mental health and mental retardation. The Bazelon Center works in the courts and in the legislative and policy arenas offering legal information and assistance to consumers, advocates, and policy makers. Its initial purpose was to halt abuse and neglect in state mental hospitals and training schools and to prevent exclusion of disabled children from public schools. Its current agenda, however, is much more comprehensive. In addition to its basic focus on protecting patients' rights, examples of its projects have included Community Watch, a program to combat exclusionary zoning and rental policies while increasing availability of housing; advocacy for health care, social services, and income support; and lawsuits aimed at reforming state systems and generating a continuum of community-based services for persons with mental disabilities.

Community psychiatrists should also have familiarity with the National Association for Rights Protection and Advocacy (NARPA), organized in 1980 to bring together mental health attorneys and other advocates in an agenda focusing on presumptive patient abuse. NARPA's national conferences have often provided a sympathetic forum for the views of psychiatrists who oppose the common use of psychotropic medications, question the biological basis of major mental disorders, and believe that a great deal of psychiatric treatment is unnecessary or countertherapeutic. One noted speaker has even suggested that psychiatry is the most abusive institution in the United States (Breggin 1989).

At the other end of the spectrum are patient and family advocates who support a biogenic model of mental illness, favor compliance with psychotropic medications, and clearly believe that lack of psychiatric interventions, as well as institutional maltreatment, comes under the rubric of abuse.

The Family Movement

The formation of the National Alliance for the Mentally Ill (NAMI) has been listed as one of the important events in the history of psychiatry by Kaplan and Sadock (1991), who have described the organization as the most vigorous citizens group in America, advocating for the mentally ill to legislators and the public. NAMI was founded in 1979, when 284 family members from various states convened at the University of Wisconsin in Madison, with backing from the Community Support Program of the National Institute of Mental Health (NIMH). Since that time, NAMI has grown to 130,000 members, with 1,005 affiliates in all 50 states, as well as Canada, Puerto Rico, and the Virgin Islands.

NAMI's multiple activities include family support; resource development; public and self-education; education of professionals; service on mental health planning, policy, and governance boards; legislative advocacy; and training consumers and family members as effective lobbyists and patient advocates. A number of members of Congress themselves have mentally ill family members, and the family organization has been a natural matrix for coordinating efforts to initiate and promote federal legislation favorable to mentally ill individuals. Thus, NAMI has been notably successful in advocating for increased research and services funding for the NIMH and in ensuring continuity of programs such as the Community Support Program.

In the period between 1986 and 1989, NAMI helped obtain a 38% increase in congressional appropriations for NIMH research on schizophrenia. The organization launched the National Schizophrenia and Brain Research campaign, cofounded the National Alliance for Research on Schizophrenia and Depression, and has offered more than $1 million in research awards through the Ted and Vida Stanley Foundation.

NAMI influence was strong in attaining enactment of 1) the 1984 Social Security Act amendments to restore eligibility to mentally ill and other disabled individuals, 2) Public Law 99-660 to require comprehensive state plans to serve mentally ill individuals, and 3) the Fair Housing Act amendment to bar discrimination against persons with mental illness. It joined with other groups to influence passage of the 1990 Americans with Disabilities Act, which includes persons with mental illness.

NAMI was also influential in obtaining the Protection and Advocacy (P&A) legislation, initiated in 1986, which established statewide P&A programs for persons with mental illness, augmenting existing P&A programs for the developmentally disabled in institutional settings. A reauthorization of this law will permit protection and advocacy services to be extended into community settings such as group homes, as well as jails and prisons. At the urging of NAMI members, the law was also amended to require increased representation from family members and consumers on P&A governing boards and advisory councils, as well as training for advocates on the nature of serious mental illness. According to the NAMI Legislative Network News, "the new law also establishes a grievances mechanism, whereby consumers and family members can file complaints against the P&A and strengthens the ability of NAMI members to provide constructive input into the development of program rules and regulations" (National Alliance for the Mentally Ill 1991, p. 1).

The new P&A formulations may help ease a situation that has disturbed a number of family members. According to Isaac and Armat (1990), in certain states some local AMI groups feel that "P&As for the mentally ill (are) staffed largely by the mental health bar, militant ex-patients, and anti-psychiatric patient advocates. . . . They have found that many of the P&A staff see treatment itself as an abuse from which the patient needs protection" (p. 268). The balancing of patients' rights with patients' needs for housing and treatment is an ongoing debate in the advocacy movement, and as we shall see, consumers themselves are divided on many of these issues.

The Consumer Movement

In a study of 104 self-help groups for former psychiatric patients, most of them with hospitalization histories, Emerick (1990) has identified two major service models: social movement and individual therapy. The social movement model is oriented toward social change, and these groups offer services such as legal advocacy, public education, technical assistance, and information referral networking. "In contrast, the individual therapy groups are quite different. They provide their members with opportunities for more 'inner-focused' individual change through group support meetings, drop-in centers, and various types of 'alternative therapy'" (Emerick 1990, p. 402). The study found that almost two-thirds of the groups were social movement models.

Although the majority of groups in both categories permitted participation of professionals, the latter apparently did not avail themselves of the opportunity. More than 70% of the groups reported little to no interaction with professionals. Moreover, the largest proportion of groups in the sample (43%) held antiprofessional attitudes, whereas only 26% were pro-professional, and 31% were neutral. As might be expected, therapy groups were most amenable to professional alliances, and social movement groups were most antagonistic.

This study is of interest in view of the agendas of the major national consumer organizations and also in light of the growing use of consumer-run programs as adjuncts or alternatives to professional services. What Emerick terms the *individual therapy model* has been around for many years in major consumer organizations such as Recovery, Inc. or Grow, Inc. The past few years have seen the rapid growth of a major consumer organization combining both therapeutic and advocacy functions: the Depressive and Manic-Depressive Association. All of these are self-help groups whose members acknowledge that they suffer from a psychiatric disorder and whose efforts are oriented toward improving their coping skills outside of the official mental health system.

"Social movement" groups have also been around for many years. Protest groups of former psychiatric patients, such as the Insane Liberation Front (Portland, Oregon) or the Mental Patients Liberation Project (New York) were formed in the early 1970s. Later, two national organizations emerged. The National Association of Mental Patients, currently renamed the National Association of Psychiatric Survivors (NAPS), remains essentially a protest movement that adamantly opposes any form of involuntary treatment, promotes initiatives to make electroconvulsive therapy illegal, and views both psychotropic medications and hospitalization as largely harmful. The National Mental Health Consumers' Association (NMHCA), which was organized primarily to improve rather than reject the mental health service delivery system, is generally opposed to involuntary treatment but acknowledges the validity of mental illness and the need for treatment. The NAMI Consumers Council similarly strives to improve the system and is generally a strong proponent of the need for psychiatric services.

Despite the protests about hospital treatment, a well-designed survey that was planned and conducted by consumers themselves under State of California auspices found a range of opinions among formerly hospitalized patients. The respondents indicated that 50% found psychiatric hospitalization helpful, 25% found the experience helpful in some ways and harmful in others, and only 20% found hospitalization "very" or "somewhat" harmful (Campbell 1989).

There is also considerable evidence of an increase in consumer-professional alliances at local and national levels. For a number of years, consumers have presented invited papers on their experiences at state and national APA conventions. After observing the first national symposium of self-help groups and providers in March 1989 in Chicago, Illinois, Emerick (1990) predicted "a tempering both of strong antiprofessional sentiments in patient groups and of anti-self-help attitudes among professionals"(p. 406). Two self-help research centers, one at the University of California at Berkeley and the other at the University of Michigan at Ann Arbor, have been funded by NIMH as collaborative efforts of academicians and consumers to study self-help groups for persons with mental illnesses. Consumers are involved as advisors and paid research assistants in formulating survey questions, developing instruments, interviewing, and data analysis. Other national consumer groups, such as the National Consumer Self-Help Clearinghouse in Philadelphia, Pennsylvania, and the National Empowerment Center in Lawrence, Massachusetts, supply technical assistance and knowledge dissemination. These, together with a range of consumer-run services for patients, have been vigorously supported by the Community Support Program of the Center for Mental Health Services.

Twelve-Step Programs

Alcoholics Anonymous (AA) is perhaps the most successful self-help group, and many other programs based on its 12-step approach have emerged (e.g., Narcotics Anonymous, Overeaters Anonymous). With the increasing awareness that many mentally ill people are also chemically dependent, it is important that community psychiatrists have a working knowledge of the AA model and its various "spin-offs." Perhaps more than other self-help groups mentioned in this chapter, the AA approach requires anonymity and strictly limits formal collaboration with outside organizations or professionals. It uses education as a primary modality but does not engage in advocacy per se. The 12 steps themselves constitute a paradoxical conceptual model that first emphasizes powerlessness (to counteract the grandiosity and denial of the addict), followed by responsibility and self-regulation of illness based on a mixture of intrapsychic, interpersonal, and spiritual principles. Discussions of the treatment of "dually diagnosed" patients have emphasized the potential value of 12-step programs but have also pointed out some pitfalls, especially for patients who must remain on psychotropic medications (Minkoff 1991; Osher and Kofoed 1989).

Simple referral to a 12-step program may not work as well as careful timing of the referral with the phase of treatment/rehabilitation and careful selection of a specific group for the patient to attend. It is often necessary for the psychiatrist to discuss the 12 steps in detail and to help the patient understand their implications. This may include a discussion of spirituality and its meaning to the patient. Many substance abuse programs formerly required that all patients participate in 12-step groups as a therapeutic modality. However, this has been curtailed by legal decisions that mandatory attendance conflicts with patients' rights to freedom of religion, as 12-step programs require acknowledgment of a belief in God "as we understood Him." Psychiatrists should be aware of this and discuss in advance whether this 12-step requirement will interfere with any religious belief before a referral is made.

Twelve-step approaches may be very effective from a psychiatric perspective, but this often depends on how well they are integrated into the overall treatment approach (Galanter et al. 1990). Alanon can be very helpful for family members of patients with substance dependency, but more than simple referral is often required. For example, a parent of a person with schizophrenia must be educated about the mental illness and its treatment/rehabilitation in some detail before the Alanon approach of "disengagement" can be constructively used. Also, the concept of codependency, although often useful, can directly conflict with the "no-fault" concept of mental illness and, in some family members, can trigger a self-blame cycle that is counterproductive. Use of the 12-step approach for eating disorders and other compulsive disorders is less well established and needs further study. Other self-help and "psychoeducational" approaches, some inspired by AA, show much promise and need further development and study. The historical development of AA is fascinating and instructive, and its study should yield many new and useful approaches.

Community Psychiatry Principles and Practice Implications for Working With Advocacy, Support, and Self-Help Groups

As we have indicated, a number of books have recommended liaisons between mental health professionals and self-help or advocacy groups but have failed to offer guidelines for accessing them and for developing appropriate role relationships. An NIMH monograph by Silverman (1978), however, is particularly relevant. The author concluded by recommending four ways professionals can cooperatively interact with such groups:

1. Making a referral
2. As consultant to a mutual help group
3. As a member of an advisory board
4. As an initiator of a mutual help group

In this section we expand on these recommendations and relate them specifically to community psychiatric practice.

Several key features of community psychiatry practice (Brown et al. 1992) suggest principles for collaborating with self-help and advocacy/support groups. In the following sections, six such principles are given, each one followed by several practical suggestions for implementation.

Viewing Patients in the Context of Their Social Networks

Although psychiatrists currently give much lip service to the biopsychosocial model, few actually practice a systems approach (Fink 1988; Hartmann

1991). Community psychiatrists by definition (Brown et al. 1993) view patients in the context of their social and cultural surroundings, which includes the growing tendency of patients and their families to join mutual help groups. Silverman (1978) pointed out that such groups may form "in response to professional failure" (e.g., AA [Alcoholics Anonymous], AMI [Alliance for the Mentally Ill], and ARC [Association for Retarded Citizens]), "in reaction to technological advances" (e.g., groups of cancer victims or ostomy patients or support groups for patients improving on clozapine), or "in reaction to social change." Lieberman (1990) described similarities and differences among a variety of self-help groups, warning that it is erroneous to assume that the ingredient responsible for positive outcome in one group is the same in another. In any case, clinicians must be aware of such groups and take them into consideration as they assess and plan their approach to their patients, just as they take into consideration patients' memberships in church or social groups.

Practice implications

- Routinely ask patients and families about their knowledge of support groups, their past and present involvement, and their intentions to participate.
- Learn which support groups are active in your area; the daily newspaper is one good source; self-help clearinghouses, or information exchanges, also exist in some areas.
- Keep a file of names and telephone numbers of support groups such as AMI, SHARE, GROW, Depressive/Manic-Depressive Association, Alanon, AA, Compassionate Friends, and others.
- Use support and advocacy groups (e.g., AMI) as sources of information about treatment and rehabilitation resources (and their absence!) in your area.

Forming Collaborative, Negotiated Helping Alliances With Patients and Their Families

To effectively treat the most severe and chronic psychiatric conditions, clinicians must be able to form treatment alliances (Goering and Stylianos 1988). Rehabilitation and treatment adherence principles dictate that such alliances be mutual and collaborative and include the patient's significant others when possible. Kleinman (1988) has suggested that psychiatrists learn the "explanatory model" used by their patients, make their own explanatory model explicit, and discuss with the patient (and significant others) common goals and expectations, as well as differences, in a process that respects all parties' beliefs. When the patient and/or family belongs to a self-help group, it is most helpful for the psychiatrist to be familiar with the views and expectations of the group, which may be relevant in a negotiation process.

Practice implications

- Assume a consultative or "coach" role with patient/family when appropriate; limit the authoritarian "expert" role to emergencies or very specific circumstances.
- Adopt a "psychoeducational" approach; stay up to date on the latest helpful information about mental illness etiology, diagnosis, course, and treatment; rehabilitation strategies; self-regulation techniques; family adaptation; and community resources (Anderson et al. 1986; Bernheim and Lehman 1986; Bisbee 1991; Falloon et al. 1984; Liberman 1987). Become familiar with the "survival" book most widely used by AMI families (Torrey 1994).
- Do not be afraid to admit ignorance or to share the boundaries of what is known (and not known) in the field; be open to learning from patients and their families.
- Learn the philosophy and tenets of the most important self-help/advocacy groups in your area; attend meetings of these groups; minimally, attend AA, Alanon, and AMI meetings.
- Engage patients and families in in-depth discussions about their explanatory model of mental illness and its treatment; keep an open mind and actively look for areas where you agree and disagree.
- Translate areas of agreement and disagreement into implications for treatment adherence; negotiate a mutually acceptable treatment plan based on patient's/family's explanatory model.
- Where the support group philosophy reinforces treatment and/or rehabilitation principles, use these in discussions with the patient/family (e.g., actively discuss the 12 steps with AA or Alanon members; actively reinforce the nonblaming coping/adaptation model of mental illness with AMI members).
- Actively raise issues of self-blame and stigma and allow patient and family members to express their fears and grief in a supportive atmosphere.

Encouraging Self-Efficacy and Self-Determination of Patients

Especially in working with patients with severe, chronic illness, positive outcome often depends on the positive attitude, initiative, and constructive action of the patient and family. The clinician's treatment and rehabilitation goals and efforts should enhance these attributes. Self-help groups tend to empower members, instill hope, and reverse demoralization—all of which are essential for the most successful rehabilitation outcomes. In addition to forming collaborative alliances as outlined earlier, community psychiatrists should actively promote membership in self-help groups and may even initiate the formation of such groups through bringing interested consumers together. A related goal of community psychiatry is to strengthen the community itself (i.e., "natural" folk healing systems) through supportive yet minimally intrusive efforts to enhance natural supportive elements of social networks (Caplan 1990).

Practice implications

- Actively refer patients and families to appropriate self-help groups; keep current brochures and telephone numbers.
- Be aware of powerful informal helpers in the community; encourage their efforts and support them if they seem willing to organize a group.
- Form personal relationships and active liaisons with leaders of existing support/advocacy organizations; offer them consultative assistance and ask them for help in engaging isolated patients and families. Some advocacy groups will do outreach, and some patients or family members will require this if they are to get involved.
- In consulting with support/advocacy groups, be aware that your clinical training and experience are not sufficient; you should seek additional training in community organization, group facilitation, and mental health (systems) consultation.
- Silverman (1978) has suggested that volunteer group members particularly want "permission, perspective and appreciation" from consultants; she also suggested that the effectiveness of the professional is maximized when he or she is a volunteer, rather than on a salary or fee basis. Lieberman (1990) stressed that professionals can "legitimize" self-help groups but should not attempt to professionalize them by directly training group leaders in mental health technology.
- "Grow your own": Introduce patients/families with similar problems to each other, or start a support group among your own patients/families as opportunity presents. Family members or patients who have gone through early and middle stages of coping with a severe illness may be of great help to others facing a similar journey. Some people have natural helping or leadership abilities that clinicians can detect and nurture—they should not be pressured, but they may get much personal reward from such a role. Family members and even patients themselves have "come out of the closet" and are very successful in inspiring peers or even professional audiences.
- As a preliminary step, consider sponsoring educational groups for people with similar problems.

Promoting Optimal Utilization of Scarce Resources

Self-help groups are growing in number because they are effective, and also because they thrive on voluntary participation and require relatively little material resources. Increasingly, community psychiatry is concerned with the organization of very scarce resources into programs or systems that are cost-effective. For this reason alone, clinicians should facilitate self-help groups where and when they can.

Practice implications

- Similar to above, but on a larger systems level, talk with program managers and top administrators in your service system about promoting or starting self-help and consumer education groups; offer to help provide leadership and consultation.
- Support consumer-run services and training of consumers and family members as therapeutic aides or similar service roles. Offer basic training and encourage agency training of interested consumers and family members in shared elements such as long-term mental illnesses, medications and side effects, and rehabilitation. Encourage patient and family member participation in inservice training.

Creatively Using Nontraditional Clinical and System Interventions

Community psychiatrists are especially known for their creativity and willingness to devise innovative and nontraditional approaches to vexing clinical and social problems. Despite their best intentions, however, they often plan systems based on past patterns rather than future trends (Bachrach 1991). Silverman (1978) pointed out that self-help groups may form because of gaps in services resulting from this lag in clinicians' foresight. Collaboration with self-help groups and with those in other disciplines may result in innovative interventions and in a rich source of continuing education for participating psychiatrists.

Practice implications

- Interventions are limited only by one's imagination. They may involve innovative programs for patients, community interventions, or nontraditional psychiatric education. Examples include the following:
  - One of the authors (CG) has collaborated with the South Carolina AMI group (SCAMI) to create an annual "respite camp" for 15 mentally ill adults. One psychiatrist and up to nine other volunteer staff from the state hospital, mental health centers, AMI, and

psychiatric residency program take the patients to a camp site for 5 days and 4 nights, thus giving family members almost a week-long respite and patients a recreational/socialization experience that is often the highlight of their year. The program is funded by the state AMI (SCAMI), and staff who are state employees receive official leave to attend. The experience has offered a dramatic educational opportunity reinforcing the principles listed previously. Plans are currently under way to expand the experience to twice a year and include the other residency training program in the state.

- At the University of Miami/New Horizons Community Mental Health Center in Miami, Florida, community psychiatrists for many years were involved in community organization efforts and in development of a network of nine "mini-clinics" that offered culturally appropriate services in Hispanic, Afro-Caribbean, and black neighborhoods. Systems interventions were widely used, including school, welfare, and social services systems, with an emphasis on community empowerment. The program structure offered all patients comprehensive case management utilizing community resources such as churches and neighborhood groups. Current involvement of professional staff with AMI has resulted in developing an AMI support group serving the needs of minority families (Lefley and Bestman 1991).

- At the University of Miami's Department of Psychiatry, the Director of Ambulatory Care Services, Dr. Ben Brauzer, who also directs outpatient rotations, established a linkage with the local AMI group to provide much-needed medical input for their weekly support group meetings. For a number of years, psychiatric residents have been volunteering as resource persons for local AMI support groups, playing a facilitative rather than leadership role and offering much-desired clinical education to the family participants (Lefley 1988b). In an innovative outpatient rotation, PGYII residents explore the multiple roles of community psychiatrists by visiting all components and specialized programs of the service delivery system, both institutional and community based, including meeting with mental health planners and with consumer and family advocacy groups. In the course of this, many for the first time see former crisis patients in a variety of community contexts, including consumer-run programs. Some residents have indicated an interest in working with a consumer-operated drop-in center to learn and to be of service to the members.

- Practice implications include heeding Leona Bachrach's (1991) advice in creating new programs and when working with self-help groups: "Service planners must be sensitive to the immanence of change so that questions about the future routinely become part of program planning . . . . How will the service system supplant the social support functions performed by patients' families as parents become disabled or die? What mental health services will the children of noninstitutionalized chronic patients . . . require? What services must be anticipated for the rapidly increasing population of never-institutionalized geriatric psychiatric patients?" (p. 1205). Such a future-oriented approach calls for creativity and will present opportunities for new self-help group formation.

Viewing Self as a Social Change Agent and Advocate for Disadvantaged Individuals

Community psychiatry has long been the socially active arm of the psychiatry profession. Community psychiatrists view the community in a comprehensive way, looking for patterns and problems that might be amenable to their interventions. Their prevention orientation, borrowed from public health, combined with their clinical focus, is a powerful combination. Community advocacy groups become natural allies as clinicians identify and address glaring social and clinical needs. Advocacy groups also may become actively involved in monitoring the quality of clinicians' practice and systems of care. Clinicians may be uncomfortable when an advocacy group accuses them of abuse or neglect or attacks their profession, but they should be relieved that forces exist to check and balance their power. Clinicians have given, and will continue to give, misguided advice and harmful treatments. Psychiatrists cannot always effectively police themselves, nor can they avoid action because it might be misdirected. Their support of advocacy and support organizations can only help them in the long run, even if they disagree with such organizations in the short run (harmful cults are not included in this statement).

When psychiatrists become involved in a support/advocacy group, their professional status often propels them to a position of leadership. As they participate in such a group, they must guard against three pitfalls: co-opting the self-help effort, competing with it, and losing their professional identity and special role. *Co-option* can occur when the primary members of an advocacy group become dependent on the advice and "expertise" of a professional and either overtly or "unconsciously" defer to his or her judgment or soften their tone out of sympathy for the problems of the professional or a wish not to offend him or her. *Competition* is possible when psychiatrists view the group as providing an alternative service and worry that it may keep patients from getting "proper" treatment. *Loss or confusion of professional identity* can occur when a psychiatrist joins forces with an advocacy group, especially when the psychiatrist is also a member of the primary group (i.e., is a consumer and/or family member). This is the other side of the coin of co-option and requires self-awareness, self-monitoring, and sometimes the advice and counsel of a colleague or consultant. As Halleck (1971) eloquently argued in *The Politics of Therapy,* psychiatrists' unavoidable role as social change agents means that they must carefully monitor the covert and overt political effects of their actions.

Practice implications

- Serve on advisory boards (e.g., AMI, Depressive/Manic-Depressive Association) and as formal or informal consultant to advocacy/support groups. This may result in major advances (e.g., developing the respite camp mentioned above). (Another example is the effort in South Carolina to make advocacy groups aware of such issues as psychiatrist/patient ratios in the community so they can be more effective advocates for improved services.)
- Use your influence to see that consumers and family members are included on mental health advisory and governing boards.
- Encourage recovering patients and selected family members to enter professional training programs so they can become full-fledged members of the team.
- Help form consumer advisory groups for professional training programs and invite consumers and family members to make formal presentations to students, faculty, and other professionals.
- Encourage interorganizational linkages; for example, the South Carolina Psychiatric Association has a standing committee on liaison to advocacy and support organizations (LASO Committee) where mutual goals are discussed and coordinated and mutually supportive action is taken.
- To prevent co-option and role confusion, community psychiatrists should monitor their involvement with such groups and step back at times, perhaps seeking the advice of a colleague or consultant.
- Remind the advocacy group that its primary value is its position outside "the system" and its constructive use of anger and outrage; give the group "permission" to criticize you and your colleagues. (This may require relatively thick skin, self-confidence, and utmost tact.)
- Do not compete with the group; most research suggests that members of self-help groups are very aware of alternatives and most are involved in several other helping relationships (Lieberman 1990).
- Try not to get defensive; keep collaboration going during conflictual episodes; agree to disagree while emphasizing areas of agreement; agree on goals, even if you disagree on some methods; try not to drop out, even if you must disengage for a while.

- If you must protest the actions of an advocacy group, do it in a respectful way; empathize with the group members' point of view.

Implications for Professional Training

Chapter 26 covers community psychiatry training issues in general and refers to the recent effort of the AACP to promote guidelines for curriculum development in community psychiatry (Brown et al. 1993). These guidelines emphasize the social network and systems intervention aspects of community psychiatry practice that form a foundation for developing the specific knowledge, skills, and attitudes required for effective collaboration with advocacy and support organizations. Lefley et al. (1989) have outlined some basic principles for all professional training programs to follow to become more acceptable to family members of mentally ill patients. The following examples from our experience illustrate some of the creative ways trainees (medical students and residents) can begin to appreciate the importance of consumer self-help groups.

- Residents have been involved in the operation of a respite camp for mentally ill adults (see previous discussion).
- Medical students and residents have participated in research regarding the effect of mental illness on the family and the impact of self-help groups on family members (AMI).
- Patients and their families have met on a regular basis with residents and medical students in workshops and seminars to discuss the impact of mental illness on their lives.
- Consumers and family members have participated on advisory boards to community psychiatry training programs and have been active in curriculum design and implementation.
- Residents have been invited to address groups of consumers to discuss such topics as schizophrenia and bipolar disorder.
- Consumers have been invited to address groups of residents on the phenomenological experience of schizophrenia and bipolar disorder.
- Members of advocacy groups have presented grand rounds on families' experiences with the mental health system.
- Residents and medical students have been required to attend meetings of self-help groups (AA, AMI, Alanon).
- An "adopt-a-resident" program has been initiated (University of Massachusetts) in which residents get to know a family with a mentally ill member on an intimate basis for at least a year.
- Consumers and family members have themselves become medical students and residents and in some cases have shared their unique perspectives with faculty and other students.

- Residents have functioned as resource persons in AMI support groups and in so doing have learned a great deal about the needs of persons living with mental illness in the family (see previous discussion).
- Residents have learned about local consumer support groups and drop-in centers and have referred socially isolated patients to them.
- Residents have learned how to work collaboratively with patients' families and how to deal with questions of confidentiality in a creative and therapy-enhancing manner (see Lefley 1988b).

Special Issues in Working With Consumer and Family Advocates

Working With Consumers

We have noted previously that some members of consumer and family groups may attack the profession. Many consumers remember involuntary commitment or other hospitalization experiences that they felt were dehumanizing and countertherapeutic, and some hold psychiatrists responsible. Members of consumer advocacy groups such as NAPS are likely to be categorically opposed to electroconvulsive therapy and to forced medication, and many are opposed to psychotropic medications altogether. Members of less radical groups, including even the NAMI Consumer Council, are likely to accept the need for medications but to question traditional psychiatric practice and opt for alternatives to involuntary treatment. We are entering an era in which competent patients may execute advance directives—psychiatric wills or health proxies—both to prescribe and to proscribe treatment for themselves in the event of later incompetence (Applebaum 1991).

Community psychiatrists have a very necessary role in educating consumers about major psychotic disorders, brain function, and the functions of psychotropic medications in stabilizing the behavioral disturbances that have led to their former hospitalizations. Consumers have a role in educating psychiatrists and other professionals about the phenomenology of the psychotic episode, the types of treatment that they feel were helpful or harmful, and suggested alternatives to traditional modes of crisis intervention.

Increasingly, the NIMH Community Support Program and state mental health administrations are sponsoring conferences in which dialogues can take place between consumer advocacy groups and psychiatrists. As suggested in this chapter, it would be wise for state psychiatric associations and departments of psychiatry to solicit linkages and to offer speakers and discussants at these meetings. There is a great deal of misinformation being offered to consumers, and the psychiatric "establishment" has done little to counter this. Community psychiatrists who work on an ongoing basis with consumer groups are in the best position to offer their expertise, and such an offer is very likely to be accepted.

We are also entering an era of profound changes in the service delivery system. Mobile crisis teams, supported housing, and case management are beginning to supplement and in some cases supplant comprehensive community mental health services. In lieu of clinic-based services, community psychiatrists may be involved in on-site service delivery, often in tandem with consumer aides. Psychiatrists should be mindful that accepted roles for consumers in service delivery have come about largely because of the advocacy movement. Any affiliations with the consumer movement, including education about serious mental illness, will be beneficial for all concerned.

Working With Families and Family Advocates

Community psychiatrists are likely to work with patients' families at case-centered, programmatic, and societal levels in joint planning and advocacy efforts. Community psychiatrists are likely to work with AMI families on mental health planning boards, to encounter them on the governance boards of their agencies, and to engage in joint legislative advocacy through their professional societies.

However, there is a need to discuss family involvement at the case level as well. With deinstitutionalization, it is estimated that 65% of patients are discharged to their families (Goldman 1982). Various studies have shown that at any point in time, about 40% are living in the family home (Lefley 1987; Petrila and Sadoff 1992). Yet numerous surveys of families have indicated that family members still believe they receive too little information to help them in the caregiving role (Francell et al. 1988; Grella and Grusky 1989). For example, some families of psychiatric patients have been kept in such profound ignorance regarding the nature of their relative's illness that they have had no basis on which to make judgments or develop appropriate role expectations. Thinking their relative cured after a hospital stay, they may insist on role performance that would be expected from a person of similar age but that a mentally ill person is incapable of fulfilling. Assumptions that the patient is capable of seeking competitive employment or returning to school on a full-time basis may reinforce vulnerability and lead to a cycle of psychotic reaction, family disruption, or even rehospitalization. Clear communication about the case with patient and family may well prevent this from happening. In both inpatient and outpatient facilities, there are demands for the type of patient and family education that is standard practice in serious physical illness.

Many families of long-term patients, especially those who have endured 20–30 years of illness, feel bitter toward a treatment system that in many cases failed to effect any significant improvements in their ill relatives, impoverished them financially, and excluded them from the basic education that might lighten their caregiving role. Family members were ill served by psychodynamic treatment models that refused communication and deflected their questions. They also resent family therapy models that were based on the premise that the symptoms of schizophrenia or major affective disorders would dissolve when they were no longer needed to maintain homeostasis of a dysfunctional family system. These assumptions, which resulted in many families feeling frustrated and blamed (Hatfield 1983), yielded few positive results and currently are repudiated as archaic by prominent family therapists (Anderson et al. 1986; McFarlane and Beels 1983; Terkelsen 1990; Wynne 1988).

None of these models offered the type of communication (i.e., information about the illnesses, knowledge of medications and their side effects, problem-solving strategies, and behavior management techniques) that families needed and wanted and that they felt would most benefit their relationship with the patient. It is only in relatively recent years that psychoeducational interventions have begun to fill these needs and to prove their effectiveness (Anderson et al. 1986; Falloon et al. 1984).

Today we find community psychiatrists increasingly willing to speak with families and to involve them in treatment planning. However, the issue of confidentiality continues to be a major barrier to communication. If the patient is in psychotherapy, some therapists will refuse any interaction because this might breach the therapeutic alliance. When noncommunication is explained in these terms, most families will accept this and convey their questions to another staff member. Most family members will also point out that they want information on medications, not private therapeutic disclosures.

Petrila and Sadoff (1992) pointed out that when a patient is released to family care in the community, at a minimum caregivers should know the importance of taking medications and what side effects might occur, the symptoms to look for if the patient is noncompliant, and any special needs observed in the inpatient setting. Potential for dangerous behavior to self or others should be discussed. Caregivers should be encouraged to give feedback on any significant behavioral changes. The authors pointed out that it is unfair to discharge the patient without providing comprehensive treatment information, because otherwise caregivers will lack the basis for making decisions. The authors cited two cases in which failure to share important information about medications or potential for dangerousness led to allegations of malpractice.

In most situations the therapist can discuss with the patient the family's desire and need to know and the value of these communications for effective treatment. If patients withhold consent, Petrila and Sadoff (1992) have suggested that the therapist must work to understand the reasons for the refusal. In most cases, however, the therapist can help the patient decide the scope and type of communication. Instead of a unilateral decision, this empowerment of the patient to decide fulfills two therapeutic functions: it puts patients in charge of their own confidentiality and eases bonding with a needed support system. Typically the family who wants to know is the family who cares, and this procedure establishes a groundwork for patient-family collaboration in managing the illness.

Much of family education takes place in a community or aftercare setting. This can involve one or more educational sessions, with patient and family members together or separately. In the latter case, diagnosis, prognosis, and other problematic issues are handled in the same way they are handled with the patient alone. Numerous manuals are available for working with patients and families using this model of joint understanding, whether the requirements are for individual family therapy (Selzer et al. 1989), multifamily therapy (McFarlane and Beels 1983), supportive family counseling or family consultation (Bernheim and Lehman 1986), specific psychoeducational approaches (Anderson et al. 1986; Falloon et al. 1984; Goldstein 1981), or education alone (Hatfield 1990). The benefits of psychoeducational interventions with families have been demonstrated to both lower relapse rates (Hogarty et al. 1986) and in enhancing the family's security to deal with the illness (Goldstein 1981). Comprehensive research by McFarlane et al. (1995) indicated that multiple-family groups produce significantly better outcomes than individual family interventions.

Working with families does not necessarily involve the time commitments of structured psychoeducational interventions. Many community mental health centers, psychosocial rehabilitation programs, or general hospitals with psychiatric wards offer free facilities for family support groups, with or without professional leadership. Psychiatrists can have a significant role both in giving formal presentations on requested topics or in occasionally meeting with these groups to provide psychiatric input. Frequently this participation results in bilateral education and reciprocal referrals.

Finally, we might note that psychiatrists in private practice also have been affected by advocacy developments. Self-help groups are often a boon for their patients. Private psychiatrists who work with long-term chronic patients frequently find them shut out from the day treatment programs and recreational activities of community mental health centers. Many of these private patients want nothing to do with the public mental health system and lead socially isolated lives. Consumer programs, which occur in a normalized setting, are excellent resources for these patients.

Private practitioners who are willing to devote time to lecturing or consulting with AMI groups will often find them an excellent source of referrals. They will also find the AMI groups knowledgeable about community resources. Many psychiatrists have reported being educated by these consumer groups about housing or socialization resources for their other patients. Overall, all psychiatrists who treat chronic patients in the community, whether in the public or private sector, will find it valuable to learn about and develop linkages with their local advocacy, support, and self-help groups.

Conclusions

We are entering a new era for community psychiatry, with changing loci and modes of service delivery. In lieu of comprehensive community mental health services, the public sector currently offers free-standing psychosocial rehabilitation centers, scattered-site supported housing, home-based case management, mobile crisis teams, and other decentralized components of a much looser system than existed previously. The consumer and family movements have had a strong impact on these developments as well as on mental health law, which currently requires both informed consent for psychiatric treatment and avoidance of involuntary treatment as much as possible.

As a result of consumer advocacy, community psychiatrists must look for innovative ways of treating seriously ill patients that will effect a satisfactory balance between patients' treatment needs and their civil rights. Because of the advocacy movements, mental health professionals in general must modify their old paternalistic attitudes and learn to deal with mentally ill persons and their families as co-equals in the therapeutic endeavor.

Self-help and support groups have been incorporated, and rarely with co-option, in the therapeutic armamentarium. Many substance abuse programs use 12-step programs as a therapeutic modality, either directly as a program adjunct or by referral. Many treatment agencies have provided resources for self-help or support groups. Some of these groups are willing to use professional help, whereas others meet completely on their own.

We have suggested various ways in which community psychiatrists may work effectively with advocacy groups. The model suggested by Silverman (1978) of referral, consultation, advisory, and initiating functions has been vastly expanded to include a range of collaborative relationships. Working with consumer groups involves changes in conceptualization of the therapeutic task and of the role of community psychiatrists vis à vis their patients. Practice principles include viewing patients in the context of social networks, encouraging self-determination and self-efficacy of patients and their families, promoting optimal utilization of scarce resources, creatively using nontraditional clinical and systems interventions, and viewing oneself as a social change agent. For each of these, practice implications are spelled out.

Collaborative relationships imply reciprocity, and in addition to suggesting ways in which community psychiatrists can help their patients and other mentally ill persons through collaborative relationships with their advocacy groups, we have given examples of ways in which patients and families can help present and future community psychiatrists. These include advocating for services and research; participating in clinical training; planning, monitoring, and evaluating programs; dispensing resource information; offering mutual referrals; and helping psychiatrists learn first hand the therapeutic aspects of the self-help experience.

References

Anderson CM, Reiss DJ, Hogarty GE: Schizophrenia and the Family. New York, Guilford, 1986

Applebaum PS: Advance directives for psychiatric treatment. Hosp Community Psychiatry 42:983–984, 1991

Bachrach LL: The 13th principle. Hosp Community Psychiatry 42:1205–1206, 1991

Bernheim KF: Psychologists and families of the severely mentally ill: the role of family consultation. Am Psychol 44:561–564, 1989

Bernheim KF, Lehman, AF: Working With Families of the Mentally Ill. New York, Norton, 1986

Bisbee CC: Educating Patients and Families About Mental Illness. Frederick, MD, Aspen, 1991

Blaska B: The myriad medication mistakes in psychiatry: a consumer's view. Hosp Community Psychiatry 41:993–998, 1990

Breggin P: Psychiatric abuse of children. Paper presented at the annual meeting of the National Association for Rights, Protection and Advocacy, St. Paul, Minnesota, September 1989

Brown DB, Goldman CR, Thompson KS, et al: Training residents for community psychiatric practice: guidelines for curriculum development. Community Ment Health J 29:271–283, 1993

Campbell J (ed): In Pursuit of Wellness, Vol 6: The Well-Being Project: Mental Health Clients Speak for Themselves. Sacramento, CA, The California Network of Mental Health Clients, 1989

Caplan G: Loss, stress, and mental health. Community Ment Health J 26:27–48, 1990

Diamond R: Drugs and the quality of life: the patient's point of view. J Clin Psychiatry 46:29–35, 1985

Emerick RR: Self-help groups for former patients: relations with mental health professionals. Hosp Community Psychiatry 41:401–407, 1990

Falloon IRH, Boyd JL, McGill CW: Family Care of Schizophrenia. New York, Guilford, 1984

Fink PJ: Is "biopsychosocial" the psychiatric shibboleth? Am J Psychiatry 145:1061–1067, 1988

Francell CG, Conn VS, Gray DP: Families' perceptions of burden of care for chronic mentally ill relatives. Hosp Community Psychiatry 39:1296–1300, 1988

Galanter M, Talbott D, Gallegos K, et al: Combined Alcoholics Anonymous and professional care for addicted physicians. Am J Psychiatry 147:64–68, 1990

Goering PN, Stylianos SK: Exploring the helping relationship between the schizophrenic client and rehabilitation therapist. Am J Orthopsychiatry 58:271–280, 1988

Goldman HH: Mental illness and family burden: a public health perspective. Hosp Community Psychiatry 33:557–560, 1982

Goldstein MJ: New Developments in Interventions With Families of Schizophrenics. San Francisco, CA, Jossey-Bass, 1981

Grella CE, Grusky O: Families of the seriously mentally ill and their satisfaction with services. Hosp Community Psychiatry 40:831–835, 1989

Gruenbaum H, Friedman H: Building collaborative relationships with families of the mentally ill. Hosp Community Psychiatry 39:1183–87, 1988

Hahn SR, Feiner JS, Bellin EH: The doctor-patient-family relationship: a compensatory alliance. Ann Intern Med 109:884–889, 1988

Halleck SL: The Politics of Therapy. New York, Science House, 1971

Hartmann L: Humane values and biopsychosocial integration. Am J Psychiatry 148:1130–1134, 1991

Hatfield AB: What families want of family therapists, in Family Therapy in Schizophrenia. Edited by McFarlane WR. New York, Guilford, 1983, pp 41–65

Hatfield AB: Family Education in Mental Illness. New York, Guilford, 1990

Hatfield AB, Lefley HP (eds): Families of the Mentally Ill: Coping and Adaptation. New York, Guilford, 1987

Hogarty GE, Anderson CM, Reiss DJ, et al: Family psychoeducation, social skills training, and maintenance chemotherapy in the aftercare treatment of schizophrenia. Arch Gen Psychiatry 43:633–641, 1986

Hyde AP, Goldman CR: Family issues that may interfere with the treatment and rehabilitation of schizophrenia. Paper presented at the 41st Institute on Hospital and Community Psychiatry, Philadelphia, PA, October 19, 1989

Imber-Black E: Families and Larger Systems. New York, Guilford, 1988

Isaac RJ, Armat VC: Madness in the Streets: How Psychiatry and the Law Abandoned the Mentally Ill. New York, Free Press, 1990

Kaplan HI, Sadock BJ: Synopsis of Psychiatry, 6th Edition, Revised. Baltimore, MD, Williams & Wilkins. 1991

Kleinman A: The Illness Narratives. New York, Basic Books, 1988

Leete E: The treatment of schizophrenia: a patient's perspective. Hosp Community Psychiatry 38:486–491, 1987

Lefley HP: Aging parents as caregivers of mentally ill adult children: an emerging social problem. Hosp Community Psychiatry 39:1296–1300, 1988a

Lefley HP: Training professionals to work with families of chronic patients. Community Ment Health J 24:338–357. 1988b

Lefley HP: Family burden and family stigma in major mental illness. Am Psychol 44:556–560, 1989

Lefley HP, Bestman EW: Public-academic linkages for culturally sensitive community mental health. Community Ment Health J 27:473–488, 1991

Lefley HP, Bernheim KF, Goldman CR: National forum addresses need to enhance training in treating the seriously mentally ill. Hosp Community Psychiatry 40:460–462, 470, 1989

Liberman RP: Psychiatric rehabilitation of chronic mental patients. Washington, DC, American Psychiatric Press, 1987

Lieberman MA: A group therapist perspective on self-help groups. Int J Group Psychother 40:251–278, 1990

McFarlane WR, Beels CC: Family research in schizophrenia: a review and integration for clinicians, in Family Therapy in Schizophrenia. Edited by McFarlane WR. New York, Guilford, 1983, pp 311–323

McFarlane WR, Lukens E, Link B, et al: Multiple family groups and psychoeducation in the treatment of schizophrenia. Arch Gen Psychiatry 52:679–687, 1995

Mental Health Law Project: Summary of Activities 1989–1990. Washington, DC, Mental Health Law Project, 1991

Minkoff K: Program components of a comprehensive integrated care system for serious mentally ill patients with substance disorders. New Dir Ment Health Serv 50:13–27, 1991

Mosher LR, Burti L: Community Mental Health: Principles and Practice. New York, WW Norton, 1989

National Alliance for the Mentally Ill: Protection and advocacy for the mentally ill. NAMI Legislative Network News 1(4):1, 1991

Osher FC, Kofoed LL: Treatment of patients with psychiatric and psychoactive substance abuse disorders. Hosp Community Psychiatry 40:1025–1030, 1989

Panzetta AF: Whatever happened to community mental health: portents for corporate medicine. Hosp Community Psychiatry 36:1174–1179, 1985

Petrila JP, Sadoff RL: Confidentiality and the family as caregiver. Hosp Community Psychiatry 43:136–139, 1992

Ruocchio PJ: How psychotherapy can help the schizophrenic patient. Hosp Community Psychiatry 40:188–190, 1989

Selzer MA, Sullivan TB, Carsky M, et al: Working With the Person With Schizophrenia. New York, New York University Press, 1989

Sharfstein SS, Beigel A: How to survive in the private practice of psychiatry. Am J Psychiatry 145:723–727, 1988

Silverman PR: Mutual Help Groups: A Guide for Mental Health Workers. Rockville, MD, National Institute of Mental Health, 1978

Terkelsen KG: A historical perspective on family-provider relationships, in Families as Allies in Treatment of the Mentally Ill: New Directions for Mental Health Professionals. Edited by Lefley HP, Johnson DL. Washington, DC, American Psychiatric Press, 1990, pp 3–21

Toro PA, Rappaport J, Seidman E: Social climate comparison of mutual help and psychotherapy groups. J Consult Clin Psychol 55:430–431, 1987

Torrey EF: Surviving Schizophrenia: A Family Manual, Revised Edition. New York, Harper & Row, 1994

Toseland RW, Rossiter CM, Labrecque MS: The effectiveness of three group intervention strategies to support family caregivers. Am J Orthopsychiatry 59:420–429, 1989

Wynne LC: Changing views of schizophrenia and family interventions. Family Therapy News, May–June 1988, pp 3–4

Yee WK: Psychiatric aspects of psychoeducational family therapy. Psychiatric Annals 19:27-30, 33–34, 1989

Chapter 21

Multiple-Family Groups and Psychoeducation: Creating Therapeutic Social Networks

William R. McFarlane, M.D.
Karen "Kip" Cunningham, M.D., Pharm.D.

P sychoeducation is a method for educating families and other natural social groups, one of whose members has a disabling chronic illness resulting from a functional impairment of the brain. The goal of this training is to enable these groups to create environmental interactions that foster correction and/or compensation of the ill members' functional disability and promotes a sustained remission from symptoms. Although clearly this goal could be applicable to many disabling illnesses, the most tested and refined forms of psychoeducation relate to schizophrenia. Therefore, in this chapter we will focus on relevant theoretical issues and clinical techniques of psychoeducation for persons with schizophrenia and their social networks.

Development of antipsychotic medications allowed progressive deinstitutionalization of schizophrenic patients in the 1960s. Despite the expansion of residential and rehabilitation services, the prognosis for schizophrenic patients has changed little (Yolles and Kramer 1969). Most still experience a life plagued by mental and emotional dysfunction and isolation from their family as well as from society in general, and they often suffer abject poverty because of an inability to tolerate the workplace (Bourdon et al. 1992). The person with schizophrenia, even with well-controlled symptoms, lives under the specter of intermittent psychotic relapses. In addition, the support such patients receive from others is often variable and inconsistent.

Prior to our current understanding of the disorder's biological nature, psychoeducation in families of schizophrenic patients often consisted of 1) "educating" the family that they had somehow caused the illness and 2) working to change the families' illness-creating behavior. Families naturally resented the notion that they had evoked this devastating illness in one of their own. In addition, even clear articulations of the supposed link between the illness and the family's dynamics did not allow the patient to shed his or her symptoms. As current knowledge would predict, results were dismal in clinical and human terms.

Although the biological reality of schizophrenia has since emerged and gained acceptance, an appreciation of its overwhelming impact, both acute and chronic, on families has come much slower. The field tends to ignore the devastating impact of watching one's child or sibling deteriorate into an essentially incapacitated stranger. Families face becoming de facto caretakers without having knowledge of the illness or coping skills specific for this disorder. The crucial role of families became apparent to clinicians. Families deal with a wide range of issues, such as providing food, clean clothing, and shelter; managing the money of an adult family member; monitoring symptoms; managing interactions with the medical community; and managing dangerous/bizarre behavior (including substance use/abuse), as well as the impact of the illness on non-ill family members. Family psychoeducation can be most simply understood as an attempt to deal with these realities. Investigators, instead of blaming families for the patient's woes, began working in collaboration with families. Methods of sharing information regarding the illness were developed along with practical behavioral strategies and coping mechanisms that fostered recuperation and a reduced sense of burden (Falloon and Liberman 1983). By providing the required knowledge, training, resources, and support, clinicians can enable families to address the complex burden imposed by schizophrenia.

Multiple-Family Group Therapy in Schizophrenia

Antipsychotic medications clearly decrease active symptoms of schizophrenia. However, as patients, families, and clinicians know, these medications do not cure schizophrenia. Some patients have at best only partial symptom control. Relapse rates, even with compliance ensured through depot medication, remain at approximately 40% during the first year following an acute episode (Hogarty et al. 1974). While research continues, other methods of assisting families are needed.

Multiple-family group (MFG) psychoeducation is based on the assumption that schizophrenia is a brain disorder (Weinberger 1987) that is usually only partially remediable by medication, and families, clinicians, and others in a social network can facilitate or impede their relative's recovery. Psychoeducational approaches, one part of which is the use of antipsychotic medications, are remarkably effective in decreasing the rates of illness relapse when rigorously evaluated in experimental outcome studies (Hogarty et al. 1986; McFarlane 1990). More will be said about this later.

MFGs initially began as a means of addressing inpatient management problems (Detre et al. 1961; Laqueur et al. 1964). Unexpected advantages quickly became apparent as patients' symptoms decreased and family morale improved. On closer examination, it was discovered that in MFGs, patients and families provided direct emotional support by trading ideas, empathizing with burdens, and suggesting and fostering behaviors that promoted recuperation. Importantly, the group allowed a framework in which a family could more clearly establish a balance between the needs of an individual and those of the family (Falloon and Liberman 1983).

Psychosocial Factors and Illness Course

By focusing on the determinants of the course of the illness rather than on its etiology, it has been possible to clarify further how family interaction and other social processes might influence an established mental illness (Breier and Strauss 1984). Through these studies we have achieved a better appreciation of what happens to families as they attempt to cope with a member who is mentally ill. Many studies have demonstrated that a reduction in the level of expressed emotion in a family has accompanied improvements in the course of the illness (Hogarty et al. 1986). For example, families with knowledge about negative symptoms of schizophrenia who understand that periods of lethargy, passivity, and social withdrawal typically follow an episode of more active, positive symptoms, are better equipped to create a lower key convalescent environment that promotes natural recuperation from a major psychotic episode. Thus, reducing environmental interactional stress is one of the primary goals of all psychoeducational MFGs.

Background work for psychoeducational MFGs also examined the ill member's effect on the family. The devastating effects on families when faced with a mentally ill member in their midst over long periods of time have been clearly documented. The burdens include chronic tension, sleep disruption, financial drain, resentment, confusion, limitation of social contacts, interference with daily routine, deprivation of attention for siblings, marital conflict, overt depression, and exacerbation of medical condition (Johnson 1990). Families often complain of feelings of guilt, anger, fear, and eventually rejection of the patient following their own demoralization (Hatfield 1983).

Another important area of investigation in the development of MFGs has been that of social networks and social supports of schizophrenic patients and their families. One finding has been harshly consistent: people with schizophrenia are more isolated than their peers. This holds true for their families as well, although somewhat less intensely. It appears to be more true for people and families dealing with schizophrenia than for those dealing with other mental disorders (Pattison 1979). Also, social network changes are progressive. At first admission, patients have a more constricted social network and are more family based when compared with medical patients. The entire network decreases even more thereafter. The explanation for this process includes withdrawal of contact and support by friends and extended kin, as well as reduced social initiative by family members, secondary to shame and/or preoccupation with the patient. Attenuated social support leads to the loss of adaptive coping capacity for family members and exacerbates the effect of caretaking burdens. The social processes surrounding the relentless course of mental disability leave families isolated. Normal family stresses are magnified by the burdens imposed by a chronic mental illness and the loss of the usual attenuating support systems (e.g., friends, community social groups, sports, school). These stresses reverberate within the family, causing further stress and, at times, dysfunction.

Assuming medications are maintained throughout, risk of relapse declines appreciably over 2 years, such that at the end of that period the risk is one-third the risk of relapse at the time of hospital discharge. These findings suggest that a slow restitution process may naturally occur when relapse does not intervene. A clinical strategy thus emerges: create a social environment, supported by antipsychotic medication, that compensates for the vulnerabilities specifically inherent to schizophrenia and allows the natural tendency for recovery to flourish in the absence of relapse.

Assumptions in MFG Psychoeducation

A clinical approach that combines antipsychotic medication with evolution of the family to a less complex and emotionally labile structure has as its

Table 21–1. Psychoeducation: basic assumptions

- Schizophrenia is a chronic biological disorder of the brain.
- Schizophrenia is characterized by long episodes of positive and/or negative symptoms. These symptoms tend to diminish slowly in the absence of stress.
- The schizophrenic patient suffers from a specific deficit involving attention, arousal, and executive cognitive functions such that the patient has an impaired ability to gate stimuli. This most likely results from underfunctioning of the dorsolateral prefrontal cortex.
- Families can influence this biological process. They may protect the patient from further relapses or inadvertently exacerbate a relapse.
- Behaviors of families can be most parsimoniously described as "natural" responses to difficult situations. Behaviors do not necessarily indicate anything about the functional level of the family.
- Living with an ill relative has negative consequences for the family.
- The illness itself negatively impacts on social support networks for both the family and patient.

primary aim to delay, reduce the severity of, and perhaps prevent relapse. This approach requires education of the family members about the details of schizophrenia and support and guidance provided over a prolonged period (Beels 1975). The approach has several basic assumptions (Table 21–1):

- Unless evidence proves otherwise, the family is functioning normally.
- Mental disorders tend to elicit responses in concerned others that are self-defeating in nature.
- The compensatory adjustments that the family makes are at once 1) abnormal activity for this family, 2) are dictated by the unique properties of schizophrenia in the ill member, and 3) have as the goal an improved outcome for the whole family.

Clinical Aims in Psychoeducational Treatment

Community integration (the ability of an individual with schizophrenia to function within normal societal expectations) is also an important therapeutic goal. To accomplish it, at least two other aims must be met first: 1) prevention of relapse and 2) social and vocational rehabilitation. Psychoeducation explicitly pursues those aims in a clear sequence, assuming that preventing relapse is essential to rehabilitation and that rehabilitation is essential to community integration. Several types of intervention are necessary to achieving these aims. They include enhancing the family's knowledge and coping skills, limiting stimulation experienced by patients, adjusting communication, and establishing clear relationship structures.

Enhancing Knowledge and Coping Skills

Living with schizophrenia is at least as difficult and confusing as treating it. Thus, families and patients need to be armed with 1) the available knowledge about the illness and 2) specific coping skills. A core principle in psychoeducational work is that it is unrealistic to expect families to understand such a mystifying condition, much less to know what to do about it. To be adaptive, families require a means of accessing needed information. The treatment system is a crucial source of that information. Families often develop, through painful trial and error, methods of dealing with the desperate state of their ill relatives. These successes, however, are few and far between. Thus, it is critical that families have access to a means of developing skills that achieve a more satisfactory outcome in the day-to-day challenges of managing schizophrenia at home and in the community.

Limiting Stimulation

Particularly in cognitive and attention capabilities, disruption in mental functioning seems directly related to the level of arousal. Regulation of the experienced stimulus load is thus a primary focus of the psychoeducational approach. In general, the amount of stimulation from the social and physical environment is limited to that which is tolerable and rehabilitative. Anderson (1986) has described this concept as "erecting barriers to over stimulation." Certain types of stimuli, especially criticism in men and abrupt withdrawal of affection and companionship in women, appear to be nearly universally destabilizing. Because of variation between patients and within a given patient over time, some very fine and flexible yet consistent tuning is required by family and clinical programs alike. It becomes apparent that stimulation that may be overwhelming to one person may simply be entertaining to another. An overly calm environment is not, however, conducive to rehabilitation and personal growth. The need for protection from environmental stimulation is phasic, being greatest in the immediate postpsychosis period and diminishing with the natural course of recovery. The clinician's task is to gauge what is excessive and find strategies that enable both family and clinical systems to avoid those stimuli. The clinician watches carefully for indications that resilience and resistance to stimulation is improving and adjust demands and expectations accordingly, upward and sometimes downward again as life events intervene.

Adjusting Communication

Because of the cognitive impairments in schizophrenia, the method and manner of communication must be addressed. Communication, especially in the early posthospitalization period, should be clear, straightforward, concrete, and moderately specific. Abundant literature demonstrates that positive comments and a calm, supportive tone are crucial in getting through to an ill relative. Requests should be made directly and simply. Being able to comprehend what is trying to be to communicated and, on the other hand, feeling one is heard often provide remarkable tension relief for the involved parties. Experience has shown that low-expressed-emotion families tend to be markedly low-key, warm, tentative, and nonpressuring in their communications to the patient, often waiting for the patient to take the initiative in conversation. On a purely practical note, family members should acknowledge the statements of others directly, as well as take responsibility for their own statements (Anderson 1986). Although this may initially be felt as a burdensome task, individuals with attentional dysfunction will find it easier to track conversations if it is clear who is saying what and why he or she is saying it.

Establishing Clear Relationship Structures

The family with a mentally ill member should have a clearly demarcated hierarchy in which necessary rules are established and respected. Well members of the family benefit from a structure that supports carrying out their caretaking duties. A clear structure tends to allay tension and prevent nagging and anxiety-driven excessive interaction. Clarity and predictability exist in the family life and defines a framework for resolving disputes and squabbles in a reasonable and timely manner. The family with a clear hierarchy that has as its overall goal the good of the family and that is backed by the clinical team is a calmer, more therapeutic family. Structure and limit setting are very important for medication compliance: the hierarchical leader may decide that the patient's using medication as prescribed is necessary for the family's well-being and may require its continuation as a condition for living at home. The same is true for dealing with violence and bizarre behavior: setting limits often is the only way to extinguish these behaviors and to preserve a semblance of normality at home.

MFG Psychoeducation: Clinical Operations

MFG psychoeducation is designed to enable families to create environmental interactions that foster correction of and/or compensation for an ill member's functional disability and that promote a sustained remission. In this section we will explain the concrete technical tasks necessary to accomplish these goals. Each phase of the approach differs depending on the needs of the specific patient and the phase's treatment goals. There are four sequential phases:

1. Engagement, which usually occurs with the family at the time of an acute psychotic decompensation
2. An educational workshop, in which the clinicians present information and describe key behavioral guidelines didactically
3. A reentry period, focused on stabilizing the family and patient after hospitalization
4. A rehabilitation phase, during which the goal is to raise the patient's level of function

MFG Psychoeducation Phase 1: Engagement of the Patient and Family

The clinicians involved in long-term treatment, usually two in number, engage families one at a time. Schedules allowing, it is desirable that both clinicians meet for a joint session with the individual family during this phase. To assist with alliance formation, each clinician involved in forming a MFG gathers about half of the participating families.

Typically, during the initial joining period, three to five meetings occur at short intervals. These generally take place in a hospital setting but, not uncommonly, may take place in an outpatient setting. The meetings have a flexible schedule, occurring generally once per week and lasting approximately 1 hour. The patient is not included in these sessions unless he or she is particularly well compensated and capable of tolerating a frank discussion of schizophrenia as an illness. Because the greatest chance for successful family engagement seems to exist in the early days of an acute psychotic exacerbation, patients rarely are able to participate in the family meetings. The clinician holds brief, less frequent sessions with the patient during this time, also with the intent to foster a treatment alliance.

The meetings' focus is on the creation of an alliance between the clinician, the patient, and his or her significant relatives. During this period, the clinician attempts to understand the family's experiences and their reactions to them. The clinician should convey a willingness to be a resource and advocate who is offering to embark with the family on an extended period of treatment. The relationship with the family is fostered by the clinician's genuine concern for the patient and family, acknowledging the family's loss and their need to mourn and not blaming the family for obvious (to the clinician) errors. The clinician focuses on the present crisis to help the family muster order out of apparent chaos. The engagement phase should accomplish one major goal: the creation of a collaborative treatment system in which family members become engaged as partners with their ill relative and the clinician.

The structure for the meetings is straightforward. All family members with whom the patient has frequent interaction are contacted by the clinician, who invites them to meet at a convenient time. Special attention is paid to ensure that those most frequently involved with the patient attend. Before each meeting, the clinician ensures that he or she has communicated with other staff engaged in treating the patient in order to be aware of the latest clinical status of the patient. The assessment with the family can be conceived as a triad: 1) evaluating the present crisis, 2) eliciting family reactions to the illness and the treatment system, and 3) evaluating the family and social system.

1. *Evaluating the present crisis.* The initial task is to determine the present state of affairs. Each family member is asked about what they have observed during the patient's decompensation, what they think might have triggered the relapse, and what they see as early prodromal signs of decompensation. This allows the clinician to gather important information about coincidental events that are stressful to the family members as well as the family system and to understand how these impact the family's coping with the psychosis. This process of identifying patterns also introduces a sense of containment for the family: that their relative's behavior, bizarre and frightening as it may seem to them, does not seem so to the clinician experienced with this disorder. The idea of contracting is introduced by asking what help the relative would like from the treatment team.

2. *Eliciting family reactions.* The clinician takes a history of the specific emotional effects the patient's illness has had on each family member. The technique used is straightforward, empathic inquiry. The clinician listens with an awareness to each individual's means of coping with these stresses while at the same time assessing the personal resources in the family. Families usually find great relief in the permission to unburden themselves about fears, anger, confusion, and their sense of loss. A great

range of responses may be expected. The most common responses center on the patient, including denial of illness severity; suppressed grief; the sacrifice of time, pleasures, personal resources; ambitions to provide protection and control; and anger or frustration with the patient and the treatment system. Because of the last, it is important to communicate to family members that the MFG program deals with family members only in a respectful, supportive, and collaborative manner.

3. *Evaluating the family and social system.* The MFG clinician has as a goal reducing the ambient stress within the family system. To foster this, the clinician should have a general sense of the family's interactional style, structural alliances, communication patterns, and coping strategies and their social network resources. This requires taking a brief family network "sociogram": asking about who tends to interacts with whom; watching for difficulties or strengths in communication between family members; asking about contacts with friends, relatives, and outside social or community groups; and gathering information on recent life events and changes in household membership, whether these are desirable or not. It may be expected that the family's overall sense of distress is high at this time. Pain is taken to avoid any implication that the patient's episodes are being triggered by the family. The family can misinterpret a well-meaning clinician's enthusiasm about them having a better future as criticism about their current behavior.

Finally, if the family is interested in joining an MFG, brief inquiry should be made into feelings about this format. Generally, most families will not readily plunge into sharing their experiences with strangers, particularly at a time of crisis. Also, it is important to explore any current or past experiences, positive or negative, with groups, including self-help groups. The clinician should inquire, with sensitivity, about feelings of shame regarding any aspect of family life. The picture that emerges can then guide the clinician in deciding how best to frame the MFG as useful to the specific needs of a given family, and whether to recommend continuation on a single-family basis.

Goals and contracts.   A salient feature of the psychoeducational MFG model is that the goals of treatment are explicit and negotiated with all participants. The overriding goals remain the same: to prevent relapse and gradually integrate the patient into the highest possible degree of community participation. These provide a unifying point when negotiating a specific family's goals.

Several secondary goals apply in almost all cases. These include the following:

- Key family members form part of a treatment team that addresses the above clinical goals.
- Family burden is minimized through management of family interactions and outside stresses.
- Information about the psychiatric disorder is provided.
- Clear, workable guidelines are established by which family members achieve their goals.
- Continuity of care for patient and family is provided.
- The MFG creates a network that supports overall clinical and individual family goals.

Once key family members agree both with the general objectives and to work in a treatment team, the clinician implements the next set of goal setting. The clinician gathers from all family members, including the patient, what they hope to achieve through this teamwork. Some goals may be unrealistic (e.g., to be without symptoms or to resume full-time school), and respectful negotiation between clinician and family members is needed. This not only is important in establishing more attainable versions of the family's goals, but also provides an opportunity for the clinician to model (and the family to practice) the negotiation process. Fortunately for most families, agreement about goals is readily achieved, because they usually want what the approach is designed to do: prolong remission and enhance day-to-day functioning. Families learn that other goals need not be discarded but may require postponement until the patient has a functional niche in the community.

A contract emerges through the process of goal setting. The frequency of sessions, who attends meetings, an approximate length of treatment, and treatment goals are agreed on. The clinician reemphasizes that he or she is available to the family for a variety of needs, including crisis intervention; representing the family's interests and concerns to the rest of the treatment system; and, either directly or by supervision, providing the patient and family a case manager.

MFG Psychoeducation Phase 2: Educational Workshop

The MFG clinician then presents an educational workshop after engaging a small number of families. Experience suggests that the optimal size is from four to seven families (which coincidentally seems to be the ideal range for an ongoing psychoeducational MFG). The workshop usually lasts about 8 hours and therefore is generally held on a weekend. The workshop is specifically for family members and friends of the patient; patients usually are not invited unless they are exceptionally well compensated and are not delusional or denying having an illness.

Workshops are not therapy sessions; this is immediately communicated and is an important reason for a dramatically different format. A formal classroom setting is used for informal lecture and discussion sessions. Extensive use is made of audiovisual aids to illustrate concepts of brain function, medication effects, and signs and symptoms of illness. Information, particularly of the more "scientific," biological sort, may best be presented using a professional-quality videotape in conjunction with frequent breaks for questions and discussion. Information about the way in which the clinician and the family will continue to work together is also presented. MFG clinicians then present guidelines—"survival skills," as coined by Anderson et al. (1986)—for managing schizophrenia (Table 21–2). These behavioral instructions for the family members integrate the biological, psychological, and social aspects of the disorder, along with recommended responses aimed at helping to maintain a home environment that minimizes relapse-inducing stress. During breaks and over lunch there is ample opportunity for informal social contact between families, as well as between families and clinicians. The opportunity to interact with other families in similar situations greatly enhances the power of this phase of the intervention.

The advantage of having the clinicians carry out this educational function is enormous. Clinicians have an opportunity to demonstrate their authority as experts. This fosters confidence and lowers families' anxiety levels. Because each clinician has had initial contact with but a few of the families in attendance, they can begin to form alliances with the rest. The value of involving the treating physicians cannot be overstated, because families continue to see them as crucial to illness management.

MFG Psychoeducation Phases 3 and 4: Reentry and Rehabilitation

Session structure in the phases after the workshop is also relatively strictly specified. The first meeting follows the workshop by one or two weeks. The same families who attended the workshop together constitute the MFG. These families, with the patients present and actively participating, begin meeting with both clinicians on a regular basis in meetings lasting approximately $1\frac{1}{2}$ hours. MFGs usually meet weekly for 4 to 6 weeks to establish cohesion. Meetings thereafter take place every 2 weeks and continue for at least 12 months, although better functional outcomes occur if the group meets for at least 2 years.

Table 21–2. Survival skills: family guidelines

Everyone's actions are important in helping things run smoothly. Below are a list of items that can help:

1. *Go slow.* Recovery takes time. Things will improve, but only at their own pace. Rest is important for all family members.
2. *Keep it cool.* Enthusiasm is normal. Tone it down. Disagreement is normal. Tone it down also.
3. *Give them space.* It is OK to offer something; it is also OK to refuse the offer. Nerves get frayed on occasion, and a time-out is important for everyone.
4. *Set limits.* A few good, consistent rules keep things clear. Everyone needs to know the rules and agree to follow them.
5. *Ignore what you can't change.* Some things are better to let slide. However, don't ignore violence.
6. *Keep things simple.* Good communication starts with being clear, calm, and positive.
7. *Follow doctor's orders.* Take medications as prescribed. Take only medications prescribed.
8. *No street drugs or alcohol are allowed.* They make symptoms worse. Family members affect one another, so no one is exempt.
9. *Pick up on early signs.* Note changes. Consult with your family clinician.
10. *Carry on business as usual.* Stay in touch with extended family and friends. Reestablish family routines as quickly as possible.
11. *Solve problems step by step.* Work on one thing at a time. Changes that last often occur on a steady, gradual course.
12. *Start at the beginning and build.* Lower expectations, temporarily. Use a personal yardstick. Compare this month to last rather than this person to another person.

The first work period concentrates on problems being experienced by the patient in the immediate postexacerbation phase. The goal is to prevent relapse. To the degree possible, families are all encouraged to institute a relatively simple, low-demand, low-intensity milieu. The MFG seeks to maintain remissions by systematically applying the group problem-solving method, addressing (on a case-by-case basis) the difficulties families have in achieving this environment.

Two special techniques are used: 1) formal problem solving and 2) communications skills training. The application of these permeates each session.

Clinicians use the problem-solving approach to demonstrate an adaptive method of controlling affect and tracking conversation. The process of bringing errant participants back to the topic or calming overly intense participants is repeatedly demonstrated by the clinician.

Psychoeducational MFG sessions follow quite strictly the format shown in Table 21–3. Experience demonstrates that a standardized, predictable structure is beneficial, because it allows the clinician to maintain benign control over sessions and enhances the group's ability to develop a likely solution for the problem under discussion. This structure serves to reduce the chance that meetings will turn into emotional, nonproductive gripe sessions that do not prove helpful to families.

All steps in the session format are essential; beginning clinicians often underestimate the importance of steps 1 and 5. In step 1 the clinician makes an emphatic attempt to avoid the session beginning with laments about any negative events or feelings. Active, engaged involvement is essential on the part of the clinicians. Specific inquiry about enjoyable events or novel occurrences in the family's life, even seemingly trivial, are essential here. Clinicians may sometimes take the lead by describing such events in their own lives. Importantly, clinicians take care to ensure that everyone is heard from, even if a given person can make only a brief, superficial contribution. The emphasis is on setting an optimistic, accepting, warm, and inclusive tone. This critical portion of each session builds unity, and thus resilience, for the sometimes more stressful attention on illness-induced problems.

Table 21–3.   Structure of MFG psychoeducational sessions

1. Socializing with families—15 minutes
2. Review of events since last session—20 minutes
   a. Week's events
   b. Relevant biosocial information
   c. Applicable guidelines
3. Selection of a single problem—5 minutes
4. Formal problem solving—45 minutes
   a. Problem definition
   b. Generation of possible solutions
   c. Weighing pros and cons of each possible solution
   d. Selection of preferred solution
   e. Delineation of tasks and implementation strategies
5. Socializing with families—5 minutes

Total time: 90 minutes

Step 2 reviews the success or difficulties of the previously assigned task, the basis of which was implementing the family guidelines for fostering recovery and remission. Unforeseen stresses may have limited the family's ability to complete the task; an empathic inquiry by the clinician assesses this possibility. Then, each family should report whether they have experienced progress or untoward occurrences. This allows the clinicians to make an informed decision on which family to focus that session's problem-solving efforts on.

Step 3 involves placing the selected family's problem, whether reported explicitly or implicitly, in a perspective that relates it to the realities of schizophrenia as an illness. In general, this involves relating psychosocial phenomena to their likely consequences for an individual with schizophrenia. This depends on the clinician's knowledge of effective strategies for managing various aspects of the recovery and rehabilitation process. If a symptomatic or functional disability aspect of the disorder creates a problem, then the general approach to solving the problem may be offered by one or more of the guidelines presented during the educational workshop. A number of clinically reliable methods exist with which to address problems that result from the effects of the disorder. In time, clinicians will find that they can ask other members to propose relevant guidelines. This fosters a sense of clarity, confidence, and self-reliance, setting an optimal tone for the specific problem solving that comes next.

Step 4 follows established problem-solving and communication skills approaches. One family is the focus. This family selects a single problem they have experienced when trying to implement the family guidelines or otherwise foster recovery. This problem is the focus of this session. The entire MFG then participates in problem solving with all participants contributing suggestions and ideas. Once accomplished, the affected family, with more limited input from the other families and clinicians, then reviews the relative advantages and disadvantages of the proposed solutions. The one that appears most attractive to the affected family is then reformulated as an appropriate task for trying at home. This becomes the homework assigned to the family.

Step 5, like step 1, is crucial. Families need time to solidify the social, interpersonal relationships developing in the group. This is enhanced by a final period of socializing.

As the stability of the patient and family increases, the MFG provides a unique resource; operating as an auxiliary social and vocational rehabilitation effort, the MFG provides a supportive, encouraging environment for each patient to begin a gradual resumption of responsibilities. The clinician continues to use problem-solving techniques to assist the MFG as the families assist their ill members to increase their social activities and find jobs.

Once the rehabilitation phase has reached a plateau, usually after 18–24 months, the frequency of sessions can be reduced to monthly. Most MFGs find it helpful to continue at this lower level of intensity for an extended period of time. Many, if not most, MFGs evolve into quasi-natural social networks with interpersonal relationships developing and extending from the group. Such support networks, increasingly recognized as one of the critical achievements of MFG, appear to be essential to preserving and enhancing the gains made during the active therapeutic phases.

Antipsychotic Medication Maintenance

It must be stated explicitly that antipsychotic medication is a key part of the psychoeducational MFG and therefore plays a crucial role in this approach's procedural and technical aspects. During each phase, the assumption that medication is the cornerstone for successful recovery and rehabilitation is consistently reinforced. Resilience in the face of environmental stimulation, whether external or internal, is greatly enhanced by antipsychotic medications. Most patients require the protection afforded by medication to lead any semblance of a normal life; this explains why medication noncompliance is the leading reason for relapse. The clinician, in an ongoing effort, assists the family and patient to understand that medication is critical for facilitating and achieving their own specific goals. Much of the educational material of psychoeducational MFG focuses on the rationale for drug treatment; medication issues often become the focus of problem solving in the ongoing sessions. At first, family members, including the person taking the medication, may not be willing to accept the need for chronic medications. Family members often need assistance in understanding the value of medication. Once they have accepted the prescribed regimen, support is then needed in dealing with the side effects that characterize chronic antipsychotic treatment. Often the improved psychosocial environment allows the use of much lower doses, thereby reducing side effects and exaggeration of negative symptoms.

Psychoeducational Treatment: Outcome Studies

McFarlane (1990) was the first to assess experimentally the outcome of psychoeducational MFGs and to delineate the contributions of its various elements. The first study was designed to test two treatment elements— psychoeducation and social network expansion—with the hope of distinguishing separate and possible additive effects. Forty-one recently admitted patients diagnosed with either schizophrenia or schizoaffective disorder and taking the lowest effective dose of medication were randomly assigned to a psychoeducational MFG, dynamically oriented multiple-family therapy, or psychoeducational single-family treatment. After 4 years, the time to first relapse was significantly longer for the psychoeducational MFG than for single-family treatment. Final 4-year relapse rates were 50% for the psychoeducational MFG, 57.1% for the dynamically oriented MFG, and 76.5% for the psychoeducational single-family treatment (Cox's coefficient/ stad. err. = 2.09; P = .01). In one of the earlier psychoeducational MFG cohort of 10 patients, 6 remained in remission for 5 years or more. Thus, the data suggest that there is an effect in the MFG, separate and independent of the educational content, that acts to prevent or forestall relapse.

Functional capacity, like relapse rate, was shown to be favorably affected. At the beginning of the study 32.5% of all studied patients were functionally occupied. At 2 years, this had increased to 51.6%. Although differences across treatment types were not significant, the psychoeducational MFG registered the highest increase.

Confirmation of these results was provided by the New York State Family Psychoeducation in Schizophrenia Study (McFarlane et al. 1995). The study cohort consisted of 172 patients with a DSM-III-R diagnosis of schizophrenia, schizophreniform, or schizoaffective disorder (American Psychiatric Association 1987). The cohort included a wide range of patients in terms of chronicity, race, ethnicity, social class, and geographic area; there were no significant differences at baseline between the treatment conditions on any of the measured variables. Psychoeducational MFG therapy was compared with psychoeducational single-family treatment over a 2-year period. Study design carefully addressed project staff training and supervision and used a standard-dose medication strategy. Based on the Brief Psychiatric Rating Scale (BPRS) symptom criteria, relapse rates at 1 year were 19.0% for the multiple-family group and 28.6% for the single-family treatment; at 2 years the respective rates were 28% and 42%. This was a statistically significant difference when controlled for cases completing the treatment protocol (80% of the initial sample) or medication compliance. Over the 2 years, the rates of clinically significant relapses were 16.3% and 25.6%, respectively. The clinically significant relapse rate of less than 10% per year in the MFG compares quite favorably to a relapse rate of approximately 40% when using medication, whether alone or with supportive therapy, or of about 70% when using placebo (Hogarty et al. 1979).

The expenditure of staff time in implementing a treatment is used as a measure of effectiveness. Because the MFG approach not only yields a better outcome and requires one-half the staff time expenditure of the single-family treatment, the cost-benefit ratio (1:2.5) strongly favors the MFG format. If the cost of hospitalization is compared during MFG psychoeducation versus during prior treatment, the cost-benefit ratio is 1:34. These studies thus indicate that MFG therapy combining medication and psychoeducation yields not only better outcomes, but also a very favorable cost-benefit ratio.

Rigorous testing has illustrated the remarkable efficacy of psychoeducational treatment models. Outcomes are unusually consistent, pointing to a valid, reliable, and quite robust main effect. The main effect is, in fact, equivalent to that observed in most studies comparing maintenance antipsychotic medication to placebo. Thus, family intervention, when combined with medication, is as powerful as the addition of the medication itself. No other psychosocial intervention has achieved this level of impact and consistency while retaining an outpatient, low-intensity treatment format.

The social networks that evolve within MFG therapy allow patients to develop relationships across families. This provides them an opportunity to expand and rebuild their social skills within an accepting and supportive environment. Through cross-parenting, intense family relationships can be eased, further diffusing excess affect and anxiety. Ill family members are validated, as are their relatives, through their own positive relationships with ill members of other families. The MFG clinical approach exploits the social network inherent in these groups to enhance the illness-coping skills of family members and patients.

Conclusion

MFG psychoeducation, in combination with maintenance medication, could become a standard of treatment in schizophrenia, particularly in cases of markedly or persistently symptomatic patients and/or especially distressed and isolated families. In addition to the benefits for patients and families, its combined efficacy and simplicity have potentially enormous implications for cost-effectiveness. It is possible that the very course of the illness could change, given the decrease in frequency of destructive relapses. It is hoped that through practice of these approaches, the next generation of schizophrenic patients and their families will suffer a much less disabling course of illness.

References

American Psychiatric Association: Diagnostic and Statistical Manual of Mental Disorders, 3rd Edition, Revised. Washington, DC, American Psychiatric Association, 1987

Anderson C, Hogarty G, Reiss D: Schizophrenia and the Family. New York, Guilford, 1986

Beels CC: Family and social management of schizophrenia. Schiz Bull 13:97–118, 1975

Bourdon KH, Rae DS, Locke BZ, et al: Estimating the prevalence of mental disorders in U.S. adults from the Epidemiologic Catchment Area Survey. Public Health Rep 107:663–668, 1992

Breier A, Strauss JS: The role of social relationships in the recovery from pyschotic disorders. Am J Psychiatry 141:949–955, 1984

Detre T, Sayer J, Norton A, et al: An experimental approach to the treatment of the acutely ill psychiatric patient in the general hospital. Conn Med 25:613–619, 1961

Falloon IRH, Liberman RP: Behavioral family intervention in the management of chronic schizophrenia, in Family Therapy in Schizophrenia. Edited by McFarlane WR. New York, Guilford, 1983, pp 117–137

Hatfield A: What families want of family therapists, in Family Therapy in Schizophrenia. Edited by McFarlane WR. New York, Guilford, 1983, pp 41–68

Hogarty GE, Goldberg S, Schooler N, et al: Drugs and social therapy in the aftercare of schizophrenic patients. Arch Gen Psychiatry 28:54–63, 1974

Hogarty G, Schooler N, Ulrich R, et al: Fluphenazine and social therapy in the aftercare of schizophrenic patients. Arch Gen Psychiatry 36:1283–1294, 1979

Hogarty GE, Anderson CM, Reiss DJ, et al: Family psychoeducation, social skills training and maintenance chemotherapy in the aftercare treatment of schizophrenia. Arch Gen Psychiatry 43:633–642, 1986

Johnson D: The family's experience of living with mental illness, in Families as Allies in Treatment of the Mentally Ill. Edited by Lefley HP, Johnson DJ. Washington, DC, American Psychiatric Press, 1990, pp 31–64

Laqueur H, LaBurt H, Morong E: Multiple family therapy: further developments. Int J Soc Psychiatry, Vol 69, Congress Edition, 1964

McFarlane WR: Multiple family groups in the treatment of schizophrenia, in Handbook of Schizophrenia. Edited by Nasrallah HA. New York, Elsevier, 1990, pp 167–189

McFarlane WR, Lukens E, Link B, et al: Multiple family groups and psychoeducation in the treatment of schizophrenia. Arch Gen Psychiatry 52:687–697, 1995

Pattison E, Llama R, Hurd G: Social network medication of anxiety. Psychiatric Annals 9:56–67, 1979

Weinberger D: The implications of normal brain development for the pathogenesis of schizophrenia. Arch Gen Psychiatry 44:660–670, 1987

Yolles SR, Kramer M: Vital statistics, in The Schizophrenic Syndrome. Edited by Bellack L, Loeb L. New York, Grune & Stratton, 1969, pp 66–113

Chapter 22

Cultural Issues in Community Psychiatry

H. Steven Moffic, M.D.

A 23-year-old married man is referred to a community mental health center
with the chief complaint of feeling "mad."

What's missing, if anything, from this not uncommon description? Doesn't
this appear like a typical brief patient introduction? What's missing is a fuller
description of this patient's sociocultural background. Is this man of Euro-
pean, Hispanic, Asian, African, subgroups or combinations of these, or other
cultural background? Is he poor, as he is coming to a community mental
health center, or are there cultural reasons why a wealthier man would not
seek care in the private sector?

Why might this sociocultural information be important anyway? Assuming the patient is an Hispanic male, we might note the tendency of such
males not to seek help for a psychiatric problem. Why the referral occurred
is important to build an initial working alliance. Cautious and more casual
interviewing questions might be less threatening. How acculturated is the
patient, and how does he view his cultural identity? If the primary language
was Spanish, a primarily Spanish-speaking clinician would be preferable to
using an interpreter. If there are language complexities, as there are with
many cultural groups, does "mad" in this case suggest anger or psychosis?
The answer will influence the diagnosis and treatment. For treatment, how

acculturated to the United States is he? If not very acculturated, the important traditional role of Hispanic women in health care might suggest the
involvement of the wife. Inquiry into whether a folk healer, or Curandero,
was already used would convey important information about prior attempts
to help. Then, are there important cultural attitudes toward medication or
psychotherapy that we need to know? The less acculturated the patient is,
the more education he will need about either treatment.

How Has Community Psychiatry Addressed Culture?

Providing improved mental health care to patients of all cultural groups was
one of the stated goals of the community mental health movement in the
1960s (President's Commission on Mental Health 1978). Prior to that,
grossly inadequate or inappropriate services to African American and other
minority groups seemed to be common (Mollica et al. 1980). Although such
questionable 19th century diagnoses as drapetomania—flight from home
madness—for runaway slaves were no longer operable (Szasz 1971), these
were replaced by the overdiagnosis of schizophrenia and underdiagnosis of
depression in African Americans (Kendrick et al. 1983) and the diagnosis of
homosexuality as a mental disease until 1974 (Campbell et al. 1983).

The community mental health movement attempted to address these
problems with several innovations (Wu and Windle 1980). These included
building centers to serve circumscribed population areas in need, involvement of community representatives on boards, training of indigenous paraprofessional clinicians, linkages with folk healers such as Curanderos, and
the training of more minority professionals.

How well, then, has the community mental health movement done since
the 1970s to address these culturally related problems? By all accounts, considerable gains have been made in providing improved treatment to previously underserved cultural groups, not only by community mental health
centers themselves, but also by other mental health institutions and clinicians. However, there is still much room for improvement (Flaskerud and
Hu 1992). Although cultural minorities are no longer "warehoused" in state
hospitals, psychotherapy is still inappropriately or underutilized (Sue 1977).
There is greater cultural diversity among professionals, but adequate education for all clinicians concerning cultural influences occurs in much less
than half of all training programs (Moffic et al. 1987). Although there are

innovative programs such as culture-specific inpatient wards or clinics, how and when they are better than heterogenous settings is unclear. Furthermore, although the importance of culture is increasingly recognized, research that incorporates how best to address the cultural variable is quite sparse (Cheung and Snowden 1990).

The Concept of Culture

Exactly what culture means in psychiatry has been controversial (Moffic et al. 1987). Although it is often used in referring to ethnic minority groups, a broader perspective may be more clinically useful. Cultural psychiatry, in its broadest sense, can refer to any segment of social reality that the psychiatrist likes or dislikes. Included, then, would be such social groups as ethnic minorities, poor persons, celebrities, "Yankees," Southerners, homosexuals, aged individuals, deaf persons, and so on.

Exactly what names to use for cultural groups is also controversial and clinically relevant (Moffic 1989). The Hispanic male in our initial example may prefer to be called "Hispanic," "Latino," "Chicano," "Mexican American," or any related term. Similarly, whether "black," "African American," "colored," or "Negro" is preferred depends on individual preference, values, and age.

Exactly what is relevant about culture in psychiatry has also been unclear (Moffic et al. 1983). For example, a new psychiatry student posed these two general questions:

1. Why are you trying to brainwash us with all this cultural stuff? Psychiatry is psychiatry.
2. Aren't we all more the same than different?

For another student more perceptive of the relevance of culture, two other questions arose:

1. How can I possibly learn all the relevant characteristics of the patients I am treating?
2. Doesn't each individual patient uniquely reflect his or her cultural background?

Another student, who did not give up considering culture at this stage, soon asked two more specific questions:

1. If you are a white clinician working with a black patient, would you introduce yourself with the "soul" handshake or the "usual" one?

2. If you are working with Asian Americans whose primary language is Japanese, shouldn't you really learn the Japanese language?

Finally, the clinician who hasn't employed denial, regressed to an omniscient stance, or encountered performance anxiety may then ask these two questions:

1. Does it matter what culture I come from?
2. What is my ethnicity anyway?

Guidelines for clinicians wanting to apply culturally appropriate practice must try to address these questions.

The Patient's Culture

The first task in analyzing the influence of the patient's culture is to determine the patient's cultural identity. As usual in psychiatry, this may not be such an easy question to answer as it seems on first glance. Although it might seem self-evident on appearance that a patient is black, that patient might consider him- or herself Cuban or Nigerian. Moreover, the existence of multiple subcultures in the United States produces significant complexity: One may be a Southern Jew, religiously orthodox, and even black simultaneously. When does a person change from Russian to Russian American to American? Especially important for clinicians, uprooting and immigration may cause an identity crisis that will result in "the creation of a new form of cultural identity . . . specific for the individual and for his unique situation of uprootment" (Mostwin 1976, p. 105). Even when the cultural identity is clear and misleading reductionism is avoided, clinicians' knowledge of the specific content and values of most cultures is usually limited. Returning to the prior question of handshake, the clinician could provide the opportunity to the patient to use either or both types.

How, then, should clinicians ascertain a patient's culture? For most patients we can sensitively ask what they consider to be their cultural background. However, caution must be used, especially with patients from a minority culture, as the clinician's interest in their culture can be at once flattering, seductive, and exploitative (Wintrob and Youngsook 1981). Ironically, in these cases, a more rigid, ethnocentric clinician can initially be more comfortable and familiar. Moreover, because psychiatric patients are answering, the answer must be considered a hypothesis. The psychiatric problem that necessitates treatment may alter the patients' perception of his or her culture. For example, black patients may psychotically consider themselves to be white but appearing dark because of the "devil's influence." To complicate things further, if the family secret of this patient was that there was a white great-grandfather, what does this imply for the patient's cultural identification, and will that influence the patient's preference for a clinician who is black or white? Cross-checking with immediate family, who presumably share a cultural identity, will help test the hypothesis. After determining the patient's cultural identity, clinicians need to know the intensity, purity, and variation of that culture. To question these variations, instead of asking "How Polish or Catholic is this patient?," clinicians should ask the more revealing question, "How is the person Polish or Catholic?" (Stein 1979).

Following these questions about cultural identity, the clinician should also obtain a more formal cultural history as part of the evaluation. This cultural history would help translate cultural values into the specific issues relevant to that patient. Included would be a cultural genogram, a description of early family life, the role of the parents, communication (verbal and nonverbal) styles, child-rearing practices, and values. The typical mental status examination requires cultural consideration, especially on informational questions. For example, a new immigrant to the United States from an African village should not necessarily be expected to know the previous president. Also, proverbs vary in cultures as to content, idiomatic understanding, and interpretation.

How the patient relates to the clinician may be culturally influenced. Any major differences in the culture of patient and clinician may create some wariness. Alternatively, ethnic difference can also elicit idealization and security regarding objectivity and confidentiality. Unfortunately, devaluation of minority clinicians solely because of their cultural background is still not rare. The patient's comfort with the cultural background of the clinician should be elicited before and during treatment.

After analyzing culture during the evaluation, the usual treatments must be culturally congruent to achieve a reasonable degree of compliance. Folk medical beliefs are often influential (Snow 1974). Opportunity should be taken to ascertain the patient's view of the problem, prior remedies, influential members of the social network, and treatment conceptions. For example, the chronic schizophrenic patient of Hispanic background who holds the cultural belief that medication should cure after one dose will have difficulty with the concept of maintenance. Consultation with cultural experts in psychiatry, anthropologists, or indigenous clinicians can be invaluable for any needed adjustments in treatment techniques. Appreciating atypical treatment requirements, such as lower dosage antidepressants in Vietnamese refugees (Kinzie 1981), may prevent clinical mistakes.

The Clinician's Culture

With all the complexity involved in therapeutically evaluating the culture of the patient, it may be even harder to evaluate the culture of the clinician. Why is cultural self-analysis of the clinician important to community psychiatric practice? First, even for those who are attracted to cross-cultural work, good motives may be suspect. Clinicians who are dissatisfied with their own culture may be attracted to such work and may then externalize internal conflict relating to their cultural identity (Bergman 1979). Grandiosity, intellectual condescension, and moral self-righteousness may also ensue. For those who feel consciously neutral about cultural issues, cultural differences may become a repository for the stimulation of unresolved conflict (Moffic et al. 1979). For those clinicians who consciously avoid or denigrate particular cultures, an internal negative cultural identity is likely (Erickson 1966). Even for those clinicians who avoid such problems, two extremes of routine discomfort are likely. Comparatively sophisticated cultural relativists can be greatly influenced in cross-cultural work by the clinician's "own sense of strangeness in an unfamiliar setting," and regressive tendencies akin to stranger anxiety commonly develop and affect the initial therapeutic alliance (Wintrob and Youngsook 1981). On the other hand, the objectivity necessary for a fair interpretation of the patient's problems may be compromised by too close a cultural match between clinician and patient (Gottesfeld 1978). In addition to alleviating such potential countertransference problems, cultural self-analysis may improve treatment in other ways. Although most research indicates increased compliance with similar ethnic patient-clinician matches, there is also some indication that training in cultural similarities and differences improves cross-cultural clinical interactions (Lefley 1984).

How, then, can clinicians achieve this cultural self-awareness? Unfortunately, typical psychodynamic psychotherapy and psychoanalysis have been as ethnic-blind as the rest of psychiatry, so personal therapy is likely to be of limited help (Prince et al. 1968). Because cultural identity may have many unconscious components, conscious perception can be deceiving. However, active recall of grandparents or elders of the clinician regarding questions of ethnicity or economic experiences may elicit some of the unconscious aspects. These familial attitudes may have become early intrapsychic feelings and memories within the clinician, thereby influencing implicit and explicit assumptions and perceptions. For example, the experience of grandparents with economic depression may produce repression of anger in grandchildren and later avoidance of poor patients. If some of the clinician's best childhood friends were in fact from different sociocultural backgrounds, an increased capacity for accurate empathy with those ethnic groups may ensue. Alternatively, the lack of early cross-cultural exposure may have a different effect, as in the case of a traditional Mexican American patient designated and treated as white by a resident who said that he had never seen or heard of Mexican Americans while growing up in a small Montana town. In addition to conducting such personal cultural histories, a culturally sensitive supervisor can be helpful. Although not very common currently, ethnotherapy groups, which analyze and stimulate cultural identity development, have proved adaptable to a variety of ethnic and cultural populations.

The Institution's Culture

With the continuing examination and reexamination of racism, sexism, and ageism in the United States, it should not be surprising that institutions may convey certain cross-cultural attitudes that could affect community psychiatric practice. A community mental health center that is supposed to serve a poor black population but is located away from major bus routes and has no black staff may be conveying a sense of unwelcomeness to those patients. A simple lack of bilingual reading material in waiting areas may indicate cross-cultural insensitivity.

When we find that black inpatients spend less time in the hospital; obtain fewer privileges; and are given more medications, seclusion, and restraint; this suggests that some form of cross-cultural bias is compromising treatment (Flaherty and Meagher 1980). If blacks are absent from research wards in a community mental health center, how will clinicians ever know if their practice guidelines are cross-culturally valid (Weiss and Kupfer 1974)? This problem of institutional and organizational cultural bias may be so pervasive that it even influences our reputedly more reliable diagnostic system. Both DSM-III and DSM-III-R (American Psychiatric Association 1980, 1987) seem inadequate to help the clinician distinguish between pathological and normative behaviors in ethnic minorities and omit cross-cultural symptoms of mental problems (Mezzich et al. 1992) (e.g., auditory hallucinations may occasionally be a normal religious phenomenon, whereas somatic syndromes may be a mask for depression). There has been some improvement in this area in DSM-IV (American

Psychiatric Association 1994). To know for sure, cultural norms must be part of the information pool.

Summary

Providing optimal, cross-cultural psychiatric practice may seem like a paradox. It is virtually impossible for most clinicians to have in-depth knowledge of multiple cultures. As an enthusiastic psychology student spending a part of a year studying San Francisco Chinatown noted, "What I don't know about Chinatown could fill many volumes. The main thing I know firsthand is that it was hard for me to learn very much about Chinatown firsthand" (Harris et al. 1976, p. 21).

If this experience is multiplied in a multicultural practice, then although enhanced cross-cultural knowledge is possible, definitive cultural knowledge is usually a grandiose delusion. It may be harder to master the varieties and effects of culture than the varieties and effects of medications. The effect of this relative ignorance on the narcissistic ideal of clinicians can readily cause denial or stereotyping.

An appropriate attitude may be even more crucial than knowledge and a way to resolve the paradox. With an attitude that appreciates and respects cultural diversity, determining the culture of the patient, obtaining a cultural history, adjusting treatment to make it culturally appropriate, improving the cultural self-awareness of the clinician, and watching for institutional bias will all seem more relevant.

In effect, the clinician must become a participant-observer in cultural negotiation with each patient. Because culture may have various degrees of influence on each clinician encounter, it must be assessed anew for each patient and for each clinician.

References

American Psychiatric Association: Diagnostic and Statistical Manual of Mental Disorders, 3rd Edition. Washington, DC, American Psychiatric Association, 1980

American Psychiatric Association: Diagnostic and Statistical Manual of Mental Disorders, 3rd Edition, Revised. Washington, DC, American Psychiatric Association, 1987

American Psychiatric Association: Diagnostic and Statistical Manual of Mental Disorders, 4th Edition. Washington, DC, American Psychiatric Association, 1994

Bergman R: The mental hygiene of staff in cross-cultural psychiatry. Paper presented at the annual meeting of the American Psychiatric Association, 1979

Campbell HD, Hinkle DO, Sandlin P, et al: A sexual minority: homosexuality and mental health care. Am J Soc Psychiatry 3(2):26–35, 1983

Cheung FK, Snowden LR: Community mental health and ethnic minority populations. Community Ment Health J 26:277–291, 1990

Erickson EH: The concept of identity in race relations: notes and inquiries. Daedalus 95(Winter):145–176, 1966

Flaherty JA, Meagher R: Measuring racial bias in inpatient treatment. Am J Psychiatry 137:670–682, 1980

Flaskerud JH, Hu L: Racial/ethical identity and amount and type of psychiatric treatment. Am J Psychiatry 149:379–384, 1992

Gottesfeld ML: Countertransference and ethnic similarity. Bull Menninger Clin 42:63–67, 1978

Harris MR, Kalis B, Schneider L: Training in community mental health in an urban setting. Am J Psychiatry 133 (suppl):20–29, 1976

Kendrick EA, McMilliam MF, Pinderhughes CA: A racial minority: black Americans and mental health care. Am J Soc Psychiatry 3(2):11–18, 1983

Kinzie JD: Evaluation and psychotherapy of Indochinese refugee patients. Am J Psychother 35:251–261, 1981

Lefley HP: Cross-cultural training for mental health professionals: effects on the delivery of services. Hosp Community Psychiatry 35:1227–1229, 1984

Mezzich JE, Fabrega H, Kleinman A: Cultural validity and DSM-III (editorial). J Nerv Ment Dis 180:4, 1992

Moffic HS: Labelling and group tensions in the United States. International Journal of Group Tensions 19:152–164, 1989

Moffic HS, Cheney CC, Barrios FX, et al: Culture primary care, and community mental health. Int J Ment Health 8:89–107, 1979

Moffic HS, Silverman SW, Adams GL: General clinical considerations for minority group patients. Am J Soc Psychiatry 3(2):70–74, 1983

Moffic HS, Kendrick EA, Lomax JW, et al: Education in cultural psychiatry in the United States. Transcultural Psychiatric Research Review 24:167–197, 1987

Mollica RF, Blum JD, Redlich F: Equity and the psychiatric care of the black patient, 1950 to 1975. J Nerv Ment Dis 168:279–286, 1980

Mostwin D: Uprootment and anxiety. Int J Mental Health 5:103–116, 1976

President's Commission on Mental Health: Report to the President of the President's Commission on Mental Health, Vol I. Washington, DC, U.S. Government Printing Office, 1978

Prince R, Leighton AM, May R: The therapeutic process in cross-cultural perspective—a symposium. Am J Psychiatry 124:1171–1183, 1968

Snow LF: Folk medical beliefs and their implications for care of patients. Ann Intern Med 81:82–94, 1974

Stein H: The salience of ethno-psychology for medical education and practice. Soc Sci Med 13B:199–210, 1979

Sue S: Community mental health services to minority groups—some optionism, some pessimism. Am Psychol 32:616–624, 1977

Szasz TS: The sane slave. Am J Psychother 25:228–239, 1971

Weiss B, Kupfer D: The black patient and research in a community mental health center: where have all the subjects gone? Am J Psychiatry 131:415–418, 1974

Wintrob R, Youngsook KH: The self-awareness factor in intercultural psychotherapy: some personal reflections, in Counseling Across Cultures. Edited by Peterson P. Honolulu, University of Hawaii, 1981, pp 108–132

Wu I-Hsin, Windle C: Ethnic specificity in the relative minority use and staffing of community mental health centers. Community Ment Health J 16:156–168, 1980

Chapter 23

Practice Styles in Rural Psychiatry

Deborah Reed, M.D.
Arthur Merrell, M.D.

T he national shortage of rural health care providers has been recognized for decades. Rosenblatt and Lishner (1991) reported that despite the continued increase in the total number of practicing physicians in the United States, there are still 10 times as many physicians in urban as in rural areas. In the 1960s the federal government enacted legislation for the construction of community health centers to provide primary health care in both urban and rural medically underserved communities. With the passage of the Community Mental Health Center Act (Public Law 88-164) in 1963, federal funding was appropriated for the establishment of mental health centers to address the psychiatric needs of people in these communities. Deinstitutionalization of chronically mentally ill persons necessitated a comprehensive system of care for this population in their own communities. In 1981 funding of the community mental health program was transferred to the states via Section 901 of the Omnibus Budget Reconciliation Act (Public Law 97-35). Unfortunately, despite these programs, many rural communities continue to have significant difficulties in attracting and retaining primary care physicians, psychiatrists, and other mental health care providers.

The National Health Service Corps (NHSC) was established in 1970 (Public Law 91-623) to aid in the financing of education for various primary health care providers, with the agreement that these medical personnel would then work for a designated period in underserved communities throughout the United States. In more recent years, the NHSC has requested that all psychiatrists fulfill their obligations in rural areas. A study by Pathman et al. (1992) showed that the retention of rural NHSC physicians has been quite poor.

Statistics from a 1980 National Institute of Mental Health (NIMH) report indicate that states with large rural populations, particularly in the midwestern, southern, and mountain states, have significantly fewer psychiatrists per capita than the national average (Muszynski et al. 1983). Winslow (1979) has described a national exodus of psychiatrists from community mental health centers. This change has had important ramifications for rural communities where psychiatric services are generally delivered by the community mental health centers. A study of the community mental health work force in Nebraska between 1981 and 1988 indicated that, in contrast to urban clinics, rural agencies had significantly fewer full-time-equivalent positions filled among all staff (Stuve et al. 1989).

More recently the federal government has once again focused on the mental health needs of rural Americans (Human and Wasem 1991). In response to the apparent increased psychiatric morbidity in rural agricultural communities as a consequence of the farm crisis, the NIMH in 1987 offered competitive grant applications to states to develop comprehensive, community-oriented mental health services. In 1989 and 1990, the NIMH provided incentives to promote research on rural mental health issues in academic centers, with a particular focus on epidemiology and plans of service delivery (Hutner and Windle 1991).

In his article on an NIMH-funded program to train psychologists for rural work, Hargrove (1991) discusses some of the reasons why professionals with advanced degrees tend to avoid practicing in rural community mental health centers. He notes that rural areas need generalists rather than specialists and that clinicians tend to advance rather quickly up the administrative ladder, which creates a dearth of treatment providers available for direct service. In addition, impoverished rural areas provide little or no opportunity for private practice so that those mental health clinicians who do choose to practice in rural areas will likely be in the community mental health centers.

Although rural community mental health centers frequently lack staff from all disciplines, the psychiatrist plays a crucial role in the provision of services to these communities. If the most basic mission of the community mental health center system is to provide care for chronically mentally ill persons, adequate psychiatric coverage is imperative for these clinics.

In the 1970s various university-based psychiatric residency programs focused their attention on the need to train physicians for rural service (Kofoed and Cutler 1982; Tucker et al. 1981). Typically, new psychiatrists seek employment situations that mirror their residency training experiences. If rural work is valued and rural experience is offered with adequate guidance, perhaps more psychiatrists will be willing to staff rural community mental health centers. These training programs emphasized the importance of adequate supervision to aid the psychiatric resident in adapting to the cultural milieu and gaining acceptance as a valued member of the team of clinicians. Also emphasized was the need for the psychiatrist to learn how to function within both the social service and the medical models of practice. Certainly, a continued liaison with a university program would help deter the professional isolation that many rural psychiatrists face.

The Concept of Rurality

In her article on rural psychiatric services, Bachrach (1983) emphasized that rurality is more aptly conceptualized in sociological terms rather than defined purely by population concentrations or geographic location. In contrast to their urban counterparts, rural individuals tend toward homogeneity in terms of behavior, political and religious beliefs, and activities. However, rural communities can differ sharply from one another. Commonly, a certain degree of pessimistic acceptance of life exists in rural populations; this seems to be a natural consequence of the dependence on the physical environment. Mental illness among members of rural locales can certainly interfere with their capacity to conform and be accepted by the community. A fatalistic attitude toward one's predicament and life experience can at times interfere with treatment acceptance and compliance, even if adequate psychiatric resources exist within a given community. Through this perspective on rurality, one can better appreciate the potential challenges a rural psychiatrist may face.

Designing a Rural Practice

In the late 1960s and especially in the 1970s, mental health clinicians began to examine the challenges and pitfalls of practice in the rural community mental health center (Clayton 1977; Gurian 1971; Jeffrey and Reeve 1978). In their article on rural mental health, Human and Wasem (1991) discuss the concepts of availability, accessibility, and acceptability as a framework for the delivery of mental health services to rural communities. In essence, decent care in this setting necessitates an adequate number of trained generalist clinicians who have an understanding and a willingness to address the geographic, financial, and cultural barriers that interfere with patients obtaining needed treatment.

In this discussion we will focus on two psychiatrist's efforts at improving accessibility and acceptability in rural communities in Kentucky and Wyoming, hopefully thereby encouraging other clinicians to provide more availability in terms of manpower to rural communities throughout the nation. It is extremely important for the psychiatrist interested in rural practice to have a keen awareness of his or her particular personal needs, both socially and professionally. Furthermore, those needs must be balanced with the community's psychiatric resources and its demands for psychiatric services. In this chapter we would like to outline more specifically various challenges and potential obstacles in rural practice and our own attempts to manage them. We will focus on different practice styles that can be modified to suit the particular needs of the individual psychiatrist in hopes of attracting more psychiatrists to rural practice.

It is highly likely that the psychiatrist who does choose a rural practice will be employed either part time or full time by a community mental health center. Commonly, however, the local mental health center may come to be viewed as the provider of all social services for the rural community. Financial hardship and economic deprivation unfortunately are rather common in many rural areas, and consequently, a full-time private practice is rarely an option.

Certainly, the lack of adequate numbers of staff contributes to the professional isolation and increased workload of the psychiatrist who chooses to practice in the rural setting. This very basic fact forms the cornerstone for an understanding of the problems and stresses of rural practice. Moreover, once the psychiatrist commits to a community and is recognized and accepted, there will likely be an increase in referrals, which may stretch the limits of the most dedicated provider. Several authors (Cutler and Madore 1987; Heiman 1983; Loschen 1983, 1986; Reed 1992) have described methods of providing psychiatric services in rural areas through extending the concept of service provision to members of the local community. Specifically, local law officers, clergy, and family practitioners can help address some of the mental health needs of the community through collaboration with the psychiatrist.

The relationship with local family practitioners deserves special attention. Typically these physicians will have already been treating mentally ill persons in the community and will welcome the new psychiatrist with open arms. Because many of these physicians have long-standing relationships with their patients, some may want to continue to provide psychiatric treatment for their more stable patients. Through availability and consultation, the new psychiatrist can aid the family practitioner, support his or her practice, and create a broader network of psychiatric services for the community.

Depending on the psychiatrist's availability and reputation, he or she may be called on to deal with numerous dilemmas beyond the purview of psychiatric practice. It is essential that the psychiatrist practicing with few other colleagues learn to set limits in those nonclinical areas without alienating community members, yet participate, if possible, in those areas that may bear directly on the treatment of psychiatric patients within the community (e.g., task forces on mental health issues, commitment legislation, etc.).

If the psychiatrist does not reside in the rural community and therefore is unavailable after hours to handle emergencies, the family practitioners or local emergency department physicians will assume the bulk of this workload. In addition, the psychiatrist in solo practice who does reside in the community but has no psychiatric coverage will rely on others in his or her absence. Because of the professional isolation and the lack of opportunity to obtain continuing medical education locally, it is extremely important for the rural psychiatrist to be away from the community periodically. Furthermore, the difficult nature of the work, coupled with the workload, will also necessitate that the psychiatrist have adequate vacation time. Much like the family practitioner, the psychiatrist in a rural community will frequently be called at home regardless of whether a formal on-call system is in place. A variety of on-call systems can be implemented depending on the resources available in the community. It is preferable that this issue be negotiated prior to employment (i.e., during the interview process), as the community may have some unspoken expectations about the psychiatrist's availability after hours.

The psychiatrist, other mental health professionals, local family physicians, and emergency department personnel can meet and establish consistent and appropriate guidelines for triage and disposition of psychiatric patients that can be implemented in the psychiatrist's absence. Cooperation among the professionals in the community is especially important when treating difficult, recidivistic, or severely characterologically disordered patients, as these patients may overly tax already limited psychiatric resources. With collaboration and limit setting, these patients will have less opportunity to "doctor shop," and acting out behaviors can be significantly reduced. In this regard, the absence of mental health care providers can at times be viewed as advantageous. Moreover, when problems develop in the therapy between patient and therapist or when the therapeutic approach is in question, another professional's personal knowledge of the therapist can be helpful in defusing the situation and in avoiding behaviors associated with splitting. Resistance in treatment can thereby be more readily identified and confronted. An ongoing dialogue between the professionals involved in the client's care is frequently more easily implemented in a rural practice.

One significant advantage to being a lone provider in a rural practice is having the opportunity to pursue one's own interests within the field and tailor, to some degree, a practice to one's particular needs. Although rural practice demands that one be a generalist, there is certainly opportunity to focus on areas of special interest and expertise (e.g., substance abuse, geriatrics, child and adolescent, and gender issues), with less concern for problems of competition that occur in larger urban settings. Even though the rural psychiatrist must establish priorities in terms of the services a community requires, the individual practitioner has the option of choosing a practice style that suits his or her desires and needs. All can agree that some psychiatric services, incomplete and disjointed as they may be, are better than no psychiatric services. Unquestionably, the clinician must balance the general psychiatric needs of the community with his or her special interests, and it is precisely this mix and balance that can be the crucial factor in job satisfaction for the rural mental health care provider. Creativity and flexibility on the part of the mental health clinician will allow for a better adjustment in the rural setting.

Various authors have drawn attention to the issue of burnout for mental health clinicians (Hargrove 1982; Pines and Maslach 1978). The rural setting, with its inherent difficulties and stresses, provides a ripe environment for burnout, which has been described as a syndrome of physical and emotional exhaustion, negativity, humorlessness, cynicism, detachment, irritability, and hopelessness. Burnout can be viewed as a consequence of an overdependence on a demanding work environment that does not meet the personal and professional needs of the clinician. In addition to the isolation, the professional and emotional demands of the rural setting can be overwhelming at times, and to survive, the clinician must be adaptable and flexible, yet able to set realistic limits for him- or herself.

Emergencies and Hospitalization

As previously stated, although the day-to-day workload of a rural practice can at times be burdensome, the psychiatrist is often additionally challenged by the handling of emergency situations and patients requiring psychiatric hospitalization. The shortage of mental health clinicians will most certainly be felt in this arena. Depending on the psychiatrist and the available community resources, these challenges can be dealt with in various ways. Whether the psychiatrist resides in the rural community will also determine how emergencies are handled. Another important consideration is the presence of psychiatric versus primary medical beds in the local hospital.

If the psychiatrist lives in or near the community, he or she may decide to start an inpatient unit within the local community hospital. There may be considerable support in this endeavor from the hospital, other physicians, the local community mental health center, and the community at large. Although the creation of an inpatient unit has significant advantages for the care of psychiatric patients in a local setting, there may be subtle potential pitfalls that need to be considered. In addition to the obvious issues of adequate psychiatric coverage, appropriate nursing staffing, and the physical plant, there are several specific questions that need to be addressed. For example, how will the psychiatric unit deal with the probable mixture of patients under emergency commitment and those whose commitment is voluntary? Should the ward be completely locked or partially locked? How will the unit deal with a potential mixture of child, adolescent, and geriatric patients? Clinical issues such as these may not be apparent until the unit is functioning, and it is often difficult to refuse admission to certain patient groups when the unit is "the only game in town." Financial concerns may also become major issues if the community has a high percentage of uninsured psychiatric clients or if there are significant restrictions on funding from government entitlement programs. In spite of some of the above potential roadblocks, a small inpatient unit can frequently improve the psychiatrist's comfort level in his or her practice and allow for better follow-up and continuity of care.

For some psychiatrists it is neither feasible nor desirable to hospitalize their own patients locally, particularly if the psychiatrist is employed full time by a community mental health center, if the outpatient workload is already excessive, or if no contractual arrangements have been negotiated with the local hospital. In addition, the rural psychiatrist commonly travels to several different locations in surrounding counties, and thus, treating hospitalized patients may be impractical. Again, the individual practitioner must balance the needs of the community with his or her own needs. State hospitals and distant community hospitals in larger population areas can be used for hospitalizing psychiatric patients. Transportation difficulties are a given complication in rural settings, particularly if the patient is under commitment, is unwilling to cooperate with needed treatment, or requires transfer to another county or state. In addition, the local police or ambulance drivers may be reluctant to transport psychiatric patients about whom they have little knowledge. The psychiatrist can help the drivers anticipate difficulties in transportation through consultative education and attention to strategic planning. The rural family's insistence on privacy and secrecy and its need to handle family problems without outside intervention may also interfere with hospitalization. Anxiety and fear about traveling far from home can be overwhelming for a rural patient in crisis. The psychiatrist must be aware of these particular issues and tailor the approach to hospitalization accordingly.

The discontinuity of treatment is also a significant problem for the rural psychiatrist who may have some trepidation about handing over the care of patients to an unknown colleague in a distant locale. For this reason, the psychiatrist who does not hospitalize patients him- or herself must make a concerted effort to meet and establish working relationships with hospitalizing physicians as well as with the emergency department staff who form the frontline. In his article on providing rural psychiatric services, Loschen (1983) discussed the development of formal staff relationships in local community hospitals, regional state hospitals, and distant tertiary care or academic settings to extend quality service provision. Relationships can be maintained through periodic meetings, frequent telephone contact, and correspondence. The importance of 24-hour telephone availability on the part of the rural psychiatrist has been stressed by other authors as well (Heiman 1983; Reed 1992).

In addition, if the psychiatrist remains in close contact with the treatment team in the hospital, treatment planning will be more meaningful and can truly help to curb future hospitalizations and ensure good aftercare. Efficient discharge planning can help reduce the length of inpatient stay, which is certainly an important consideration in these days of limited insurance benefits and economic hardship. Effective liaison relationships help to ensure that the tremendous amount of time and energy that can be expended in the referral for hospitalization are worthy of the psychiatrist's effort. The frustration of a denied admission or an inappropriately early discharge because of inadequate information transmittal can be defeating for the rural practitioner.

When firmer relationships with hospital personnel do not exist, the psychiatrist must at times relegate the responsibility for involuntary commitment to less experienced physicians. Flexibility and a tolerance for ambiguity are essential for the psychiatrist in this situation. Networking with effective community referral sources who understand the limitations inherent in rural practice is essential. The psychiatrist will then be rewarded when especially difficult situations arise (e.g., the homicidal or suicidal patient who refuses hospitalization or the patient who presents differently to various clinicians).

Legal Issues

Because the laws governing the psychiatric commitment process are enacted by each state's legislature, the actual process of involuntary hospitalization can become quite cumbersome in certain locales. For example, if the initial hospitalization or 72-hour psychiatric reevaluation requires that a judge preside or that more than one psychiatric clinician evaluate the patient, a number of practical difficulties may arise in the rural setting. Commonly, the local and county judges preside over several jurisdictions and may not necessarily be available for emergency commitments. The psychiatrist must then make other arrangements to ensure the patient's safety while attempting to provide necessary psychiatric treatment. The commitment laws are generally constructed to provide treatment in the least restrictive setting, in terms of both location as well as length of stay in the hospital. Although these requirements may easily be met in urban areas, this is often not the case in less populated communities with limited medical and judicial resources. It is imperative that the psychiatrist find effective methods of working within the existing legal system to ensure patient safety and provide treatment while simultaneously protecting the rights of the patient. Again, if the psychiatrist is willing to make a concerted effort to network with and educate the legal professionals and law officers in the rural community, appropriate care can be provided and liability can be reduced.

The rural psychiatrist also interfaces with the legal system with regard to how psychiatric patients are identified and managed in the community. It is not uncommon for a mentally ill person who engages in bizarre and sometimes criminal behavior to be jailed rather than hospitalized initially, as this behavior may be viewed as willful and illegal. Only when the patient is observed for several days by the jail staff will significant psychiatric, substance abuse, or even medical problems sometimes be identified. Again, it is imperative that the psychiatrist develop collegial relationships with workers in the local criminal justice system and offer telephone consultation in order to quickly identify and provide access to care for those in need.

Confidentiality and Privacy

A rural practice may lead to unique pitfalls in dealing with patient confidentiality; this has been discussed by numerous authors (Jeffrey and Reeve 1978;

Loschen 1986; Reed 1992). Certainly, although it is helpful to the mental health professional to form strong alliances with local authorities, one must be persistently conscious of the importance of privacy and confidentiality, which is required by law. Small towns lend themselves to overfamiliarity, which can at times be helpful and at other times be quite disruptive and potentially unethical, particularly in a psychiatric practice. Commonly the community mental health center or the psychiatrist's office is in the center of town, and some patients do not want to be seen entering the office and having other townspeople "know my business."

In the rural setting, community members may feel free to inquire about one another or about other family members in the treatment system. One must become keenly aware of the local mores regarding confidentiality and adopt a flexibility in handling these issues while following the American Psychiatric Association's guidelines in this area. These situations may also have important legal ramifications (e.g., in terms of one's duty to report suspected abuse). Commonly family members may call to inform the psychiatrist about a patient who may have stopped his medication and begun to decompensate after missing appointments. A telephone call to the patient may be a helpful intervention to prevent further decompensation.

In addition to concerns about the privacy of one's patients, the mental health clinician in the rural setting may face problems with maintaining his or her own sense of privacy. The rural psychiatrist will frequently see current and past patients outside the office when he or she attends social events, goes shopping, etc. These contacts are varied in nature, and the response of the patient to the psychiatrist will vary as well. In some cases the patient may not acknowledge or speak to the psychiatrist because of 1) failure to recognize him or her outside the familiar office setting, 2) embarrassment about being in treatment, or 3) because of the patient's individual psychological reaction or particular psychopathology. In these cases it is prudent to avoid interacting with the patient in public.

In other instances patients may exchange the normal social amenities in customary and appropriate ways. At other times patients may want to be overinvolved with the psychiatrist and may pursue discussions about medication issues or even intimate psychological concerns in spite of the presence of third parties nearby. This may be acted out in a somewhat exhibitionistic fashion, which can be uncomfortable for the clinician. Appropriate boundaries must be set in these situations, which can present challenges to the psychiatrist's flexibility and adaptability.

An example of one of these dilemmas involves the spouse of a patient who was employed at the local auto dealership where the psychiatrist's car was serviced. The patient's spouse informed the psychiatrist that the patient had not yet been "fixed" despite treatment, and consequently there was a perceived reluctance on the part of the spouse to "fix" the psychiatrist's car. This scenario can be played out in various settings and may parallel the transference dynamics of treatment and affect therapy either positively or negatively. It is essential that the psychiatrist who encounters these situations remain open to exploring all the possible meanings and implications of these everyday interactions for the patient.

Interfacing With the Culture

As previously stated, the concept of rurality is not defined by census or geography alone. The psychiatrist who resides in the rural community will likely come to embrace some particular aspect of the culture that suits his or her personal and family needs. The cultural and ethnic diversity and the opportunity for varied experiences that are readily available in urban areas are difficult to match in most areas of rural America. However, the rewards of community involvement and the feeling of belonging can bring a remarkable sense of satisfaction. The rural mental health professional is often highly respected in the community and has the opportunity to provide leadership and guidance for effective community projects and developments with fewer bureaucratic headaches. The role of visible leader also affords the professional the opportunity to educate the community about mental illness and advocate on behalf of patients, thereby improving the local mental health care delivery system. The impact of the mental health professional in this setting cannot be overestimated.

The familiarity and closeness common to many small towns may certainly suit the needs of some. Typically, religious organizations in rural communities play a significant role in addressing the problems of residents in need. Congregations are often willing to provide housing, food, and support to local townspeople, some of whom may have significant mental illnesses. Religious beliefs and church membership provide hope and sustenance to many disenfranchised persons in rural areas. Their actions and beliefs can be greatly influenced by the minister and the congregation. When the psychiatrist feels comfortable in developing collegial relationships with the local clergy, access to care for patients can be greatly enhanced.

Depending on the level of education, experience, and cultural beliefs within the community, persons with mental illness will be dealt with in a variety of ways. Unfortunately, in some more isolated, less educated rural communities, odd behavior resulting from severe mental illness is sometimes attributed to a lack of religious involvement or, worse, to demonic influence. For example, in one rural Southern community, a female patient with undiagnosed temporal lobe epilepsy was ostracized by her family and her church for years because her seizures were thought to be clear evidence of possession by the devil. She became extremely depressed and isolated and was initially highly resistant to any other interpretations or medical intervention. Her loss of self-esteem and guilt became incapacitating until she finally received treatment with the encouragement of her family physician.

Many rural communities embrace specific stereotypical values that affect how individuals deal with psychiatric illness. For example, rural Appalachians have been described as highly individualistic, antiauthoritarian, opinionated, and stubborn (Weller 1966). Since the 1700s these traits have served to protect community members struggling to create a new existence for themselves in the rugged terrain of West Virginia and Kentucky. During the 19th century, lumbering and coal mining were chief industries in these areas. Many families felt cheated out of their wealth by the land companies, which bought land cheaply and developed large, lucrative operations in the mountains. Many Appalachians came to mistrust all outsiders in order to protect their interests.

The frontier ideology prominent in Wyoming and other western states advocates an independent approach to living that can lead to isolation and limit access to needed medical and psychiatric care. A commonly espoused cultural ethic is to "take care of yourself no matter what," as turning to others for aid is often seen as a sign of weakness. This attitude can certainly deter patients from seeking psychiatric as well as medical help in the rural West. Such insistence on stoicism and personal strength is particularly notable among the geriatric population, many of whom choose to suffer through episodes of major depression or other psychiatric illness in silence and isolation. Unlike the Appalachian community's culturally experienced fear, it is more likely the rural western patient's personal experience of fear that causes him or her to endure severe illness in isolation and without treatment. Fortunately, the younger members of these communities appear to be relinquishing this tendency and are less resistant to pursuing treatment.

These personal perceptions and character styles have significant implications for psychiatric practice and for psychotherapy in particular. The psychiatrist may initially be seen as yet another outsider who cannot be trusted. Psychiatric treatment may be perceived as intrusive and quite foreign by members of rural communities. As psychotherapists, our work is based on the tenet that the process of understanding the dynamic roots of a problem holds the possibility for true change in the course of one's life. Therapy is not particularly helpful unless the patient maintains the expectation that understanding can ultimately lead to a true sense of control over one's path in life. These ideas may run counter to the basic beliefs of some rural communities. In their article on powerlessness and natural support systems in rural communities, Murray and Kupinsky (1982) discussed the impact of alienation and learned helplessness on the mental health of members of various rural communities.

The lack of education, with resultant illiteracy and poverty, plagues the lives of many rural patients, much as it does urban mentally ill individuals. A basic sense of the possibility and potential for gaining a sense of control may be harder to find in remote rural settings. In some rural communities there may not be the usual middle-class expectation that children will move on to a better life than their parents. Instead, there may be a strong, existence-oriented, sometimes regressive approach to life.

In his 1971 book, *The Relevance of Education,* Jerome Bruner discussed the specific aspects of an education that are capable of transforming a life. The experience of self-consciousness and the concomitant acknowledgment of a subjective versus an objective reality for a child are essential as he or she learns to observe, think abstractly, and problem solve. Rural cultures traditionally do not promote an experience of self-consciousness, but tend to uphold the universal perception of a shared, permanent, objective reality. Alternative modes of perceiving a situation are simply not entertained. This method of perceiving the world was initially helpful to the Appalachian society of the 1700s as they attempted to form a cohesive group. Yet this perception no longer seems useful and in fact usually impedes adaptation and growth. Psychological growth and maturation stem from the capacity to explore one's subjective reality and to develop an objective perspective on the origins of one's feeling states and thoughts. Without this distance, a patient will continue to feel helpless, immobile, and unable to act. A sense of competency and control emerges through the process of identifying varied viewpoints, evaluating the relevancy of each to one's personal situation, and then choosing a course of action. It is extremely difficult to help an undereducated adult with limited experience in problem solving to cultivate this essential flexibility of thought and action. However, the psychiatrist or mental health professional in a rural community is in a unique position to stimulate change and growth in both the individual and the community at large.

Conclusion

The rural experience in delivering mental health services can be unique and challenging, yet it offers a remarkable opportunity for personal and professional growth through strategic planning with other professionals and various community members. By taking a thoughtful approach to the demands and pitfalls common to rural practice, the individual clinician may reap the rewards of offering essential, high-quality psychiatric services to an appreciative population.

References

Bachrach LL: Psychiatric services in rural areas: a sociological overview. Hosp Community Psychiatry 34:215–226, 1983

Bruner JS: The Relevance of Education. New York, WW Norton, 1971

Clayton T: Issues in the delivery of rural mental health services. Hosp Community Psychiatry 28:673–676, 1977

Cutler DL, Madore E: Community network therapy in rural settings, in Innovations in Rural Community Mental Health. Edited by Murray JD, Keller PA. Mansfield, PA, Mansfield University Press, 1987, pp 75–89

The Emergency Health Personnel Act: P.L. 91-623, 1970

Gurian H: A decade in rural psychiatry. Hosp Community Psychiatry 22:56–58, 1971

Hargrove DS: An overview of professional considerations in the rural community, in Handbook of Rural Community Mental Health. Edited by Keller PA, Murray JD. New York, Human Sciences Press, 1982, pp 169–182

Hargrove DS: Training PhD psychologists for rural service: a report from Nebraska. Community Ment Health J 27:293–298, 1991

Heiman EM: The psychiatrist in a rural CMHC. Hosp Community Psychiatry 34:227–229, 1983

Human J, Wasem C: Rural mental health in America. Am Psychol 46:232–239, 1991

Hutner M, Windle C: NIMH support of rural mental health. Am Psychol 46:240–243, 1991

Jeffrey MJ, Reeve RE: Community mental health services in rural areas: some practical issues. Community Ment Health J 14:54–62, 1978

Kofoed L, Cutler D: Issues in rural community psychiatry training, in Training Professionals for Rural Mental Health. Edited by Dengerink H, Cross HJ. Lincoln, NE, University of Nebraska Press, 1982, pp 70–81

Loschen EL: Providing psychiatric services in a rural setting. International Journal of Mental Health 12:118–129, 1983

Loschen EL: The challenge of providing quality psychiatric services in a rural setting. QRB Qual Rev Bull Nov 12:376–379, 1986

The Mental Retardation Facilities and Community Mental Health Centers Construction Act: P.L. 88-164, 1963

Murray JD, Kupinsky S: The influence of powerlessness and natural support systems on mental health in the rural community. In Handbook of Rural Community Mental Health. Edited by Keller PA, Murray JD. New York, Human Sciences Press, 1982, pp 62–73

National Institute of Mental Health: Mental Health. Washington, DC, U.S. Government Printing Office, 1983

Omnibus Budget Reconciliation Act: P.L. 97-35, 1981

Pathman DE, Konrad TR, Ricketts TC: The comparative retention of National Health Service Corps and other rural physicians: results of a 9-year follow-up study. JAMA 268:1552–1558, 1992

Pines A, Maslach C: Characteristics of staff burnout in mental health settings. Hosp Community Psychiatry 29:233–237, 1978

Reed DA: Adaptation: the key to community psychiatric practice in the rural setting. Community Ment Health J 28:141–150, 1992

Rosenblatt RA, Lishner DM: Surplus or shortage? unraveling the physician supply conundrum. West J Med 154:43–50, 1991

Stuve MA, Beeson PG, Hartig P: Trends in the rural community mental health work force: a case study. Hosp Community Psychiatry 40:932–936, 1989

Tucker GJ, Turner J, Chapman R: Problems in attracting and retaining psychiatrists in rural areas. Hosp Community Psychiatry 32:118–120, 1981

Weller JE: Yesterday's People: Life in Contemporary Appalachia. Lexington, KY, University of Kentucky Press, 1966

Winslow WW: The changing role of psychiatrists in community mental health centers. Am J Psychiatry 136:24–27, 1979

Chapter 24

Community Consultation

Richard U'Ren, M.D.
David L. Cutler, M.D.
David A. Pollack, M.D.

C ommunity consultation continues to be a crucial element in public mental health work, yet in relatively recent years the attention given to it has declined. This no doubt reflects the fall from grace of the community mental health movement, begun with such enthusiasm in the early 1960s, as well as the domination in psychiatry of biological models since 1980. Whatever the reason, we view this development as unfortunate from the standpoint of community consultation, not only because it reduces its importance and status, but also because it blunts attention to the great need many community organizations have for competent psychiatric input.

In any event, community consultation skills continue to be taught in the Public Psychiatry Training Program at the Oregon Health Sciences University (see Chapter 26). The texts we use (Caplan 1964, 1970) envision consultation primarily as a method of primary or secondary prevention, but tertiary prevention is taught as well. Bloom (1975) conceptualized consultation as an offshoot of the community mental health movement, differentiating it from the kind of consultation that physicians are more familiar with in which an outside medical expert formulates a diagnosis and treatment plan for specific medical or psychiatric problems. Also, in this traditional model, the treating physician and the consultant share responsibility for the case:

in essence, they collaborate. In mental health consultation, as described by Caplan (1970), the consultant is more interested in the consultee than in the client. The consultant's primary goal is to improve the skills, knowledge, and objectivity of the consultee, not to treat the individual client or patient. In the real world, of course, mixed models are common, but the distinction between these two paradigms can be useful.

Certain problems are common in community consultation. Perhaps the most common these days is lack of knowledge and/or skills in what must be considered an undertrained work force. To a large extent, of course, this is driven by the need to save money by hiring younger and less well-trained professionals, paraprofessionals, and nonprofessionals to do tough jobs in tough settings with difficult patients. Psychiatric consultants are often called on to do basic skill building in areas such as interviewing, diagnosing, and treatment planning. Our expertise can be of considerable help to staff in various settings, including nursing homes, primary care clinics, and day-care centers.

What Caplan (1970) called *theme interference* is another problem. The term refers to transference- or countertransference-like issues in the consultee-client relationship that interfere with the former's objectivity. These issues, however, are not as exotic as they are in classic Freudian analysis. Instead, they represent various prejudices and negative attitudes that result from a lack of experience or from training that is inappropriate to particular target populations. It is our belief that if one makes an effort to provide training, education, and consultation to various groups and organizations within the community that deal with mentally ill persons, negative attitudes can be reduced and requisite skills enhanced. As a result, the morbidity associated with mental illness may be attenuated. There is no evidence that earlier hopes of reducing the incidence and prevalence of mental illness through community consultation have been realized, but reduction of morbidity is and remains a worthy goal.

In their book, *Community Mental Health: Reflections and Explorations,* Karno and Schwartz (1974) point out that it is not necessary for psychiatrists to be administrators and supervisors of all nonpsychiatric mental health professionals. It is, however, necessary to understand the roles of these providers in order to offer leadership with respect to treatment. Especially in settings where providers of mental health services are demoralized, lacking in knowledge and skill, or imbued with negative attitudes, there is much that psychiatrists can do. There are many examples. Psychiatric consultation has been described in relation to halfway houses (Budson 1979), to police (Reiser 1979), to schools (Berlin 1979), and to facilities that serve individuals with mental retardation and developmental problems (Robinowitz 1979). Some target populations that are currently of most concern include chronic and/or severely mentally ill individuals; people of low socioeconomic status, such as minority groups or immigrants; nursing home residents; and severely mentally ill children. In this chapter we will describe two examples of community consultation—one to primary care clinics, another to a nursing home—and emphasize the consultants' experiences of working in these settings. The examples we present do not use classic "Caplanian" methods because they are not pure consultee-centered or client-centered models. Rather, they are a mixture of these types and also include a certain amount of direct service. Because client-centered and consultee-centered case and/or administrative consultation have been described by Caplan in three books (Caplan 1964, 1970; Caplan and Caplan 1993), we will not address those issues here. The reader is encouraged to look up the more detailed descriptions of method there and elsewhere (Schwab 1986).

Consultation to Primary Health Care Clinics

Theoretical models that help us understand linkages between mental health care and primary care clinics can be useful (Pincus 1987; Strathdee 1987), but more often than not they help us understand what we have done after the fact rather than serve as neat blueprints at the beginning stages of consultation. The example here illustrates the point.

The two primary health care clinics described in this account are part of a multisite county health care system. Clinic A, with a full-time-equivalent (FTE) provider staff (a combination of physicians, physician assistants, and nurse practitioners) of 3.1, receives 780 visits from 490 patients in a typical month. Ninety-five percent of the clientele is homeless. The most common medical problems are skin disorders, pulmonary diseases (primarily upper respiratory tract infections), trauma, and hypertension. Eighty-five percent of patients have a history of substance or alcohol abuse. Eighty-five percent also have a diagnosis of psychiatric disorder, though not necessarily chronic mental illness. Clinic B, with an FTE provider staff of 2.5, receives 800 visits from 660 different patients a month. Only 5%–10% of this population is homeless, and the concurrent diagnosis of alcohol/substance abuse and psychiatric disorder is much lower than in Clinic A, about 33%. The most common medical disorders are hypertension, diabetes, and upper respiratory tract infections.

In Portland, Oregon, as in many communities, there is distinct separation of mental health and primary care services. One problem with this arrangement is that patients do not differentiate between the two services as easily as administrators do. Many patients with psychiatric disorders seen in primary care clinics also need mental health attention but, for one reason or another, do not seek or receive it. They seem to fall into one of four categories:

1. Patients with mental illness whose disorder is not acute enough, chronic enough, or severe enough to meet established eligibility criteria (e.g., patients with dysthymia, impulse disorder, and generalized anxiety)
2. Individuals who deny the existence of a psychiatric disorder and their need for care
3. Individuals who have had negative experiences with mental health clinics and refuse to return, although they remain eligible for care
4. Mentally ill patients who are no longer welcome in mental health facilities because of past troublesome behavior

Also in Portland, as in many communities, there are few individuals in primary health care settings who possess the psychiatric expertise to help these unfortunate patients. Furthermore, there remains a stigma about mental illness that causes some health care workers to shy away from psychiatric patients, to use dismissive labels, or to attribute problems to laziness or malingering. Also, they often express a sense of futility about psychiatric treatment.

Consultation to the two primary care clinics in the Portland inner-city area began with an invitation to the mental health clinic director, a psychiatrist, to present a 4-hour seminar to the staffs of the two primary care clinics. The need was acute. Providers in the primary care clinics found themselves caring for an increasing number of psychiatric patients discharged from the state hospital. They felt inadequate to diagnose them or manage psychotropic medications and were frustrated by the scarcity and inaccessibility of mental health services. The initial consultation sessions provided by the psychiatrist focused on psychotropic medications. The sessions were so useful, appreciated, and necessary that the consultant agreed to return to each clinic for $1^{1}/_{2}$ hours each month. These consultations, initiated more than 4 years ago, are ongoing at the present time.

Consultation has broadened, however, to include not only education but also case consultation and, occasionally, direct service. No payment was offered to, or any fee demanded by, the psychiatric consultant, as the arrangement was of a quid pro quo nature: the primary care clinics received psychiatric consultation and improved access to psychiatric care, and the mental health consultant was instrumental in facilitating referrals of psychiatric patients to the primary care clinics. Furthermore, because of his affiliation with the medical school's psychiatry department, he was able to attract several third- and fourth-year residents to take electives in his public mental health clinic. As part of their jobs, they were encouraged to provide several consultations to five other primary care clinics within the county during their 6- to 12-month rotations.

From the standpoint of the providers working in the primary care clinics, psychiatric consultation arrived none too soon. One of the physician assistants working in Clinic A, whose training was in family practice, estimated that fewer than 40% of her caseload consisted of medical patients; more than 60% were psychiatric. Major diagnoses, excluding diagnoses of alcohol and drug abuse, were major depression, bipolar illness, personality disorder, posttraumatic stress syndrome, dementia, mental retardation, and schizophrenia.

Also in Clinic A, a psychiatric nurse kept track of 47 consecutive patients referred to her during a 7-month period while she was working there 4 hours a week. Thirty-four were men, and 13 were women. Seven were from minority groups. Thirty-five (74%) had a history or a current diagnosis of substance abuse, primarily alcohol. The diagnostic breakdown was

Affective disorder	18
Schizophrenia	10
Posttraumatic stress syndrome	6
Personality disorder	6
Organic mental disorder	3
Generalized anxiety disorder	1
Other	3

All providers agreed on several points after psychiatric consultation was established. First, their feeling of confidence in managing psychiatric problems was enhanced. Second, cooperation between the two agencies was improved: the level of communication about cases rose and accessibility for selected patients to the mental health clinic was facilitated. Third, patients began to keep their appointments more often once they were referred to the mental health clinics. As one psychiatric nurse said, "Since I appear to be part of the primary health care system, clients were able to slide over into getting mental health services without first having to define themselves as mentally ill." Fourth, patients got better care. Countless numbers of patients with mood disorder, for example, had been receiving either lithium or antidepressants for years, and nothing else: no psychotherapy, counseling, or case management. With better access to the mental health facility, they received these services more often.

From the consultant psychiatrist's viewpoint, the staff at the primary health care clinics clearly became more confident about their ability to diagnose mental illness and use medication appropriately (more antidepressants, fewer benzodiazepines). Also, they learned when and how to refer patients for mental health consultation or services and were more comfortable managing the mental and emotional problems of patients who refused referral to mental health.

Several examples illustrate the ways patients were treated in the primary care and mental health clinics after the liaison was established. In the first three instances the individuals were patients in the primary care clinics:

A 37-year-old male recovering from drug and alcohol addiction presented with a severe depression that initially responded to antidepressants. He suffered a relapse, however, and even with trials of different antidepressants remained unimproved. A consultation referral to the visiting psychiatrist was initiated and further recommendations for therapy (the addition of lithium to the medication regimen, in this case) were made. The patient improved and continues to be followed by the nurse practitioner in the primary care clinic.

A 31-year-old woman, also recovering from alcohol and drug abuse, complained that a microchip had been implanted in her brain at birth and that thousands of women could talk to her through it. A diagnosis of schizophrenia was made by the primary health care provider, a neuroleptic was started, and the patient was then referred to the mental health clinic for case and medication management. She continues to be followed in the primary care clinic for gynecological care and disulfiram (Antabuse) monitoring.

A 54-year-old woman, a long-standing patient in the primary care clinic, was delusional and perhaps showing early evidence of dementia. Because of temper outbursts, she was in danger of losing her subsidized housing. She was referred by the primary care clinic to the mental health clinic for medication consultation. She did not trust the mental health system, however, and would not accept the referral. A physician's assistant at the clinic, after case consultation over the telephone, is currently prescribing fluphenazine for her.

Reciprocally, the following cases are examples of patients who were referred from the mental health facility to the primary care clinics:

A 41-year-old schizophrenic man was referred with a persistent cough. He was discovered to have asthma and is being treated for it by a primary care provider.

A 29-year-old man with bipolar affective disorder was noncompliant with his medications and drinking heavily. He was dismissed from the mental health clinic as unmanageable and referred to the primary care clinic for adminitration of his psychotropic medications(!). He has stopped drinking, is taking lithium, and is currently eligible for re-referral back to the mental health clinic.

A 33-year-old woman with bipolar disorder, posttraumatic stress disorder, and a history of drug and alcohol abuse was referred to the primary care clinic for a physical examination. She would not take lithium, which was indicated for her bipolar disorder, until a good relationship had developed between her and the physician's assistant in the primary care clinic. After several weeks and a psychiatric case consultation, she agreed to take lithium and continues to receive her medication from her primary care provider, even though she sees a counselor regularly at the mental health clinic.

These examples of cooperation are heartening. Because of improved care for patients and more satisfaction on the part of providers, one yearns for the expansion of cooperative ventures such as the modest one described here. To provide mental health consultation to a target population of 168,000 individuals served by seven primary health care clinics that in fact provide 175,000 visits to 39,400 patients in a typical year, a team with a minimum of a full-time psychiatric nurse, a half-time nurse practitioner, and 0.2 FTE psychiatrist would be required. Ideally, however, a full-time psychiatric nurse and a full-time psychiatric nurse practitioner at each site, in addition to a 1.0 FTE psychiatrist to rotate through all seven sites, would be best.

Unfortunately, even a minimal mental health team that could expand its services to the five remaining primary care centers in the Portland metropolitan area could not be established. Issues of power, control, and—not least—money intervened. The original arrangement between the mental health psychiatrist and the two primary care clinics remains at the core of the consultation arrangement described here.

Nursing Home Consultation

Nursing home residents represent another population that is underserved by psychiatry. Available data suggest that less than 1% of all patients in nursing homes receive explicit mental home interventions, although as many as 70%–90% in this setting suffer from some form of mental disorder (Borson et al. 1987; Curlik et al. 1991; Grossberg et al. 1990). The nursing home consultation described here arose the same way consultation to the primary care clinics did: in response to an urgent need. A faculty psychiatrist was called by a social worker at a nursing home and asked if he would come, just once, to the home and consult with the staff about an elderly demented woman who was agitated and aggressive. Transfer to another nursing home or a state hospital was being considered, but staff wondered if any psychiatric intervention could be helpful before such a move was taken.

The first visit turned into a 17-year, weekly continuing consultation meeting to a 124-bed nursing home that offers skilled nursing, intermediate, and residential care. A total of 200 residents live in the home each year, most of them permanently. The death rate each year is 15%. The residents' average age is 84.8 years. Seventy-nine percent are women, and 21% are men. Sixty percent are on Medicaid, and 40% pay privately.

The consultant faced two particular problems at the beginning of the consultation process. First, residents were presented without background information, so that he knew nothing about them except their current troublesome or worrisome behavior. A related problem was that no context was described for the troublesome behavior: no immediate circumstances, precipitating events, or triggering episodes. Second, the consultant felt great pressure from the staff to prescribe psychotropic medications, particularly for patients who were agitated or aggressive.

These problems were resolved only over time. Structure—organization—is critical for effective consultation. A regular 2-hour block of time each week was set aside for the meeting. The psychiatric consultant taught the staff what information was needed to make psychiatric diagnoses (U'Ren 1987), and a standard history and mental status form is currently being used. The principle that behavior rarely takes place without a context was emphasized, and over many sessions the staff became aware of the appropriate use of psychotropics, particularly neuroleptics; their side effects; and the value of social, behavioral, and environmental interventions.

Currently, the first hour and 15 minutes of the consultation period is devoted to presentation of five to eight cases. New cases are presented formally by the social work director at the rate of one every other week. The remaining 45 minutes of the session are spent interviewing two to four of the patients who have been discussed and/or talking with family members. At the end of the session, notes are dictated on patients interviewed. The consultant is available by telephone throughout the week, but in fact calls are infrequent, rarely more than two a month.

The consultant provides case consultation, direct service to the residents, and education and training for the staff. Occasional didactic sessions are held (e.g., the definition and causes of dementia, the uses and side effects of neuroleptics, and criteria for delirium), but most of the training takes place around individual case presentations, aided by liberal use of didactic questions to the staff: What do you think is going on? What do you make of that? What do you think we should do? In regular attendance at the sessions are the assistant head nurse, the head of social work, the assistant head of social work, and the nurse responsible for the resident's care. Students and residents on elective, nursing aides, and the nursing home director attend intermittently. A relatively large group of people at consultation rounds is helpful. Multiple reports on a particular patient provide the consultant with more information on which to make a considered judgment. Brainstorming about treatment issues, which is freely encouraged, is also facilitated by the larger group.

It is difficult to prescribe what tone a nursing home consultation should possess, but at least one could say that it should be cheerful rather than morbid. Coffee, pastries, and a sense of humor help. Whatever the consultant can do to bring excitement, enthusiasm, and hope to what some might mistakenly consider a dreary setting is good. The following cases are two examples of nursing home consultation:

An 86-year-old man with moderately severe dementia living in the residential section of the home was presented for medication review. Staff reported that he could not settle down for the night after he went to his room in mid-evening. He would come out of his room and insist, for example, that he be shaved, that staff call his son, or that he be taken to activities, which of course were held only during the day. He asked repetitively, "Where should I go?" "Where should I be?" His medications included digoxin, furosemide, oxazepam (15 mg at 4 P.M. and 8 P.M.), and an as-needed order for 15 mg temazepam, which he was given not more than three times a month. His digoxin level was normal. The temazepam was discontinued after consultation, and the oxazepam was tapered and discontinued within a week.

After 2 weeks his behavior remained unchanged, however, and a 2-mg dose of perphenazine was prescribed at 5 P.M. After 2 more weeks, no change in his behavior had occurred, and the dose was raised to 4 mg. There was still no change in his moderately disruptive behavior in the evenings, and in addition, he wandered out of the building on a couple of occasions. The staff, afraid for his safety, arranged for his transfer from the residential section of the home to the intermediate care facility, which provided more supervision and more company. His troublesome behavior disappeared within a few days and 10 days later the perphenazine was discontinued. In retrospect, it was clear that he needed more structure and attention during his evening bouts of disorientation than he was able to get in the residential section of the home.

An 82-year-old woman with moderately severe dementia and tardive dyskinesia secondary to previous neuroleptic use was presented in consultation rounds because she had become increasingly restless and irritable. She had begun to go into the kitchen at all times of the day demanding milk and food. She had been taking 4 mg of perphenazine to control her dyskinesia, but it was possible that her increased restlessness represented akathisia, and the neuroleptic was discontinued. Several subsequent discussions with staff focused on how to keep her out of the kitchen, as her presence there during busy times was thought to be unsafe. The possibility of having a lock installed on the kitchen door (at great inconvenience to other people) and the suggestion that no one talk to her if she was in the kitchen at an inappropriate time, thus eliminating social reinforcement, were considered. The problem was solved, however, when one staff member put a small glass of milk on a snack tray in the living room of the home in mid-afternoon. The patient's wandering into the kitchen ceased immediately.

These examples are typical of the combined pharmacological-social interventions that are usually tried in response to behavior problems.

From 1982 to 1992 (minus 1 year when the consultant was away), 197 new patients were presented in consultation rounds. Sixty-seven percent had either Alzheimer's, vascular, or mixed dementia. Seventeen percent had primary mood disorder, 5% had Parkinson's disease with behavioral or mood problems, and 11% had other diagnoses. The most common presentations of those with Alzheimer's disease alone were agitation (38%), dysphoria (17%), and delirium (9%). One study revealed that the major behavioral problems associated with dementia are agitation, withdrawal, and noisiness (Everitt et al. 1991).

During 1991–1992, a typical year, 20 new patients were presented, and a total of 49 patients (29 from the previous year) were discussed. The total number of discussions about these 49 individuals was 288; 66 (23%) of these discussions included an interview with the patient. The average number of discussions about each patient during the year was six. Each year about 15% of the patients, most of them with behavioral problems associated with dementia, take up 45% of the total consultation time.

Only one patient per year is referred to the hospital for psychiatric reasons; the vast majority of problems can be handled within the home, although one must remember that behavioral problems tend to be cyclical in nature, and some of the improvement may be due less to planned specific intervention than to other less clearly defined processes such as mutual adaptation between patient and staff (Cumming et al. 1982).

During 1993–1994, 28 (57%) of the patients presented in consultation rounds were exposed to psychotropic drugs. Medications were altered (prescribed, discontinued, or dose changed) in 36% of the consultations. The most common medications prescribed were neuroleptics (59%), benzodiazepines (14%), and antidepressants (12%); lithium, antihistamines, and anticonvulsants accounted for the remainder. When neuroleptics were initially prescribed or their dose raised (which occurred 50% of the time), improvement was observed 54% of the time; worsening, 3% of the time; and no change, 42% of the time. When the neuroleptic dose was lowered or the medication discontinued, improvement was reported 27% of the time; worsening, 16% of the time; and no change, 57% of the time. Another study elsewhere found that when the neuroleptics were discontinued in demented nursing home patients, 22% showed no change, 22% got worse, and 55% improved (Risse et al. 1987). Consultants know how helpful neuroleptics can be in selected cases of behavior disorder, but the case for discontinuing them, especially after the acute phase of disturbance has passed, is compelling.

After regular consultation was initiated, benefits to the staff fell into four categories.

1. The staff learned what constituted an adequate psychiatric evaluation and became more sensitive to diagnostic issues, particularly those that pertain to dementia, depression, and delirium. They also became more aware that medical illnesses can cause psychiatric symptoms and came to appreciate that dementia could account for troublesome behaviors that had been previously considered willful.
2. They became familiar with the specific indications for the various psychotropic drugs; the side effects of these drugs, particularly neuroleptic agents; and, perhaps most important, the limitations of psychopharmacology. After seeing the side effects of medication, especially lethargy, akinesia, and tardive dyskinesia, the outright failure of drugs to work in some situations (e.g., perseverative yelling), and the success of socioenvironmental measures in other instances, the staff became less likely to press for drug solutions to behavioral problems.
3. By sharing and generating new ideas and approaches in the treatment of problems, the staff expanded their repertoire of nonpharmacological responses to behavioral problems.
4. Staff said that they appreciated both the regularity and structure of weekly rounds that gave them access to a health care professional who knew the residents in a setting that encouraged easy exchange of information. They felt that their opinions and observations were taken seriously. They received confirmation from other staff members and from the consultant that behavioral problems were often difficult to manage, thus relieving them of feelings of personal inadequacy. Furthermore, when problems seemed at least temporarily intractable, they welcomed the chance to express their feelings about them. They viewed rounds also as

a setting in which they could discuss management problems reflectively, and they believed that as a result of consultation rounds, they knew and understood the residents better, which made for more individualization of approach, more interest in what was often difficult work, and better morale.

Concluding Comments

Both consulting arrangements, for better or for worse, were initiated in response to urgent need and were not preceded by careful planning. Structure, especially in the nursing home consultation, came afterward. Both arrangements provided some combination of case consultation, direct service, and training. All involved staff reported and demonstrated more confidence in working with their patients as a result of consultation. Their diagnostic skills improved, they felt more confident about the efficacy of psychosocial intervention, and they gained an appreciation of the benefits and problems of medications, as well as a better understanding of what psychiatrists can and cannot do. In the mental health–primary care clinic consultation, referral between agencies was facilitated. As a result, patients received better care.

Financial support for such consultation arrangements, however, remains problematic. The consultant to the primary care center took on the job because of the quid pro quo advantages of the arrangement, which meant improved access to services of both agencies. However, the absence of funding leaves the position itself vulnerable to elimination if the consultant moves on. Also, lack of funds made expansion of psychiatric services to other primary care clinics impossible. Still, from the point of view of the mental health center, the consultation established an important linkage, improved the image of the center by its offer of help, and created an atmosphere for future development opportunities, should circumstances change.

Payment was not a problem in the nursing home consultation, as the home paid the psychiatrist a retainer fee that covered 90% of his usual hourly office fee. Generally, however, payment is a problem in nursing home consultation. Compensation for nursing home work is about half that for private practice outpatient work for the same amount of time; income for a nursing home practice is not comparable to that for office work (Borson et al. 1987). Unless this is changed, it will remain a disincentive for psychiatric nursing home consultation.

For the consultants themselves, the rewards of working with groups in settings that are not traditionally the most glamorous were several. Staff appreciation was high in both settings, and seeing confidence and competence grow in a staff is pleasing, as is collaboration with a group of interested individuals trying to help others. The opportunity to share—and show—one's knowledge and expertise, as well as to improve it through experience, is rewarding. Consultations such as these add variety and, hence, interest to one's professional life; the money, if forthcoming, is welcome; and most patients that one sees personally or hears about from others improve or are stabilized often enough for optimism to be maintained. The opportunity to collaborate with, support, and influence other community agencies also broadens and deepens the community psychiatrist's work.

The place of psychiatry, after the reorganization of the American health care system has been completed, is currently unclear. Will mental health achieve financial parity with the rest of medicine, for example? What seems safe to predict, at least, is that there will be more demand for psychiatric knowledge on the part of primary care providers. This will enable such providers either to refer more judiciously or to take care of patients who require integrated care. The future of psychiatric consultation to community organizations is harder to predict. What is indisputable is the need. How it will be addressed is uncertain.

References

Berlin I: New approaches in school mental health consultation, in Mental Health Consultation in Community Settings. Edited by Rogawski AS. San Francisco, CA, Jossey-Bass, 1979, pp 1–11

Bloom BL: Community Mental Health: A General Introduction. Monterey, CA, Brooks-Cole, 1975

Borson S, Liptzin D, Nininger J, et al: Psychiatry and the nursing home. Am J Psychiatry 144:1412–1418, 1987

Budson RD: Consultation to halfway houses, in Mental Health Consultations in Community Settings. Edited by Rogawski AS. San Francisco, CA, Jossey-Bass, 1979, pp 41–57

Caplan G: Principles of Preventive Psychiatry. New York, Basic Books, 1964

Caplan G: The Theory and Practice of Mental Health Consultation. New York, Basic Books, 1970

Caplan G, Caplan RB: Mental Health Consultation and Collaboration. San Francisco, CA, Jossey-Bass, 1993

Cumming J, Cumming E, Titus J, et al: The episodic nature of behavioral disturbances among residents of facilities for the aged. Can J Public Health 73:319–322, 1982

Curlik SM, Frazier D, Katz IR: Psychiatric aspects of long-term care, in Comprehensive Review of Geriatric Psychiatry. Edited by Sadavoy J, Lazarus LW, Jardik LF. Washington, DC, American Psychiatric Press, 1991, pp 547–564

Everitt DE, Fields DR, Soumerai SS, et al: Resident behavior and staff distress in the nursing home. J Am Geriatr Soc 39:792–798, 1991

Grossberg GT, Hassan R, Szwabo PA, et al: Psychiatric problems in the nursing home. J Am Geriatr Soc 38:907–917, 1990

Karno M, Schwartz D: Community Mental Health: Reflections and Explorations. New York, Wiley, 1974

Pincus HA: Patient-oriented models for linking primary care and mental health care. Gen Hosp Psychiatry 9:95–101, 1987

Reiser M: Police consultations, in Mental Health Consultations in Community Settings. Edited by Rogawski AS. San Francisco, CA, Jossey-Bass, 1979, pp 73–83

Risse SC, Cubberley L, Lampe TH, et al: Acute effects of neuroleptic withdrawal in elderly dementia patients. Journal of Geriatric Drug Therapy 2:65–77, 1987

Robinowitz CB: Consultation in mental retardation and developmental disabilities, in Mental Health Consultations in Community Settings. Edited by Rogawski AS. San Francisco, CA, Jossey-Bass, pp 13–24, 1979

Schwab JJ: Mental health consultants: psychiatrists' roles and functions in the 1980s, in Handbook of Mental Health Consultation. Edited by Mannino FV, Trickett EJ, Shore MF, et al. Rockville, MD, National Institute of Mental Health, U.S. Department of Health and Human Services, 1986, pp 115–144

Strathdee G: Primary care-psychiatry interaction: a British perspective. Gen Hosp Psychiatry 9:102–110, 1987

U'Ren RC: Testing older patients' mental status: practical office-based approach. Geriatrics 42:49–56, 1987

Chapter 25

Ethical and Legal Issues

Gregory B. Leong, M.D.
Spencer Eth, M.D.

T he same ethical and legal mandates indigenous to the psychiatric profession as a whole also confront psychiatrists employed by community mental health centers (CMHCs). Some of the working conditions within the CMHC can affect the ability of the CMHC psychiatrist to discharge these ethical and legal responsibilities. CMHCs may not administratively adhere to the traditional medical model, but rather follow a multidisciplinary treatment team model, with clinical authority diffused or concentrated in other mental health disciplines. Such a decentralized model may bring the CMHC psychiatrist into conflict with other mental health professionals when ethical and legal issues arise concerning the treatment of psychiatric patients. Regardless of the prevailing CMHC's administrative structure, the general public and the legal system commonly view the CMHC psychiatrist as bearing primary responsibility for patient care. It is therefore imperative that CMHC psychiatrists perform their clinical duties consonant with their ethical and legal responsibilities, irrespective of the administrative leadership at the CMHC.

The CMHC psychiatrist is first and foremost a physician who specializes in psychiatry. As such, all the tenets of American medical ethics apply to the clinical practice of the CMHC psychiatrist. Psychiatrists are bound by the principles of medical ethics adopted by the American Medical Association (AMA) and the American Psychiatric Association (APA), regardless of whether they are members of these organizations. Because of the special situations encountered in psychiatric practice, the general medical guidelines have been expanded for psychiatrist, as recorded in the current edition of *The Principles of Medical Ethics With Annotations Especially Applicable to Psychiatry* (APA 1992a). In addition, the Ethics Committee of the APA has formulated opinions in response to specific questions concerning ethical problems arising in clinical practice in *Opinions of the Ethics Committee on the Principles of Medical Ethics With Annotations Especially Applicable to Psychiatry* (APA 1992b). Psychiatrists should be aware of the contents of both booklets. Alleged violations of these ethical guidelines by APA members will lead to formal ethics proceedings, which can result in admonishment, reprimand, suspension, or expulsion from the national organization and its local branches (APA 1992a). Moreover, an adverse action by the APA of suspension or expulsion resulting from an ethical complaint requires the filing of a report with the National Practitioner Data Bank, as outlined in the previously cited booklets.

CMHC psychiatrists are bound by all state statutes and codes pertaining to the practice of medicine, as well by any federal regulations that may supersede or extend state law. In many states psychiatrists are considered not only physicians, but also psychotherapists and are therefore also subject to special laws that additionally define the clinical practice of psychotherapists. For example, some states have enacted criminal sanctions for sexual contact between the psychotherapist and the patient. In this instance, a psychiatrist must conform to this prohibition, even though the behavior of other medical specialists is not similarly restricted.

Because the domain of the ethical and legal issues arising in mental health practice is so large and varied, this chapter will focus on two paradigmatic issues that have particular relevance to the CMHC psychiatrist: confidentiality and dangerousness. Other cogent ethical and legal topics are covered in works devoted to the subjects of medical and psychiatric ethics and forensic psychiatry (Appelbaum and Gutheil 1991; Beauchamp and Childress 1979; Bloch and Chodoff 1984; Rosner 1994; Simon 1992).

Confidentiality

General Considerations

The Western notion of medical confidentiality was clearly articulated by Hippocrates: "Whatsoever things I see or hear concerning the life of man, in any attendance on the sick or even apart therefrom, which ought not to be voiced about, I will keep silent thereon" (from the Hippocratic Oath [APA 1987, p. 1522]). Our current ethical guideline pertaining to confidentiality appears in Section 4 of the principles of medical ethics (APA 1992a): "A physician shall respect the rights of patients, of colleagues, and of other health professionals, and shall safeguard patient confidences within the constraints of the law" (p. 2).

Any discussion of confidentiality must begin by differentiating it from the concept of (testimonial) privilege. *Privilege* is a legal term that allows the holder of the privilege to prevent confidential communications from being admitted into a judicial proceedings (Simon 1992). For example, unless there is an automatic waiver of privilege, a psychiatrist may not testify about the contents of a patient's psychotherapy sessions unless the patient gives the psychiatrist permission to do so, because the patient is the holder of the privilege in a psychotherapist-patient relationship (in those states where such privilege exists). In their elemental forms, confidentiality is an ethical canon, and privilege is a legal right. However, informally, confidentiality and privilege are often used interchangeably.

The first medical confidentiality law in the United States did not appear until 1828 in New York state (Weinstock et al. 1990). Laws governing medical confidentiality currently are widely found in statutes governing physician-patient and psychotherapist-patient privilege and medical records, as well as in other areas of a state's business and professional codes. Case law, which is based on decisions by an appellate-level court, also helps to determine the parameters of what may remain confidential (Appelbaum and Gutheil 1991). The law, however, cannot cover every hypothetical situation, and an ethical and legal analysis may be needed in novel circumstances.

Primary ethical principles flow from one of two broad philosophical perspectives. The *utilitarian perspective* emphasizes that the benefits served by medical confidentiality outweigh any resulting harms. In this ethical framework the likely negative consequence of a violation of confidentiality between physician and patient is seen to have a deterrent effect on other patients who would avoid seeking necessary treatment for fear of a loss of privacy. In the alternative *deontological perspective*, physicians are deemed to have a moral duty to preserve medical confidentiality, because the patient was induced to reveal personal information in the context of a fiduciary relationship in which privacy is implicitly or explicit promised (Appelbaum and Gutheil 1991).

Specific Situations

Because of the interdisciplinary nature of the CMHC, many mental health care providers may be involved in a patient's treatment. The more practitioners there are, the greater the risk of a breach in confidentiality, and a heightened awareness of this issue is indicated.

The CMHC psychiatrist may be called on to assume the role of the child and adolescent psychiatrist in conjunction with a nonmedically trained child psychotherapist. Although the psychiatrist may not have completed a child and adolescent psychiatry fellowship, he or she may nonetheless be needed to provide psychiatric services to these patients. The custodial parent(s) of children and adolescents, or *minors* in legal parlance, have the legal authority to make decisions and be informed about the minor's health care, unless the minor is "emancipated" under local state law or under certain conditions granted by local state law, such as when receiving treatment for a sexually transmitted disease. Although by law custodial parents should be kept fully informed of their child's treatment, psychiatric ethics favors respecting the confidentiality interests of older, morally autonomous children, especially in instances where a limitation of parental access to treatment information protects sensitive, embarrassing, or inflammatory material. This may be especially true for patients who have already entered adolescence, whose claim for confidentiality in the treatment process parallels that of adults.

Family therapy is often prescribed as an adjunct to the treatment of the individual child or adolescent patient. Maintaining confidentiality may be especially problematic depending on which family member is the identified patient and which family members have individual CMHC medical records. Care should be taken regarding what is recorded in the psychiatric (medical) record, especially with regard to information involving other family members, as the information contained in an individual patient's chart can be released with only the consent of that patient. One suggestion for addressing this problem is to have all of the family members in treatment sign a statement prior to beginning therapy acknowledging that their records might contain information about other family members and specifying which member(s) must consent before the information can be given to others (APA 1987). This contract may have to be renegotiated when the family constellation changes (e.g., by marriage or divorce, or when a minor reaches the age of majority).

Analogous to the confidentiality problems encountered in family therapy are the dilemmas of maintaining confidentiality in the group therapy setting. In only a very limited number of jurisdictions are group therapy members legally required to maintain the secrecy of communications arising from group therapy sessions (Simon 1992). It is therefore essential for the psychiatrist to inform prospective group therapy members, especially at the time of entry into the group, about their personal responsibility to maintain confidentiality, as well as any limitations posed by law. The treating psychiatrist can minimize the risk of an unintended breach of confidentiality by safeguarding identifiable information about other group therapy patients in the medical records of group members (APA 1987). Although the psychiatrist could also choose to maintain a separate record of the group's interactions (APA 1987), depending on the jurisdiction, this extra record may not be entirely protected from confidentiality breaches, and prudent care must be exercised even when employing a separate record of overall group processes.

After a patient dies, the psychiatrist's ethical and legal responsibilities toward the deceased patient endure. However, local state law may permit access to the patient's health records by executors or administrators of the patient's estate or by the next of kin (APA 1987).

The CMHC psychiatrists may be called on to evaluate and treat patients on behalf or by request of a third party. Examples include evaluation or treatment requested (ordered) by the courts, employers, governmental agencies, military, prisons, worker's compensation boards, or employee assistance programs. Care must be taken on several fronts. First, the patient should be aware of the compromise of confidentiality imposed by the involvement of a third party. An initial warning about the limitations of confidentiality probably satisfies a legal standard (see, e.g., *Estelle v. Smith* 1981) but not necessarily an ethical one. "Slippage," or lessening of the effect of the warning, can occur as the evaluation or treatment progresses (American Academy of Psychiatry and the Law 1991), in part because of the psychotherapeutic skills of the psychiatrist in uncovering potentially damaging material. The patient may need to be reinformed at intervals over the course of therapy (Leong et al. 1990). Second, the psychiatrist should limit, in the record as well as in any communication to the third party, any extraneous material that the individual has disclosed (APA 1987, 1992a).

In a free-standing CMHC, depending on local state law, the patient's record may have a different status than a medical record. Distinguishing between a medical (health) record and a psychiatric (mental health) record may be more difficult if the CMHC has a de jure or even a de facto connection with a hospital or outpatient medical clinic. Nevertheless, there are more similarities than differences. In many jurisdictions psychiatrists are required to maintain contemporaneous and retrievable records of the patients for whom they have medical responsibility (APA 1987). For psychiatric patients, the record is especially important when questions of suicidality, dangerousness, and involuntary treatment arise (APA 1987). For the psychiatrist in the CMHC setting in which a nonphysician mental health care provider is the patient's case manager or primary clinician and the psychiatrist's contact with the patient is limited, the CMHC record may be especially significant. At the opposite end of the spectrum, limiting extraneous and irrelevant material is important, particularly in the CMHC setting, where a large staff have ready access to the record. In addition, although computers have greatly facilitated health and mental health care, they have also increased the risk of confidentiality breaches (Wolkon and Lyon 1986). It is the practice of some psychiatrists to record a second set of notes *(process notes)* for the purpose of documenting the unfolding of a dynamic psychotherapeutic treatment. Local state law determines whether this separate set of notes constitutes a part of the official CMHC record and the information contained in it is only as confidential as the CMHC record, or if the notes are granted extra protection because they are the sole property of the psychiatrist.

Although the CMHC owns the physical record (i.e., the folder and paper itself), the information contained within belongs to the patient. Unless there is a legally permitted exception, the patient retains the power to decide whether the contents of his or her record can be released to a third party. An exception includes third-party payers and legitimate accreditation surveyors. Here, as in other comparable situations of information disclosure, only the minimal amount of data required for the CMHC to accomplish the stated purpose (e.g., reimbursement) should be released. Copies of the patient's medical or psychiatric records obtained from other sources generally must have a separate authorization from the patient for their release, even though they are routinely placed in the patient's CMHC record (APA 1987).

Patients themselves may desire to read or possess a copy of their medical records. For health care records, this usually does not pose much risk. In contrast, access to a patient's own mental health record can be problematic and can negatively affect the patient. States differ as to the procedures by which patients can gain access to their psychiatric records. Although some states limit one's ability to obtain mental health records, the patient can always have the psychiatric record sent to another physician (or psychotherapist) of his or her choice (APA 1987). It is also possible to offer a patient a redacted copy of the record so as to minimize a deleterious reaction. Ultimately, the patient's attorney can subpoena the records to ensure their delivery to the patient.

Exceptions to Confidentiality

Medical and psychiatric confidentiality is not absolute. Many of the exceptions to confidentiality constitute legally sanctioned waivers of privilege. The most familiar example of an exception to the principle of psychiatrist-patient confidentiality arises in response to one of many mandatory reporting laws. Depending on local state laws, the CMHC psychiatrist may be required to breach confidentiality and report certain information about patients in his or her role either as a physician or as a psychotherapist (Leong et al. 1992). Nonpsychiatric physicians are not subject to the confidentiality exceptions operating for psychotherapists, and nonmedical psychotherapists are not subject to the exceptions operating for physicians, unless the rules specifically overlap, as in the case of child abuse reporting.

Reporting laws applicable to psychiatrists as physicians or psychotherapists include notifying the appropriate authorities regarding patients with gunshot wounds, specified communicable diseases, or lapses of consciousness and children and elders suspected of having been abused or neglected. There may be many other reporting requirements depending on local state law. Some jurisdictions require that patients diagnosed as suffering from Alzheimer's disease and related dementias be reported to the state department of motor vehicles (Eth and Leong 1992). Mandatory reporting laws have been enacted to protect dependent members of society or the public at large, despite their intrusion on the privacy of the treatment relationship.

Other exceptions to the rule of maintaining strict confidentiality may occur during involuntary hospitalization proceedings, court-ordered evaluations, will contests, child custody disputes, child abuse proceedings, or a legally required report, and when the psychiatric patient-litigant exception applies (Simon 1992). The patient-litigant exception arises when the patient places his or her mental state at issue, such as in the filing of a worker's compensation claim, personal injury suit, or malpractice action in the civil arena, or raises the insanity defense in the criminal arena. Even when an exception to confidentiality is in operation, care should be exercised in providing information relevant to the issue involved and in limiting the amount of irrelevant or extraneous information (Appelbaum 1984).

Most CMHC psychiatrists at some point in their careers will be served with a subpoena. A subpoena compels a court appearance only. A subpoena duces tecum orders that the medical (psychiatric) record be brought to court. A subpoena ad testificandum requires the psychiatrist to testify. The subpoena does not necessarily mean the patient has given permission to disclose the contents of the record. If, however, the patient has given permission or waived his or her privilege automatically, as in the case of the patient-litigant exception, then the psychiatrist must disclose the previously private information (*In re Lifschutz* 1970). However, if the information might be irrelevant and extraneous to the case at hand, then the psychiatrist, with an attorney's assistance, may request an in camera (private) review by the judge to determine whether part or all of the information is relevant for the case and should be disclosed in court.

Dangerousness

The characterization of dangerousness is driven by a legal and not a medical need. The CMHC psychiatrist will most likely evaluate a patient's dangerousness in the context of pursuing involuntary civil commitment. The standard for dangerousness—or, more accurately, the degree of danger—derives from the local state law. For example, the degree of danger needed for an emergency commitment of a CMHC outpatient differs from that required to continue the commitment of an insanity acquittee after the maximum commitment time has elapsed.

Dictionaries commonly define danger as a hazard, peril, risk, or jeopardy. Psychiatrists can describe the factors that contribute to the intensification of the threat of danger in a particular patient. In the case of emergency short-term commitment, the psychiatrist, after obtaining historical information and performing an examination, operationally determines that the patient poses a danger to self or others and proceeds with the commitment. However, this is a temporary decision only that must be reviewed by the court to sustain continuing commitment on the basis of dangerousness.

Danger to self in the form of suicidality is a more typical clinical problem than dangerousness to others. Managing a patient's suicidality usually entails careful treatment of the individual patient, as well as possible involvement of the patient's significant others. Evaluation and treatment of the patient who may harm others often provoke considerable anxiety in the psychiatrist, as the safety of third parties, perhaps even persons unknown to the psychiatrist, are in jeopardy. In this sense, there are more uncontrollable variables at play with the patient who poses a danger to others.

The psychiatrist treats a patient's mental illness to diminish the degree of danger posed by that patient; the psychiatrist does not "treat" dangerousness. Although it appears the legal system would like psychiatrists to predict future dangerousness, psychiatrists can only try to assess present dangerousness or dangerousness in the immediate future. The exacerbating and ameliorating factors that may be present one day can easily change the next day. The requisite expertise in assessing dangerousness derives first and foremost from evaluating the mental status of the patient and then describing the relationship of the present mental state to various factors that can affect the likelihood the patient will commit acts harmful to self or others. In particular, psychiatrists attempt to make informed judgments regarding the magnitude, likelihood, and imminence of the potential harm (Monahan 1981).

Although dangerousness to others encompasses more than simply the danger of physical harm to others, for practical purpose the evaluation of dangerousness involves only this domain of violent behavior. In addition, physical violence is more conducive to study, as physical injury is readily observed, unlike a psychological injury. Progress in the methodology of forecasting the risk of short-term physical violence in controlled settings has shown promise (Brizer and Crowner 1989). Moreover, research has identified several biopsychosocial and demographic risk factors for violence (Monahan and Steadman 1994). Despite the clinical utility of these findings to permit more accurate identification of patients fitting a high-risk profile for interpersonal violence, the psychiatrist should base an opinion as to a patient's degree of danger on the patient's mental condition and its relationship to case-specific variables.

When a patient presents as an immediate danger to another, the psychiatric agenda is generally clear: involuntary commitment. Even outside of the zone of imminence, there is a tendency to err on the side of pursuing civil commitment because of societal pressure (Appelbaum 1988; Petrunik 1982). In those instances when the threatening patient is not hospitalized, either on a voluntary or involuntary basis, then the duty to warn or protect, the so-called *Tarasoff*-type duty, may be considered to apply in many states.

In brief, the *Tarasoff* decision originally imposed on psychotherapists a duty to warn (*Tarasoff v. Regents of the University of California* 1974); this was supplanted by a psychiatric duty to protect after a definitive rehearing by the California Supreme Court (*Tarasoff v. Regents of the University of California* 1976). The *Tarasoff* case involved Prosenjit Poddar, a foreign student at the University of California, Berkeley, who communicated to his treating Student Health Service psychotherapist his desire to kill his girlfriend, Tatiana Tarasoff, a fellow student. After Poddar did, in fact, kill Tarasoff, her family filed a negligence action against the university contending, among other things, that the psychotherapist had failed to inform Tatiana Tarasoff of the danger posed by Poddar. In the second *Tarasoff* decision, the California Supreme Court ruled that psychotherapists in California have an affirmative duty to protect an endangered third party whenever a patient poses a serious threat of physical harm (*Tarasoff v. Regents of the University of California* 1976). The court, however, suggested that warning the third party of the patient's threat was but one method to discharge that duty to protect. Other clinical methods include reasonable inpatient or outpatient treatment interventions designed to diminish the patient's level of dangerousness.

In the years since the duty to protect was applied to California's psychotherapists, many other states have adopted similar precedents (Simon and

Sadoff 1992). Because the *Tarasoff* cases were the first to address a psychiatric duty to warn and a psychiatric duty to protect, subsequent cases that in any way pertain to this duty are often known as "*Tarasoff*-type" cases. However, local state law determines the specific confines of the duty to warn or protect. At least one state, Vermont, has extended the duty to protect to include property (Stone 1986). In some jurisdictions, *Tarasoff*-type cases have involved a psychiatric patient driving an automobile and subsequently injuring others (Felthous 1990; Pettis 1992). Such cases have intensified the apprehension of psychiatrists and other mental health clinicians treating psychiatric patients who have the potential to harm others, whether they have a homicidal mental state, as Poddar had, or merely possess the means to commit homicide, such as a car.

Because of the constant expansion of *Tarasoff*-type case law and the alarm raised in the psychiatric community fueled mainly by malpractice actions, *Tarasoff*-type immunity statutes have been enacted in several states (Appelbaum et al. 1989). However, these laws have reduced professional liability exposure at the expense of clinical flexibility (Weinstock 1988). For example, in California, to enjoy immunity from a civil action in the event that a patient physically injures the threatened person, a psychotherapist must have warned the intended victim and alerted the police (California Civil Code section 43.92). However, although these procedures protect the psychotherapist from lawsuits, the clinical option of protecting the third party by treating the patient may unfortunately be superseded by the practice of issuing *Tarasoff* warnings. Of further concern are court decisions that have allowed psychotherapists to testify against their patients in a criminal trial after a *Tarasoff* warning had been enunciated (*People v. Wharton* 1991).

The *Tarasoff*-type duty is intended to offer benefit to society by enhancing public safety at the expense of confidentiality (Mills et al. 1987). However, as noted in *Tarasoff*, American medical ethics did not prohibit physicians from violating confidentiality in the event a dangerous situation could be thwarted (*Tarasoff v. Regents of the University of California* 1974). Moreover, *Tarasoff* observed that the public health model for reporting communicable diseases could be applied to breaching confidentiality. So, what appears at first glance to be a purely legal issue finds its roots in medical ethics.

Summary and Conclusions

We have explored one primarily ethical issue (confidentiality) and one principally legal issue (dangerousness). Each is directly relevant to the work of

CMHC psychiatrists. Sound clinical practice demands the recognition of patient privacy and active involvement in strategies to identify and reduce the potential for violence of psychiatric patients. Ironically, these issues are seen to be intertwined, and each raises other ethical and legal problems, such as involuntary civil commitment, malpractice, and informed consent.

We have alluded only to some of the difficulties associated with special patient populations, principally children and adolescents, encountered in the practices of CMHC psychiatrists. Increasingly, the CMHC psychiatrist may be called on to evaluate and treat geriatric patients. Issues of competence, conservatorship and guardianship, and advance directives may be of particular importance to the older patient (Eth and Leong 1992; Weinstock et al. 1994). Finally, local forensic psychiatric patients may be referred to the CMHC for evaluation and treatment. The CMHC psychiatrist may be pressed to evaluate competency to stand trial or to treat insanity acquittees on an outpatient basis. Forensic questions generate complex problems of confidentiality as well as multiple agency, and the CMHC psychiatrist must be aware of clinical-legal dilemmas that can arise in these often convoluted professional relationships.

In closing, we reiterate that an understanding of the ethical and legal aspects of the work of CMHC psychiatrists is embedded in the larger study of the ethical and legal issues involved in the practice of psychiatry. The CMHC psychiatrist as a physician and psychotherapist is best served by acquiring a broad-based knowledge of the foundation of medical ethics and forensic psychiatry.

References

American Academy of Psychiatry and the Law: Ethical Guidelines for the Practice of Forensic Psychiatry, Revised. Bloomfield, CT, American Academy of Psychiatry and the Law, 1991. Reprinted in American Academy of Psychiatry and the Law: 1993 Membership Directory, pp xi–xiv

American Psychiatric Association: Guidelines on confidentiality. Am J Psychiatry 144:1522–1526, 1987

American Psychiatric Association: Principles of Medical Ethics With Annotations Especially Applicable to Psychiatry. Washington, DC, American Psychiatry Association, 1992a

American Psychiatric Association: Opinions of the Ethics Committee on the Principles of Medical Ethics With Annotations Especially Applicable to Psychiatry. Washington, DC, American Psychiatry Association, 1992b

Appelbaum PS: Confidentiality in the forensic evaluation. Int J Law Psychiatry 7:285–300, 1984

Appelbaum PS: The new preventive detention: Psychiatry's problematic responsibility for the control of violence. Am J Psychiatry 145:779–785, 1988

Appelbaum PS, Gutheil TG: Clinical Handbook of Psychiatry and the Law, 2nd Edition. Baltimore, MD, Williams & Wilkins, 1991

Appelbaum PS, Zonana H, Bonnie R, et al: Statutory approaches to limiting psychiatrists' liability for their patients' violent acts. Am J Psychiatry 146:821–828, 1989

Beauchamp TL, Childress JF: Principles of Biomedical Ethics. New York, Oxford University Press, 1979

Bloch S, Chodoff P (eds): Psychiatric Ethics. New York, Oxford University Press, 1984

Brizer DA, Crowner ML (eds): Current Approaches to the Prediction of Violence. Washington, DC, American Psychiatric Press, 1989

Cal. Civ. Code, section 43.92

Estelle v Smith, 451 U.S. 454 (1981)

Eth S, Leong GB: Forensic and ethical issues, in Handbook of Mental Health and Aging, 2nd Edition. Edited by Birren JE, Sloane RB, Cohen GD. San Diego, CA, Academic Press, 1992, pp 853–871

Felthous AR: The duty to warn or protect to prevent automobile accidents, in American Psychiatric Press Review of Clinical Psychiatry and the Law, Vol 1. Edited by Simon RI. Washington, DC, American Psychiatric Press, 1990, pp 221–228

In re Lifschutz, 85 Cal Rptr 829 (1970)

Leong GB, Silva JA, Weinstock R: Ethical considerations of giving Miranda-type warnings in psychiatric evaluations in criminal cases, in Ethical Practice in Psychiatry and the Law. Edited by Rosner R, Weinstock R. New York, Plenum, 1990, pp 151–162

Leong GB, Silva JA, Weinstock R: Reporting dilemmas in psychiatric practice. Psychiatric Annals 22:482–486, 1992

Mills MJ, Sullivan G, Eth S: Protecting third parties: a decade after Tarasoff. Am J Psychiatry 144:68–74, 1987

Monahan J: The clinical prediction of violent behavior (DHHS Publ No (ADM) 81-921). Rockville, MD, U.S. Department of Health and Human Services, 1981

Monahan J, Steadman HJ (eds): Violence and Mental Disorder: Developments in Risk Assessment. Chicago, IL, University of Chicago Press, 1994

People v Wharton, 53 Cal 3d 522 (1991)

Petrunik M: The politics of dangerousness. Int J Law Psychiatry 5:225–253, 1982

Pettis RW: Tarasoff and the dangerous driver: a look at the driving cases. Bull Am Acad Psychiatry Law 20:427–437, 1992

Rosner R (ed): Principles and Practice of Forensic Psychiatry. New York, Chapman & Hall, 1994

Simon RI: Clinical Psychiatry and the Law, 2nd Edition. Washington, DC, American Psychiatric Press, 1992

Simon RI, Sadoff RL: Psychiatric Malpractice: Cases and Comments for Clinicians. Washington, DC, American Psychiatric Press, 1992

Stone AA: Vermont adopts Tarasoff: a real barn-burner. Am J Psychiatry 143:352–355, 1986

Tarasoff v Regents of the University of California, 118 Cal Rptr 129 (1974)

Tarasoff v Regents of the University of California, 17 Cal 3d 425 (1976)

Weinstock R: Confidentiality and the new duty to protect: the therapist's dilemma. Hosp Community Psychiatry 39:607–609, 1988

Weinstock R, Leong GB, Silva JA: Confidentiality and privilege, in American Psychiatric Press Review of Clinical Psychiatry and the Law, Vol 1. Edited by Simon RI. Washington, DC, American Psychiatric Press, 1990, pp 83–118

Weinstock R, Leong GB, Silva JA: Competence to terminate life-sustaining care: ethical and legal considerations. American Journal of Geriatric Psychiatry 2:95–108, 1994

Wolkon GH, Lyon M: Ethical issues in computerized mental health data systems. Hosp Community Psychiatry 37:11–16, 1986

Chapter 26

Training in Community Psychiatry

David L. Cutler, M.D.
William H. Wilson, M.D.
David A. Pollack, M.D.
Sally L. Godard, M.D.

This chapter begins with a discussion of historical developments regarding the training and recruitment of community psychiatrists over the past three decades followed by a review of efforts to train psychiatrists to work in community mental health centers. In particular, highlights of some of the more successful current training programs are presented, with a discussion of the Oregon program in some detail. We also describe the Pew Foundation efforts to stimulate state/university collaboration. Finally, we comment on recommendations for training nationwide with regard to community psychiatry.

Historical Background

Vaccaro and Clark (1987) have decried the plight of community psychiatrists in the 1980s. Frustration, role conflict, and inadequate training have characterized the recent history of psychiatrists' participation in community mental health centers. Unfortunately, this country's ambivalent attitude toward the mentally ill and those who try to serve them goes back a long way. On May 3, 1854, a bill entitled "An Act Making a Grant of Public Lands to the Several States for the Benefit of Indigent Insane Persons," was vetoed by President Franklin Pierce on constitutional grounds because it would give "Congress unqualified power to provide for expenditures in the states"—in essence, interfere with states' rights at a point in history where civil rights and states' rights were rapidly moving toward a disastrous confrontation (Cutler 1992).

Dorothea Dix and the 13 physicians who founded the American Psychiatric Association helped to establish the states as the responsible governmental entity to care for the mentally ill. At Eastern State Lunatic Asylum, in 19th-century Williamsburg, Virginia, Dr. John Galt established a cottage model based on the concept of family. Patients could work in the surrounding farms and believe they were making some form of contribution. In the spirit of John Galt's innovative work, the mental health department in Virginia in 1982 created the Galt Scholarship, based on principles of collaboration between public and private entities (Bevilacqua 1986). The scholarship funds an academic mental health professional for 2-year periods; this professional is charged with the task of strengthening professional ties between the Virginia Department of Mental Health and Mental Retardation and the University of Virginia, Virginia Commonwealth University, and Eastern Virginia Medical School (Yank et al. 1991).

We begin our review of training with a look back at the state hospitals, not because of their success or failure as treatment facilities, but because of their utilization as a training ground for psychiatrists. Without them there might not be a profession of psychiatry. Nearly all psychiatrists, including psychoanalysts, trained in state hospitals prior to the middle of the 20th century (Cutler 1990). It wasn't until the 1950s—after the establishment of the National Institute of Mental Health (NIMH), which provided training grants to universities—that universities began to dominate the training scene in psychiatry (Faulkner et al. 1983). Many of these "hospital-based" training programs had terrific success in training public sector–oriented psychiatrists. Programs such as those at Massachusetts Mental Health Center, Worcester State Hospital in Massachusetts, Fort Logan Mental Health Center in Denver, and Oregon State Hospital produced publicly oriented psychiatrists, many of whom went on to become superintendents of state hospitals, directors of community mental health centers, and commissioners of state mental health offices throughout the country. However, as the locus of training moved from the hospitals to the universities, future psychiatrists began their training embedded in academic, as opposed to public sector, institutions. Consequently, through the well-recognized phenomena of modeling and mentoring, they became more likely to follow the interests and habits of their supervisors, who were academicians and private practitioners, as opposed to public inpatient and outpatient clinical psychiatrists (Cutler 1990).

Along with this process there was a loss of exposure to the care of chronic and severely mentally ill persons. In particular, psychiatrists began to lose interest in treating schizophrenia and other severe disorders (Talbott 1979) and became more interested in treating anything that responded to psychotherapy. In the 1950s and 1960s, in an attempt to get more physicians to become psychiatrists, a great deal of money was allocated to resident stipends through grants from NIMH. These stipends were provided to residency programs, but with little or no strings attached in terms of results or accountability. Consequently, universities used them to augment their training programs in a variety of ways, often excluding hospitals and mental health centers as training sites, which resulted in minimal exposure to persons with chronic mental illness. In the 1970s NIMH began to redress these policy failures and rewrote their criteria for training grants (Pardes et al. 1979). Features such as interdisciplinary training; collaboration of educational institutions, service agencies, and program administrators; and working with the chronically mentally ill in community support systems began to appear in new announcements. Nevertheless, by the 1980s training grants were being slowly phased out, so the effects of these new requirements were not very profound. Several programs took advantage of these new directions and developed new training modules for the public sector, but most did not.

Community Psychiatry Training

In the 1960s and 1970s, following the passage of President Kennedy's Community Mental Health Center Construction Act of 1963, community mental health centers became training sites for psychiatrists (Faulkner et al. 1987). There was a great deal of enthusiasm about this. In the beginning a number of these centers had psychiatrists as directors (Beigel et al. 1979). One of the earliest training models was the Harvard Laboratory of Community Psychiatry, established by Dr. Gerald Caplan in the 1960s (Caplan and Killelea 1976). The program was designed as a postgraduate fellowship and included seminars with Caplan and experiences as consultants in agencies in the surrounding areas. A similar program existed in the late 1960s and early 1970s at University of California at Los Angeles (Karno et al. 1974; Karno 1982). This program was a 2-year postgraduate fellowship leading to a Master of

Social Psychiatry degree. When federal funding ran out in 1974, the remnants of the University of California at Los Angeles social and community psychiatry training program were absorbed by the general residency. Columbia University also had a 2-year program (now a 1-year program), with a core curriculum in epidemiology and research methodology (Bernard 1964). The residency program at Albert Einstein in New York over the years has produced many dedicated public psychiatrists, including several leading figures in the American Association of Community Psychiatrists (AACP). These pioneering programs were comprehensive, broad-based, and very much ahead of their time. They received support from the federal government but were never able to secure permanent local funding. Despite their effectiveness, most declined after their grants ran out.

There were numerous other programs whose fates were dependent on the availability of federal grant money. The University of Washington in Seattle, the University of California at Irvine, the University of California at Davis, and the University of North Carolina all had effective programs in the late 1960s. Some programs were integrated with basic residency training; others have faced considerable cutbacks.

On the other hand, some programs have been resurrected, and a number of newer ones have developed. These include programs at the University of South Carolina in Columbia; Dartmouth College in Hanover, New Hampshire; the University of Kentucky in Lexington; Southern Illinois University in Springfield; Tulane University in New Orleans, Louisiana; The University of New Mexico in Albuquerque; and the University of Massachusetts in Worcester. At least four programs, however, have managed to exist uninterrupted for 20 or more years and continue to be recognized as effective models: the University of Maryland, the University of Colorado in Denver, the University of Wisconsin, and the Oregon Health Sciences University.

The Maryland program has been oriented mainly toward state hospitals and Department of Veterans Affairs facilities (Harbin et al. 1982; Weintraub et al. 1991), although there are also community mental health rotations available. It is a highly regarded, publicly oriented training program. In the Wisconsin program there is a strong community orientation. It is a model training program set in a model service system at Dane County Mental Health Center in Madison, Wisconsin. This particular system was designed to serve severely mentally ill persons outside of state hospitals, and residents have the opportunity to rotate through elements of the system, working side by side with motivated, high-quality psychiatrists (Factor et al. 1988). At the Oregon Health Sciences University, residents have had the opportunity since 1973 to work under supervision in state hospitals and mental health centers during their residency. The Oregon program differs from the Wisconsin program in that residents have both a state hospital rotation and a community placement chosen from a roster of mental health centers throughout the state of Oregon.

Community Psychiatry Training in Oregon

What began as a small program in an out-of-the-way state in the northwest corner of the country has now become widely recognized as a model program for training contemporary community psychiatrists for both rural and urban mental health programs. The program began in 1973 (Shore et al. 1979) following meetings held in 1972 between the chairman of the Department of Psychiatry and the head of the Oregon Mental Health Division. These and other key individuals agreed to advocate for funding for faculty, staff, resident stipends, and travel for a comprehensive training program in community psychiatry. A federal training grant was submitted and approved, but on February 16, 1973, the Department of Psychiatry received a telephone call indicating that NIMH was unable to fund the grant because of "recent budgetary action by the president." After that fateful event the Oregon legislature passed a bill to provide state funding for the project. Ironically, the federal grant was funded the following year. However, if not for its failure to receive federal funding in 1973, the program might never have received the crucial state support that continues to this day.

With funding secure, an advisory board was established with representatives of key agencies and departments, including the dean of the medical school and a representative from the commissioner's office. This board has overseen the program since 1973, ensuring that psychiatrists trained in Oregon are given sufficient knowledge and skill to meet the needs of public sector psychiatry in the state. The program reports semiannually to the board on its progress.

The first director of the program, Dr. James Shore, was hired shortly after local funding was established in 1973. He immediately began negotiating with county mental health programs throughout the state of Oregon to establish training sites. Local programs were paid to provide local supervision for the residents at their centers. The resident stipends were paid by the training program. In the spring of 1976 Dr. Gerald Caplan of the Harvard Laboratory of Community Psychiatry spent 3 days providing consultation and seminars with Oregon's young Community Psychiatry Training Program.

Program structure. The Public Psychiatry Training Program Board advises the chair of psychiatry in selecting the director of the program, who currently is a professor of psychiatry in the department. The board also participates in finding an associate director, who by definition is the head of psychiatric training and education for the state of Oregon. Currently this person is also the human resource development director for the state. This particular position was formerly the director of training at the Oregon State Hospital residency program. In the 1970s this residency program was free-standing, except for its collaboration with the Community Psychiatry Training Program. Now the two residency programs have merged, and the position of training director has been moved to the Oregon Mental Health Division. This position provides a "linchpin" (Godard and Hargrove 1991) between the academic institution and the mental health administration. There are other key individuals with assistant and associate director appointments—one at the state hospital and another at a local community mental health center—who are closely affiliated with the department of psychiatry. These four individuals make up the staff of the Public Psychiatry Training Program (Cutler et al. 1993).

The basic program. During training residents are required to have clinical experiences in state hospitals and community mental health centers. Didactic experiences are interspersed throughout the training program, including ongoing courses and special seminars at the state hospital and the Public Psychiatry Training Program Friday interdisciplinary seminar.

The first exposure to public psychiatry occurs in the second year, when all residents rotate through a state hospital (Wilson 1992). These rotations last 3 months and are accompanied by a multidisciplinary seminar, which focuses on the role of the hospital as a part of the overall public mental health program in the residency program. All members of the faculty take part in the seminar. However, the most important element is the care of long-term patients under the supervision of experienced academic clinicians. This rotation is the only one where residents actually work with long-term inpatients. The other inpatient units (University Hospital, Veterans Hospital) have very high turnover rates and low lengths of stay, resulting in extensive experience with workups but little with continuing care and treatment. In the state hospital rotation, residents become familiar with long-term patients and long-term treatment and rehabilitation strategies. They also take part, if they are interested, in psychopharmacological or service system research projects that are ongoing at the hospital. Residents also participate in a monthly advisory committee to the faculty and administration of the hospital. Here they provide feedback on the quality of the training, which we use to constantly improve the rotation. All in all, it is a typically staffed but well-supervised state hospital environment. Residents have been very pleased with the style, process, and orientation of the rotation. In the third year all residents are required to spend 6 months, half-time, in the community mental health program. They select a roster of county programs throughout the state of Oregon. Because there is a travel budget, residents can elect to travel to any part of the state prior to making their selection and are asked to choose two or three sites to visit. They then identify a site and begin spending 2 days a week (Monday and Tuesday), at this location. They return to Portland on Wednesdays, Thursdays, and Fridays, where they get supervision and a 2-hour seminar from the Public Psychiatry Training Program. The rest of the time is spent in child psychiatry.

The overall goal of this project is to familiarize residents with the community mental health system and the roles a community psychiatrist can occupy in a manner most comfortable and most attuned to his or her own individual interests, talents, and needs. Residents are encouraged to work collaboratively with clinical and case management staff. They are required not to spend more than 50% of their time seeing patients, so that they have adequate time to become involved in other indirect activities at or outside the mental health center, such as mental health consultation, staff or community training and education meetings, and various quality assurance and other administrative processes (Cutler et al. 1993).

Residents participate in a weekly interdisciplinary community psychiatry seminar, which includes all the staff of the Public Psychiatry Training Program and students and faculty from the School of Social Work at Portland State University and the Department of Psychiatric Nursing at Oregon Health Sciences University. These seminars include topics such as epidemiology, mental health service systems, managed care, and treatment of target populations of disabled and culturally disadvantaged individuals. In addition, all residents receive an hour of supervision from a member of the faculty of the Public Psychiatry Training Program and an hour of supervision by administrators at the local mental health clinic. We do not require the residents to be supervised by psychiatrists at the community sites. By the end of the rotations, residents are required to have developed special skills, knowledge, and attitudes (see Table 26–1).

In the fourth year residents have an opportunity to take electives in public psychiatry, either in the community or in state hospitals. They can spend 6 months full time or 1 year half-time in these electives. In addition, residents may elect to rotate in specialty clinics that focus on public patients, including a young adult clinic for chronically mentally ill patients and a clinic for Southeast Asians who are chronically mentally ill. There is also an administrative elective at the Oregon Mental Health Division, in which about half the residents choose to become involved. Regardless of whether the residents elect to do something in public psychiatry, the Public Psychiatry Training Program pays their salary for whatever rotations they choose. For

Table 26–1.   Public psychiatry training program training objectives

Skills: The ability . . .	Knowledge	Attitudes
To enter a community mental health delivery system with a working understanding of the psychiatrist's role	History of the community mental health movement	Appropriate respect for interdisciplinary mental health team members
To distinguish between levels of intervention and prevention	Basic concepts in social and transcultural psychiatry and psychiatric epidemiology, including the service delivery system, to specific ethnic groups and disadvantaged minorities	Responsibility to patients, their families, and significant others, including agency people, and appropriate respect for their opinions and welfare
To participate in and support case management activities (assessment, planning, linking, monitoring, and advocacy)		
To plan, work, and relate on an interdisciplinary team for the provision of direct or indirect services for mentally disabled persons	General principles of primary prevention, secondary prevention, crisis intervention, and tertiary prevention (the care of the chronic patient in the community)	Willingness to consider and evaluate criticism and peer review of one's professional work
To negotiate a consultation contract		Commitment to evaluation of treatment results as scientifically as possible
To conduct a mental health consultation with a community agency	The role of social, cultural, and family stress in mental adaptation	
To collaborate in mental health program planning, quality assurance, and management activities	The theory and practice of different models of consultation and the identification of the characteristics of direct and indirect service	Comfort in dealing with highly personal and emotionally charged situations
To conduct precommitment evaluations and court examinations under Oregon's commitment statute	The structure of community mental health delivery systems in Oregon	Sensitivity to and willingness to explore a variety of opinions and attitudes and ideas set forth by patients, patient advocates, and community people at large
To demonstrate a thorough understanding of the use of medications in collaboration with nonmedical staff concerning issues of compliance and informed consent	The general principles of forensic psychiatry with particular focus on the Oregon commitment process	

example, residents may choose an elective in seasonal affective disorder research, and their stipends are still paid by the Public Psychiatry Training Program. The fact that the program has the flexibility to allow residents to choose their electives freely is a tremendous advantage. Such freedom allows them to do whatever they want to do, whether it is public psychiatry, academia, or even private practice. We believe this creates good will, and residents tend to see public sector work in a positive light. The program, in its 22 years of existence, has been able to place 75% of its graduates in public sector work, and recently received an award for creativity in psychiatric education from the American College of Psychiatrists.

The program has been successful despite changes in leadership at the mental health division and other major obstructions. It has survived largely because of a very close working relationship with the Oregon Mental Health Division through multiple contractual and organizational linkages. One contract allows for three faculty members to spend 1 day a week at the mental health division providing consultation and technical assistance. Another provides a child psychiatrist as the Children and Adult Support Services Program director. The most important contract is the linkage position occupied by the program's associate director, which was mentioned earlier. These very strong ties are examples of so-called "linchpin" positions (Godard and Hargrove 1991) that have been strongly recommended by the Pew Foundation State/University Collaboration Project. The faculty was selected as training faculty for the Pew Foundation workshops in 1990 and 1991 in six different locations around the country.

The Pew Foundation Initiative

Does good training result in more and better community psychiatrists? If so, how do we get them to work in community mental health centers, and what keeps them there? The American Psychiatric Association and the National Association of State Mental Health Program Directors also asked these questions. In June 1989, the two organizations jointly received a grant from the Pew Foundation to develop a 3-year project designed to enhance the level of collaboration between state mental health offices and departments of psychiatry. The project was funded by the Pew Foundation, and representatives of the American Psychiatric Association, the National Association of Mental Health Program Directors, the American Academy of Child and Adolescent Psychiatry, the American Association of Chairmen of Departments of Psychiatry, and the American Association of Directors of Psychiatric Residency Training Programs formed a group to jointly administer the project (Talbott et al. 1991). Richard Lippincott, from NASHPD, and John Talbott, from the American Psychiatric Association, were appointed as codirectors. Six workshops were planned and delivered in cities around the United States. The Oregon faculty and the Maryland faculty collaborated in designing and conducting these workshops, which have been held in Washington, DC; Minneapolis, Minnesota; Memphis, Tennessee; Boston, Massachusetts; Cincinnati, Ohio; and Denver, Colorado. The workshops were followed by consultations in various sites that had participated in the workshops. In addition, awards were given to programs that appeared to have been making meritorious progress. The hope was to attract national attention to the idea that public-academic collaboration is worthwhile and feasible. The project has been very well received, with favorable responses to the workshops and consultations. New initiatives have begun at Tulane University, Vermont, Louisville, and South Dakota. Old programs at Arkansas, University of California at Los Angeles, New Mexico, and others have been rejuvenated. It is not yet clear how many new community psychiatrists have been created, but the project has had an impact wherever a consultation has occurred, just from the data-gathering process of assembling constituency groups and getting principal leaders in academia and public mental health to talk with each other.

Recruitment and Retention

The Pew Foundation project is an example of an attempt to improve the image of public psychiatry. Other strategies less grand in nature are also taking place. The linchpin model, which establishes an academic person jointly at the state and the university (e.g., the Galt Scholar Program in Virginia) appears to be a successful method. The Maryland program uses jointly appointed training directors who work for the state and for the university. In Oregon the associate director of the Public Psychiatry Training Program is also the medical director for the state. These kinds of collaborative arrangements and joint positions are crucial for the recruitment of younger psychiatrists to a career track that guides them into combined public and university service. Similarly, the presence of valuable and well-placed role models is important for retention in these environments. Other strategies include annual conferences for all public sector psychiatrists.

Design Principles in Community Psychiatry Training

The following principles seem to have been key to the success of those programs that have been able to produce public sector and community psychiatrists and survive over an extended period of time:

- *Strong state and local support.* It is extremely important that the highest levels of government within the state see the program as important and have some influence in the articulation of its mission. The Maryland program has been strongly supported by a series of psychiatrist mental health commissioners, who were well aware that they would have recruitment problems if they did not have a university-based program producing state hospital psychiatrists. There is also strong state support for the Wisconsin program, which, along with its model service delivery system, has been an example for the nation. The Oregon program has a broad-based board, supported by all levels of the mental health division, university, and community mental health directors association. That broad support has helped it through difficult financial times and enabled it to maintain its budget while other programs face retrenchment.

- *A strong core faculty.* Trainees will never become interested in public and community psychiatry if there are not strong and competent faculty role models. These individuals must be able to survive and prosper in the academic system, in addition to having broader clinical skills.
- *In vivo training.* Residents need to train in real community-based clinical sites. Supervision must involve helping them understand these local situations and negotiate their own individualized roles and activities. The Oregon program has been quite successful in this regard. Consequently, residents are encouraged to view community mental health centers as interesting, challenging adventures that can be mastered, as opposed to hopeless prescription mills where psychiatrists are not respected for their broad expertise.
- *Interdisciplinary training.* Working in the public sector means working with individuals from a variety of disciplines. Most residency programs operate with traditional hospital-based systems where residents learn to be totally in control. In the community this model is anachronistic. Residents must learn to work collaboratively with other professionals. Collaborating with and empowering other professionals is the key skill in social, community, and public psychiatry. Most residents do not learn this, because the opposite is what is tacitly modeled in many academic hospital settings.

Conclusions

We have tried to tie the historical roots of psychiatry training in the public sector to the evolution of community psychiatry since the 1960s and to some examples of effective modern methods of training. Developments such as the State/University Collaboration Project have given community psychiatry a "shot in the arm," so to speak. However, it is also clear from feedback from contemporary community psychiatrists that not all the problems are solved. Managed care strategies will also have a narrowing effort on the role of psychiatrists in community mental health settings. The fact that psychiatrists in the public sector now have the AACP to advocate for them is certainly a welcome development. This kind of national advocacy (especially the guidelines for community psychiatry practice) is very helpful to whatever local efforts are established.

The AACP is also beginning to put more of its energy into community and public sector psychiatry. Currently there are efforts to establish a special section on public psychiatry within the American Psychiatric Association. The AACP recently completed a national survey to determine what sort of training was already in place nationwide to prepare psychiatrists to work in community mental health programs, particularly those that serve underserved populations. They recommended that more needed to be done to spread what was already good training to other parts of the country (Goldman et al. 1993). Brown et al. (1993) have recommended guidelines for curriculum development for training residents to work in community psychiatry. Efforts such as these could certainly help to maintain a pool of involved psychiatrists and help them remain involved in public and community work after training.

References

Beigel A, Sharfstein S, Wolfe JC: Toward increased psychiatric presence in community mental health centers. Hosp Community Psychiatry 30:763–767, 1979

Bernard VW: Education for community psychiatry in a university medical center, in Handbook of Community Psychiatry and Community Mental Health. Edited by Bellak L. New York, Grune & Stratton, 1964 pp 82–122

Bevilacqua J: The Galt Visiting Scholar in Public Mental Health: a Virginia experience, in Working Together: State-University Collaboration in Mental Health. Edited by Talbott JA, Robinowitz CR, Carolyn B. Washington, DC, American Psychiatric Press, 1986, pp 111–120

Brown DB, Goldman CR, Thompson KS, et al: Training residents for community psychiatric practice: guidelines for curriculum development. Community Ment Health J 29(3):271–284, 1993

Caplan G, Killelea M: Support Systems and Community Mental Health: Multidisciplinary Explorations. New York, Grune & Stratton, 1976

Cutler DL: Training psychiatrists to work with the seriously mentally ill, in Service Needs of the Seriously Mentally Ill: Training Implications for Psychology. Edited by Johnson D. Washington, DC, American Psychological Association, 1990, pp 28–37

Cutler DL: A historic overview of community mental health centers in the United States, in Innovations in Community Mental Health. Edited by Cooper S, Lentner T. Sarasota, FL, Professional Resource Press, 1992, pp 1–22

Cutler DL, Wilson WH, Godard SL, et al: Collaboration for training. Administration and Policy in Mental Health 20(6):449–458, 1993

Factor RM, Stein LI, Diamond RJ: A model community psychiatry curriculum for psychiatric residents. Community Ment Health J 24(4):310–327, 1988

Faulkner LR, Rankin RM, Eaton JS: The state hospital as a setting for residency education. Journal of Psychiatric Education 7:153–166, 1983

Faulkner LR, Bloom JD, Cutler DL, et al: Academic, community and state mental health program collaboration: the Oregon experience. Community Ment Health J 23(4):260–270, 1987

Godard S, Hargrove D: Public-academic linkages: a "linch-pin" model. Community Ment Health J 27(6):489–500, 1991

Goldman CR, Brown DB, Thompson TK: Community psychiatry training for general psychiatry residents: results of a national survey. Community Ment Health J 29(1):67–76, 1993

Harbin HT, Weintraub W, Nieman GW, et al: Psychiatric manpower and public mental health. Hosp Community Psychiatry 33:277–281, 1982

Karno M: Teaching psychiatry and behavioral science, in Social and Community Psychiatry. Edited by Yeager J. New York, Grune & Stratton, 1982, pp 74–91

Karno M, Kennedy JG, Lipschitz S: Community psychiatry at UCLA: a decade of training. Am J Psychiatry 131:601–604, 1974

Pardes H, Sirovatka MS, Jenkins JW: Psychiatry in public service: Challenge of the eighties. Hosp Community Psychiatry 30(11):756–760, 1979

Shore JH, Kinzie JD, Bloom JD: Required educational objectives in community psychiatry. Am J Psychiatry 136:193–195, 1979

Talbott JA: Why psychiatrists leave the public sector. Hosp Community Psychiatry 30(11):778–782, 1979

Talbott JA, Bray JD, Flaherty L, et al: State/university collaboration in psychiatry: the Pew Memorial Trust Program. Community Ment Health J 27(6):425–439, 1991

Vaccaro JV, Clark GH: A profile of community mental health center psychiatrists: results of a national survey. Community Ment Health J 23(4):239–241, 1987

Weintraub W, Neiman G, Harbin H: The Maryland Plan: the rest of the story. Hosp Community Psychiatry 42(1):52–56, 1991

Wilson WH: Psychiatric education in the state hospital: a current approach. Community Ment Health J 28(1):51–60, 1992

Yank GR, Fox JC, Davis KE: The Galt Visiting Scholar in Public Mental Health: a review of a model of state-university collaboration. Community Ment Health J 27(6):455–471, 1991

Chapter 27

Demystifying Research: Applications in Community Mental Health Settings

Robert E. Drake, M.D., Ph.D.
Deborah R. Becker, M.Ed.
Stephen J. Bartels, M.D.

I deally, research and clinical work are mutually beneficial. Researchers are well aware that mental health care, even for the most disabled patients, has progressively shifted from the hospital to the community and that, as a consequence, the potential for doing research in community mental health settings has grown considerably. The great majority of patients with severe and persistent mental illness are in the community; most of the exciting and innovative work in the treatment and rehabilitation of these patients occurs in community mental health settings; and the potential for studying how service systems organize, finance, and deliver care is almost limitless.

At the same time, research can offer the clinical staff and administrators in a clinical setting many rewards. Research stimulates intellectual activity and encourages reflection, learning, and innovation, all of which can improve job satisfaction and the quality of clinical care. Research can enhance an academic environment for trainees as well as staff. By addressing key clinical questions, research can help to understand and improve clinical

This chapter was supported by Grant K02-MH-00839 from the National Institute of Mental Health.

outcomes. In this era of cost containment, research can support new programs, justify the continuance of some programs, and facilitate the transfer of limited resources to other, more effective programs. Finally, research can advance the state of knowledge. The goal of mental health services research is, in fact, to produce a mental health system that is based on empirical data rather than clinical opinion or customary practice and that has the capacity to modify itself to increase the effectiveness and efficiency of programs.

Many of these purposes can be served by research that is done on a small scale without funds or with limited budgets. Research begins with careful observation. Astute clinicians regularly make the type of critical observations that lead to productive research projects, provided they allow themselves to observe and wonder rather than be intellectually trapped by training or ideology. One clinical event can become the occasion for reviewing the literature, for putting together a case report, for gathering similar cases within a clinic to ask an important question, for questioning the validity or generalizability of the observation, for deciding to collect data prospectively in a standardized format, or for developing a new intervention. All of these steps, which precede a controlled experiment or even an open clinical trial, are important aspects of the research process. Similar comments could be made regarding administrators' roles in studying the administration and financing of services.

As clinicians and researchers in community mental health centers, we have been conducting clinical and services research in these settings for over 10 years. More recently, our group has added several academic disciplines, expanded the scope of its projects to include statewide and national studies, and been designated a psychiatric research center. Prior to seeking external grants, however, we were doing essentially the same type of work for several years without funds. In this chapter we share some of our experiences in this endeavor and attempt to provide a "roadmap" for doing research in community mental health settings. Many excellent texts (Bausel 1986; Posavac and Carey 1989; Shontz 1986) address the technical aspects of conducting empirical research in clinical settings, and we will not attempt to summarize this information. We instead discuss the practical aspects of initiating and conducting research projects in community mental health settings.

Establishing a True Collaboration

The keystone of the research enterprise is the relationship between the researchers and clinicians. In most settings the researchers will have to devote considerable attention to understanding the details of the setting; to addressing the concerns of clinicians, administrators, clients, and families; and to educating all of these stakeholders about the purposes, procedures, and ethical aspects of the research. Researchers must make certain that all stakeholders derive net benefits rather than losses by participating in research.

The easiest way to ensure that research produces positive effects is to develop a truly collaborative relationship from the beginning. If clinicians and administrators also serve as the researchers involved in planning projects, they can protect clinical and administrative interests and help to create the mechanisms that produce net benefits. In other situations clinicians may make the critical observations, identify the areas of research, participate in the project, or serve as coinvestigators. In still other cases the researchers are a separate team from outside the community mental health setting and must therefore develop these mechanisms to ensure benefits through collaborating with insiders. We give several examples of this process in the text that follows.

When researchers from academic institutions are conducting research in community settings outside of their own work environment (e.g., the arrangements that have been encouraged by the National Institute of Mental Health [NIMH] under the Public-Academic Liaison [PAL] initiative), attending to these issues of relationship is critical. Many of the PAL arrangements that we have observed appear to be failing or not reaching their potential, because the distance between the researchers and the clinical enterprise remains too great. In many cases both groups have failed to participate in the preparatory work necessary to ensure mutual benefits.

Administrators should also be included in this process. With their overview of the system, they are often best suited to identify systems issues for research and to anticipate financial and other barriers to conducting a project. All of the problems that will be encountered in a research project cannot be anticipated beforehand, and administrators must be prepared to intervene when difficulties arise. At one extreme, a research demonstration project involving random assignment and specific models of treatment may be impossible to conduct without complete support from those who control salaries, positions, and job descriptions. Even highly funded projects have been abandoned, ruined, or severely compromised when critical decisions regarding staff, money, and other resources undermine a project in mid-course. At the other extreme, small projects are often totally dependent on the cooperation of one person, such as a secretary in medical records who answers to an administrative supervisor.

Research of course requires technical expertise, including the capacity to collect, manage, and analyze data. In some cases the clinicians or administrators in a setting will be capable of handling the technical aspects of designing, implementing, and analyzing a project by themselves, but this becomes increasingly unlikely as projects become more complex. For example, in many mental health services research projects, a multidisciplinary team of experts from areas such as economics, anthropology, and biostatistics complements the mental health professionals who serve as clinical researchers. Part of building a collaborative relationship with clinicians involves explaining who these people are, what they do, and what assistance they will need.

Identifying a Specific Project

After developing a collaborative relationship, the next step is identifying a relevant question for research. This process works most easily when clinicians and researchers are part of the same team and collaborate from the beginning on developing projects. One way to start is by meeting regularly in a study group that addresses a clinical topic area. This group can review the literature in a particular area, define specific questions for study, discuss research designs, and begin to address the practical aspects of doing a study within the setting (see later discussion). For example, a group of colleagues struggling with a clinical situation may agree to report a series of cases that they have encountered or to write a review of the literature in the area. To answer a specific question, they may decide to systematically examine clinical records from several years or to collect new data on a series of cases in a standardized manner. Alternatively, the group may decide to initiate a specific clinical procedure in a group for whom it has not been carefully studied and to keep track of their clients' changes in a systematic way. Success in this sort of open clinical trial may lead to plans for a controlled experiment.

This approach to research may sound too simple, but all of our research projects have evolved from a study group of clinicians and researchers who have gathered weekly for several years to discuss clinical problems and related research projects. We have studied clinical issues related to severe mental illness (e.g., suicide, homelessness, community tenure, substance abuse, and vocational rehabilitation), precisely because these topics were of greatest concern to the clinicians in the community mental health centers in which we worked.

Developing a project when the research team and the clinicians come from separate institutions is considerably more difficult. The two parties should meet often enough to develop a sincere appreciation and respect for each other's perspectives and talents, to find an area of mutual interest that would make the collaboration worthwhile, and to agree on all the details of the collaborative project so that each party feels it is benefiting from the partnership. The relationship must be attended to from the beginning, often by one person—a clinical researcher—who serves as the liaison between the two parties. This relationship often founders if those on one side fail to understand all that is involved or to appreciate the others' perspective. For example, a project that is imposed on clinicians who are expected to cooperate often fails if they misunderstand its purpose, design, or relevance.

Developing the Infrastructure for Research

Reviewing the literature, reporting cases, or reviewing records are relatively simple projects that can usually be accomplished without creating research committees. These low-risk studies can be reviewed administratively within the clinical setting, and the protection of human subjects can be ensured by a committee from a local university. Before developing more involved research projects in a clinical setting, however, several additional safeguards must be in place. These include the appropriate committees to evaluate the impact of projects on the clinical setting, to review the scientific merit of the project, and to ensure the protection of human subjects. Committees to advise on specific projects are also helpful, but these can be established later (see later discussion).

A research committee to assess the potential impact on the clinical setting should include, at a minimum, administrators, clinicians, and researchers. This committee protects the clinical integrity of the program, not by defending the validity of current programs, but by making sure that all the details of how a project will affect staff and clients have been considered carefully. It ensures that the potential gains from a particular project outweigh the disruptions, inconveniences, or extra work that may be required.

A separate committee, which typically includes researchers as well as a broad representation of other stakeholders (e.g., clients, families, clinicians, administrators, ethicists, and lawyers) examines the scientific merit and potential ethical and legal aspects of a project. This type of committee is called an *Institutional Review Board* (IRB). All academic institutions that conduct research have an IRB, and public mental health systems that are involved in research should have their own IRB. Scientific and ethical issues are sometimes addressed by two separate committees, but they cannot be totally separated. For example, no inconvenience to patients is justified for a project that lacks potential to produce anything of scientific merit because of flaws in the design.

Conducting a Project

When a project is in process, a number of mechanisms can help to ensure success. Informal meetings with key personnel can serve to keep everyone informed on small projects. Alternatively, nearly all of this work can be done or planned in the study group meetings. For larger projects the stakeholders can be represented on an advisory board, which meets regularly to review the progress, problems, and findings of the study. The board can help with publicity, participation, anticipating problems, and solving difficulties that arise. For example, the board may identify barriers within the mental health system or community and help to develop and implement solutions.

When the research team meets regularly to discuss all aspects of the project, key representatives from the clinical setting should be included to help identify and solve problems. Alternatively, larger projects employ a project director who regularly spends time in the clinical setting interviewing key personnel to assess the process of the study. This aids the project in several ways, not the least of which is keeping track of unanticipated changes in the clinical setting that may influence implementation or outcome.

Throughout the conduct of the project, the principle of attending to the relationship between clinicians and researchers applies. Clinicians must understand the research project in enough detail to protect its integrity. For example, they cannot refer a client who is assigned to one condition to another program. Researchers should remain cognizant of the need to produce net benefits within the clinical setting. This involves much more than sharing results at the end of a study. Small contributions such as providing inservice training and listening to clinicians' views of the project are often sufficient and help to keep researchers on track as well. Clinicians may want to collaborate in writing a paper, presenting research results to conferences of their peers, or providing consultations to other mental health centers. Larger funded projects allow the research team to make a more substantial contribution, such as funding a clinical position.

Funding a Project

Research projects often operate without funds. For example, only clear thinking and a small amount of effort are required to collect information on a group of clients in a standardized fashion and follow them 6 months after treatment by a telephone call. Internal sources are often willing to fund local evaluations of innovative programs, especially those that may make a difference for future programming or expenditures. For example, shifting the orientation of a program and following all clients for a year can be accomplished with a half-time research assistant—a very modest budgetary expense for a mental health center or state mental health authority when significant policy is at issue.

Small projects (e.g., literature reviews, case studies, and open clinical trials) provide the pilot data for developing larger projects and for applications to federal agencies and national foundations for funding. These organizations have staff who can be extremely helpful in guiding aspiring researchers through the process of developing an application. If a larger project and external funding are goals of the organization, including an academic collaborator at the beginning of the process is wise. The process of funding grants is conservative, and because agencies want to be as certain as possible that projects will be completed successfully, the experienced investigator has an enormous advantage.

Examples

In this section we will describe two projects to illustrate how they were started and how they continue to be conducted. The first is a small, unfunded study initiated by a psychiatric resident who subsequently joined the mental health center staff. The second is a larger project funded by the NIMH that involves collaboration of several agencies and many researchers, clinicians, and administrators.

Subjective Response to Alcohol in Schizophrenia

As part of our group's interest in the relationship between substance use and severe mental illness, we decided to collect data on all persons in our mental health center who carried a clinical diagnosis of schizophrenia. After obtaining administrative approval from the mental health center's research committee and approval of human subjects issues from Dartmouth's IRB, two mental health center psychiatrists reviewed all records of clients with a clinical diagnosis of schizophrenia and conducted structured interviews to verify diagnoses. A psychiatric resident, Doug Noordsy, was recruited to interview the clients about their use of alcohol and drugs. His interest in the relationship between subjective experiences and substance use helped us to develop a list of psychotic symptoms, nonpsychotic symptoms, and other experiences that might be affected by alcohol use. As part of the interviews, he and the other mental health center staff asked the clients if they had had these experiences and if the experiences were influenced positively or negatively when they drank alcohol. Administrators supported the staff time involved in collecting data because of the importance of the topic.

These interview data have led to several publications on the relationship between alcohol and schizophrenia (Bartels et al. 1992; Drake et al. 1990, 1991), among them an article on subjective experiences (Noordsy et al. 1991) that addresses the popular self-medication hypothesis. Moreover, these baseline assessments have been used to evaluate 4-year outcomes of our clinical program for dual diagnosis (Drake et al. 1993) and as pilot data for several successful grant applications. This project was conducted without funding, using only our mental health center staff, and with all of the planning, administration, and data analysis accomplished in the course of our weekly study group.

Vocational Rehabilitation of Severely Mentally Ill Persons

In contrast to the previous study, one of the psychiatric research center's current projects is an NIMH-funded vocational research demonstration that involves a collaboration among several agencies: the New Hampshire Division of Mental Health, the New Hampshire Division of Vocational Rehabilitation, the Boston University Center for Psychiatric Rehabilitation, the Mental Health Center of Greater Manchester (a community mental health center), the Central New Hampshire Community Mental Health Center, Employment Connection Specialists (a private vocational rehabilitation vendor), and the New Hampshire–Dartmouth Psychiatric Research Center. The project entails a controlled clinical trial of two models of supported employment for individuals with severe mental disorders in two New Hampshire cities. With so many collaborators, mechanisms to facilitate communication among the researchers are extensive. We will detail here only the connections between the researchers and the two participating mental health centers to illustrate the process of administrating the project, nurturing the relationship, sharing resources, involving clients and families, and developing products.

Researchers and mental health staff developed several administrative vehicles. Along with the vocational specialists who initiated the project, they met regularly to plan the study, to discuss the details of implementation, and to write the grant. The two mental health centers' research committees as well as the Division of Mental Health's IRB and Dartmouth's IRB approved the project. Since beginning the project, the research project director has met weekly with the clinical staff, and the research center director has met quarterly with clinicians to discuss the course of the study and to learn from their perspective and observations. Finally, an advisory board, which was established before the project began, has met quarterly. It includes all of the participating organizations plus clients, family members, and employers from the two cities.

Additional mechanisms support the relationship between the research center and the two mental health centers. The organizations had a history of working together on other research projects related to case management, dual diagnosis, and management information systems prior to beginning the vocational project. The research staff regularly attend clinical staff meetings in the two centers to explain the project, to provide educational materials and inservice training on vocational rehabilitation, and to encourage case managers and other clinicians to refer their clients to the project. Other researchers conduct site visits and focus groups to study the process.

The research project explicitly provides several financial benefits to the centers. The NIMH grant pays for clinical positions (vocational specialists) in each center. The research center helped each center to purchase a computer and developed the programs for data entry related to services provided through the project. The project pays for clinical training related to vocational rehabilitation and case management from national experts throughout the course of the project. Finally, the research center makes its biochemistry laboratory available to all mental health centers that participate in research projects to provide free laboratory tests for clients who are unable to afford critical tests, such as blood levels of neuroleptics.

Researchers, along with mental health center clinicians, meet throughout the project with groups of clients and with families to explain exactly what the project is about, what clients should expect from participating, and what researchers are hoping to learn from the project. In addition, all clients who are interested in joining the project are required to attend a weekly group that is co-led by the research project director and a member of the mental health center vocational team to discuss the details of participation. Clients must attend at least four meetings of this group before they can enter the study. This process ensures that clients not only meet study criteria but also are truly informed and consenting.

Researchers and clinical staff share in developing and using research data. The project director from the research center meets weekly with vocational staff in each center to share implementation data, to discuss model implementation, and to help solve any problems that are occurring in the course of the study. She is also on call to the staff full-time as concerns arise.

Research center staff and mental health center staff have collaborated in writing a treatment manual that specifies the novel intervention and in presenting the model and the research project at local and national meetings.

Conclusions

Community mental health settings are excellent arenas for conducting clinical and mental health services research. Having research in a clinical setting offers enormous potential for cross-fertilization between clinicians and researchers. The research team gains the advantages of working in ecologically valid settings, and the clinical and administrative team potentially gain knowledge, skills, and opportunities. Attending to the relationship is critical, however, and we have discussed several of the mechanisms that can help the participants to develop and conduct a project of mutual interest in a way that enhances all stakeholders. We anticipate further development of community mental health–research liaisons and refinement of the mechanisms that we have described.

References

Bartels SJ, Drake RE, McHugo GJ: Alcohol use, depression, and suicide in schizophrenia. Am J Psychiatry 149:394–395, 1992

Bausel RB: A Practical Guide to Conducting Empirical Research. New York, Harper & Row, 1986

Drake RE, Osher FC, Noordsy DL, et al: Diagnosis of alcohol use disorder in schizophrenia. Schizophr Bull 16:57–67, 1990

Drake RE, Wallach MA, Teague GB, et al: Housing instability and homelessness among rural schizophrenics. Am J Psychiatry 148:330–336, 1991

Drake RE, McHugo GJ, Noordsy DL: A pilot study of outpatient treatment of alcoholism in schizophrenia: four-year outcomes. Am J Psychiatry 150:328–329, 1993

Noordsy DL, Drake RE, Teague GB, et al: Subjective experiences related to alcohol use among schizophrenics. J Nerv Ment Dis 179:410–414, 1991

Posavac EJ, Carey RG: Program Evaluation: Methods and Case Studies. Englewood Cliffs, NJ, Prentice-Hall, 1989

Shontz FC: Fundamentals of Research in the Behavioral Sciences: Principles and Practice. Washington, DC, American Psychiatric Press, 1986

Index

*Page numbers printed in **boldface** type refer to tables or figures.*

Chronic mental illness *(continued)*
  combining psychosocial and
    pharmacological therapies,
    182–184
  defined, 174
  diagnostic and symptomatic
    assessment, 176–177
  evolution of treatment, 173–174
  family intervention, 180–181
  functional assessment and
    rehabilitation planning, 177
  HIV infection incidences and,
    244–245
  models of care, 175
  neuroleptics and rehabilitation,
    184–186
  patient education on
    medication, 183
  psychopharmacology and
    rehabilitation, 184–185
  Public Law 99–660, 175
  relapse prevention strategy, 184
  relapse rates, 175
  social skills training, 178
  substance use disorders
    diagnosis, 222–223
  symptoms and signs preceding
    relapse in schizophrenia,
    184
  vocational rehabilitation,
    178–179
Civil rights, patient, 119. *See also*
  Confidentiality; Legal issues
Clomipramine, depression, 246
Clonazepam
  nonresponsive patients, 186
  violence treatment, 284
Clonidine
  nonspecific maladaptive
    behaviors, 164
  opiate withdrawal, 196–197

Clozapine, patients nonresponsive to
  traditional neuroleptics, 186
Clubhouse programs, psychosocial
  rehabilitation, 84–85
Clustered Apartments, Santa
  Clara County, California, 99,
  101, 105, 107
CMHCs. *See* Community mental
  health centers
CNS. *See* Central nervous system
Coconut Grove fire (Boston,
  1942), 71
Cognitive disability, theory of,
  84
Cognitive remediation, 83–84
Colorado Division of Mental
  Health, 96
Columbia-Presbyterian CTI
  Mental Health Program for
  the Homeless, 267
Commission on Accreditation of
  Rehabilitation Facilities
  (CARF), 337
Commission on Mental Health
  (1977), 7
Commitment. *See also* Legal issues
  dangerousness and, 454
  involuntary, 455
  laws in rural communities,
    425
Community consultation
  decline and rise of, 433
  financial support, 444
  nursing home consultation,
    439–444
  primary health care clinic
    consultation, 435–439
  rewards, 444–445
  theme interference, 434
Community integration, 156–158
Community involvement, 30–31

Developmental disabilities and
    mental illness *(continued)*
    medications, 164–166
    obtaining reliable information,
    158
    psychotherapy, 162–163
    team approach, 157–158
    treatment planning, 161–162
Diazepam
    alcohol withdrawal, 196
    elderly and, 316
    vs neuroleptics, 94
Didanosine (ddI), 244
Dideoxycytidine (ddC), 244
Digoxin, anxiety, 319
Diphenhydramine, side effects of
    antipsychotic agents, 316
Disability, defined, 78
Disasters. *See also* Crisis resolution
    and emergency psychiatry
    child psychiatrist role in,
    146–149
    providing services at times of,
    71–73
Discharge planning, 129
Disulfiram, 197, 283
Disulfiram-alcohol reaction
    (DER), 197
Dix, Dorothea, 462
Domestic violence, 294–297,
    298
Drop-in care, alternative treatment
    care, 110
Drug abuse. *See* Substance use
    disorder
Drug Abuse Screening Test, 201
Drug Use Screening Inventory,
    145
Drugs. *See* Medications; individual
    drug name
Drummer, Elizabeth, 136

DSM-IV
    chronic mental illness
    diagnostic system, 176
    dementia criteria, 322
    diagnostic classification system,
    37
    differential diagnosis in
    immediate treatment plan, 62
    mental retardation criteria, 155
    substance use disorder criteria,
    192, 222
Dual diagnosis
    acute stabilization/
    psychopharmacology, 224–
    225
    addiction and mental illness
    parallels in recovery process,
    214–217
    alcohol and drug use
    assessment, **220–221**
    areas of special preparation for
    patients to utilize twelve-step
    programs, **230**
    assessment, 145, 213–222
    barriers to care, 211–212
    common features of psychosis
    and addiction, **213**
    community mental health
    program, system model for,
    232, 234
    course and outcome, 211
    disease and recovery model,
    212–213
    emergence of, 30
    engagement, 214, 224–227
    Epidemiologic Catchment Area
    (ECA) study, 191–192
    policy and contract
    development for patients in
    treatment, **228**
    prevalence, 209–211